Cultural Competence in Trauma Therapy

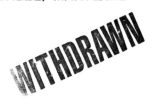
Cultural Competence in Trauma Therapy

Beyond the Flashback

Laura S. Brown

American Psychological Association
Washington, DC

First Printing January 2008
Second Printing March 2009

Published by
American Psychological Association
750 First Street, NE
Washington, DC 20002
www.apa.org

To order
APA Order Department
P.O. Box 92984
Washington, DC 20090-2984
Tel: (800) 374-2721; Direct: (202) 336-5510
Fax: (202) 336-5502; TDD/TTY: (202) 336-6123
Online: www.apa.org/books/
E-mail: order@apa.org

In the U.K., Europe, Africa, and the Middle East, copies may be ordered from
American Psychological Association
3 Henrietta Street
Covent Garden, London
WC2E 8LU England

Typeset in Goudy by Stephen McDougal, Mechanicsville, MD

Printer: United Book Press, Inc., Baltimore, MD
Cover Designer: Naylor Design, Washington, DC
Technical/Production Editor: Marian Haggard

The opinions and statements published are the responsibility of the authors, and such opinions and statements do not necessarily represent the policies of the American Psychological Association.

Library of Congress Cataloging-in-Publication Data

Brown, Laura S.
    Cultural competence in trauma therapy : beyond the flashback / Laura S. Brown.—1st ed.
        p. ; cm.
    Includes bibliographical references and index.
    ISBN-13: 978-1-4338-0337-6 (hardcover : alk. paper)
    ISBN-10: 1-4338-0337-2 (hardcover : alk. paper)
    1. Post-traumatic stress disorder—Treatment—Cross-cultural studies. 2. Psychic trauma—Treatment—Cross-cultural studies. I. American Psychological Association.
II. Title.
    [DNLM: 1. Stress Disorders, Post-Traumatic—therapy. 2. Cultural Diversity.
3. Psychotherapy—methods. WM 170 B878c 2008]
    RC552.P67B764 2008
    362.196'8521—dc22   2007043650

British Library Cataloguing-in-Publication Data
A CIP record is available from the British Library.

Printed in the United States of America
First Edition

CONTENTS

ACKNOWLEDGMENTS

This book owes large debts of gratitude to my colleagues who have thought long and hard about trauma and identity. I particularly wish to thank Pamela Hays and Maria Root, whose paradigms for understanding identity have deeply influenced my own thinking and work as a psychotherapist, teacher, and writer. Special thanks are also due to my friends and colleagues Judith Alpert, Lillian Comas-Diaz, Christine Courtois, Jennifer Freyd, Steve Gold, Beverly Greene, Ken Pope, and Melba Vasquez, all of whom have personally and professionally enriched me with their writing, thinking, and friendship. There are many other colleagues whose work informs and educates me, but to attempt to remember and list all of them would take up an entire volume. Among them are the leadership and workshop presenters at the annual meetings of the International Society for Traumatic Stress Studies and the authors publishing in the *Journal of Traumatic Stress*, *Dissociation*, *Journal of Trauma and Dissociation*, and *Journal of Trauma Psychology*. My associates in the Society for the Psychology of Women; the Society for the Psychological Study of Ethnic Minority Issues; the Society for the Psychological Study of Lesbian, Gay, and Bisexual Issues of the American Psychological Association (APA); and the Division of Trauma Psychology of APA as well as the many colleagues who have consulted with me in the last 3 decades are all influences on my writing and thinking.

My research assistant, Tracy Bryan, was an invaluable contributor to this process. Her diligent search for the scholarly literature on culture and trauma was eye-opening for us both (in large part because of how hard it was to find anything that I hadn't read already on this topic, although I'm sure that publishing this book will bring those whose work we didn't find yet in touch with us). Tracy is a gifted writer whose work psychotherapists will all be seeing in a few years, including an article coauthored with me in 2007 on feminist therapy and self-inflicted violence (Brown & Bryan, 2007).

None of this would have been written without the privilege of having known and met many survivors of trauma in my roles as psychotherapist and forensic psychologist. These people have been willing to tell me their stories, have allowed me to be witness and participant in their healing processes, and have taught me everything I know about being a psychotherapist. The people I work with are amazing human beings. Despite confusion, pain, and terror, they have struggled to have lives of dignity and decency, practicing compassion for others, although initially they struggle to do this for themselves. They are my heroes because in the face of endless invitations from life to become violent and abusive or simply callous and nihilistic, they are instead kind and loving. I can name none of them because to all of them I owe a debt of confidentiality, but I thank each one of them; they know who they are.

Finally, no writer exists in a vacuum. My partner, Lynn, has been unfailingly supportive of the activities that made this book happen, including those that temporarily took me away from home or from her while I holed up in my study or on the couch and wrote for hours. My beloved dog, Schmulik, who has worked as my copsychotherapist since he arrived in my life 12 years ago, has shown me repeatedly that what trauma survivors benefit from most is hope and the desire to connect, something he offers to clients every working day. Finally, my thanks to APA's Books Department, especially Susan Reynolds, who solicited this manuscript and was patient with my somewhat delayed production of it.

Cultural Competence in
Trauma Therapy

INTRODUCTION: TRAUMA, A MULTICULTURAL REALITY

Trauma and its psychic aftereffects have a texture. The experience conveys meanings that derive from personal histories; cultural heritages; and the social, political, and spiritual contexts in which the painful event happens. Even such an apparently neutral trauma as a natural disaster or a car accident can have a complex and multidetermined meaning structure, because the emotional impact of trauma is not merely about what happened in the moment but also reflects what occurred before and what transpires next. A psychotherapist's ability to understand how a trauma survivor's multiple identities and social contexts lend meaning to the experience of a trauma and the process of recovery comprises the central factor of culturally competent trauma practice. This volume is an extended discussion of how psychotherapists can develop such understandings that are sophisticated, thoughtful, and reflective of the current paradigms of identity and culture.

At the core, trauma is simply trauma. An assault, an earthquake, and combat are all recognizable as events that threaten safety and shatter assumptions about the nature of the world and one's relationship to it. Trauma of some sort is extraordinarily common even in a supposedly safe place, with research on the U.S. population suggesting that as many as one half of all residents have experienced exposure to a major traumatic stressor, most commonly some kind of interpersonal violence (Briere & Scott, 2006).

Trauma, no matter how endemic, is never generic and never the same for any 2 people. Each experience of an encounter with a traumatic stressor is unique and is given unique meaning by the life history of the person to whom it occurs. Some of that unique meaning arises from the cultural and group memberships in which a person participates and from the multiple, intersecting identities defining each person's individual sense of selfhood. When the trauma is of human design, the most common type, some of the meaning ascribed to the trauma by its targets will arise from the cultural and group memberships and identities of the perpetrators. The relationships of those reference groups, both in the present day and historically, will also give color, texture, and specificity to the trauma; those social and contextual factors can make a wound deeper, extend suffering, become obstacles to healing, or allow even the worst of psychic wounds to heal quickly.

RESPONDING TO TRAUMA COMPETENTLY

Responding to trauma in a culturally competent manner requires the psychotherapist to understand how those added meanings that derive from context and identity make each instance of trauma unique. It also requires the psychotherapist's awareness of her or his own identities, biases, and participations in cultural hierarchies of power and privilege, powerlessness and disadvantage, as well as personal experiences of trauma. Failure to bring cultural competence to the table can lead to missteps in genuinely helping trauma survivors or worse can result in deepening the wounds of trauma, creating secondary and tertiary traumas that are more painful than the original because they are correctly appraised by victims and survivors as unnecessary wounds.

This volume reflects my long interest in two topics and their convergence in my own work. I have worked since the beginning of my career as a psychologist with survivors of trauma. At first I did so accidentally, not realizing how common trauma was in the lives of people in emotional distress. By the early 1980s I was intentionally engaging with trauma survivors, with a deepening focus on what Judith Lewis Herman (1992) called "complex trauma." Complex trauma represents the inter- and intrapersonal effects of multiple and repeated exposures to varieties of interpersonal violence and violation, an experience that is becoming recognized as far more common in the United States than the one-episode traumatic stressor initially envisioned by diagnostic manuals.

As a psychologist trained in the early 1970s, a period in which trauma was virtually never considered a component of distress, I had to learn to uncover and listen to the hidden and silenced stories of trauma that my clients carried to me. I frequently did not know what I was seeing and hearing when people told me about trauma. I did not yet know the ways in which people communicated their traumatic experiences before they could name them and use language to talk about them. My training as a psychologist had taught me to ignore or trivialize experiences of trauma or to interpret the distress that people shared with me as evidence of something entirely other than the aftermath of trauma exposure, thus the accidental nature of my specialization. It was only because I had the good fortune to be able to hear those stories that I was then willing to intentionally pursue trauma as a topic.

Additionally, since the beginning of my career I have been involved with the development of feminist practice, which in turn has led me to an interest in broader visions of cultural competence in psychology. Feminist psychology has been uniquely situated within the realm of clinical practice as a result of its attention to issues of power and social location and to how people's experiences of gender, culture, social class, sexuality, and other experiences that denote inter- and intrapersonal power or powerlessness might affect both distress and resilience in response to traumatic stress. Because one core aspect of how trauma functions as a source of psychic wounding is that trauma induces powerlessness and loss both of real control and self-protective illusions of control, a theory of therapy that centers its attention on power is likely to have much useful to say to its practitioners and others about trauma.

Like other similar critical psychologies, including multicultural psychologies, queer psychologies, and liberation psychologies, feminist psychology and the psychotherapists informed by it have also been more likely than psychotherapists of other orientations to knowingly and intentionally encounter the survivors of traumas. This is because feminist psychotherapists' theories exposed narratives of trauma even in eras when such stories were forbidden or hidden in the larger psychological discourse (Comas-Diaz & Jacobsen, 2001; Fox & Prilleltensky, 1997). As psychotherapists open to telling truths about the human experience of powerlessness, critical psychologists created the psychological spaces where trauma survivors could speak their truths. This is what happened for me and many of my feminist psychotherapist friends and colleagues; we communicated our willingness to hear truths, and people told us about their hidden experiences of terror and violation. It is not surprising that almost all of the authors who first wrote about the traumas of interpersonal violence, the most hidden yet pervasive of human traumatic stressors, were pioneers of feminist therapy such as Judith Lewis Herman, Florence Rush, and Lenore E. Walker.

In the wake of Hurricane Katrina (which blew through the U.S. Gulf Coast a month after I proposed this book to the American Psychological Association [APA], making my work more urgent and, sadly, timely), the intersection of culture and trauma has become increasingly visible to everyone in the mental health field as well as to anyone who could turn on a television or open a newspaper in the United States since the fall of 2005. One of APA's many humanitarian responses to that disaster was promotion of the awareness that the mostly poor, mostly African American and Acadian victims of that storm would need not simply posttrauma support from mental health professionals but specifically required culturally competent posttrauma support that avoided reenacting wounds rooted in racist and classist assumptions about the world (Dass-Brailford, 2006). Even the apparently neutral trauma of a hurricane does not have neutral meaning for its victims; nor do the outcomes of such a trauma fail to aggravate old wounds of oppression and discrimination or underscore and enhance old histories of privilege.

THE SECONDARY TRAUMA OF CONTEXT AND CULTURE

Additionally, as the entire culture gained access to Katrina survivors' stories through such media presentations as Spike Lee's (2006) post-Katrina documentary *When the Levees Broke: A Requiem in Four Acts*, people also got to see how an already devastating yet apparently morally neutral act of nature can be more traumatizing when it is disruptive to culturally based coping and resiliency strategies that were dependent on the presence of coeval communities now scattered to every part of the continent. There is no accident in the fact that this event, experienced by all who lived on the Gulf Coast, has had differential impact on survivors based almost solely on interlocking issues of ethnicity and social class.

Speaking of the impoverished Katrina evacuees sheltering in Houston who had suffered grievous losses of home, family, culture, and connection, former First Lady Barbara Bush commented to a news reporter during her visit to the Houston Astrodome,

> What I'm hearing, which is sort of scary, is that they all want to stay in Texas. Everyone is so overwhelmed by the hospitality. And so many of the people in the area here, you know, were underprivileged anyway, so this [is] working very well for them. ("Barbara Bush Calls Evacuees Better Off," 2005)

Perhaps intending well, she wounded the evacuees and many of those simply hearing her words on TV in a way that the hurricane alone could not have. She seemed to be implying that the lives and experiences of the poor and disenfranchised survivors of the storm were lacking in value. Imagine being told that living as a displaced person in makeshift accommodations is an upgrade for your life. The presence of this secondary, tertiary, and additional trauma connected to the trauma of the flood was revealed to the entire American public. Mrs. Bush appeared to be delivering a clear message to Katrina survivors that what was important about their lives—their unique cultures and communities; their rich traditions; the homes, no matter how small, that they had struggled to own and to build—were of little value in an American society that regards lives in poverty as lives lacking in worth. The destruction of those communities by the floodwaters was apparently seen by her as a good thing, rather than as the heartbreaking drowning of a culture as rich in traditions as it was poor in cash.

What is striking about this episode was not that it happened nor that secondary institutionalized trauma was heaped on the pain of another traumatic stressor as a result of cultural insensitivity, but rather that it was done publicly and so was visible to all. Secondary trauma inflicted by agencies, researchers, and mental health providers as a result of absence of cultural competence has been painfully common but rarely is committed and broadcast on the national news; it usually happens in private, behind the doors of therapy offices and social service agencies, in shelters that define families to exclude family members not related by blood or law, in funding for posttrauma care that has arbitrary end dates reflecting some generic sense of how long trauma recovery should take, in research that fails to ask about identity while inquiring into symptom frequency and then interprets those numbers out of context. How trauma survivors are responded to by their helpers and the biases held by those who purport to assist them make a difference in whether and how those survivors will heal. When a psychotherapist lacks cultural competence, the capacity to understand the complex human identities that inform each survivor's relationship to trauma, that psychotherapist is at greater risk to unintentionally inflict secondary traumas on clients; cultural competence, conversely, may speed healing by connecting trauma survivors to their own resources and honoring the inner and outer realities informing trauma and its meanings.

The Katrina disaster thus also made more generally visible, but did not invent, the necessity for thinking about trauma within a framework of cultural competence. Human beings are entirely human and share a universal DNA, brain structure, and capacity for language and meaning making, each of which is implicated in the trauma response. Humans, trauma survivors and not, are also entirely the individual, unique, infinite intersections of their cultures, their genders, their ethnicities and phenotypes, and all of the other many factors that contribute to multiple and overlapping identities held by each and every person. Trauma does not happen to a generic human being any more than it is generic itself, and the ways in which humans translate their inner biological states of posttraumatic disequilibrium into outward expressions of distress are strongly affected by culture and context.

To date, few of the excellent psychotherapeutic models that have been developed for working with trauma survivors have intentionally taken into account this diversity and complexity of human identity and experience as it informs the encounter with trauma. Although the list in the *Diagnostic and Statistical Manual of Mental Disorders* (4th ed., text rev.; *DSM–IV–TR*; American Psychiatric Association, 2000) of so-called "culture-bound syndromes" is replete with posttraumatic responses framed in culturally specific manners, no editor of that important volume has connected the dots in writing. A trauma-savvy or culture-savvy reader may do so; but in the absence of those intellectual frameworks, the relationship of trauma to such phenomena as *ataque de nervios* is submerged, requiring skills at uncovering and contextualizing to be correctly understood as a form of posttrauma response. Additionally, although psychotherapists working with specific target group populations have occasionally proposed culturally specific paradigms for working with trauma in those settings (e.g., Marsella, Friedman, Gerrity, & Scurfield, 1996), few of those interventions have been mainstreamed into the work of trauma experts in North America; they are special treatments for special populations.

THE DISCONNECTION BETWEEN TRAUMA STUDIES AND CULTURAL COMPETENCE

It is surprising and ironic that this disconnection between the fields of trauma studies and cultural competence exists. Although the mental health disciplines have had at best an uneasy and ambivalent relationship with trauma as a topic, the modern field of traumatic stress studies in psychology and related disciplines was founded largely by social justice activists like me who cut their teeth in the 1960s and 1970s in movements against the Vietnamese War and for women's equality and by European and Israeli colleagues living in the aftermath of World War II and the Nazi Holocaust. The very diagnosis of posttraumatic stress disorder (PTSD) was lobbied into the *Diagnostic and Statistical Manual of Mental Disorders* (3rd ed.; American Psychiatric Association, 1980) by a somewhat uneasy coalition of antiwar Veterans Administration staff, some of them veterans of Vietnam themselves, and feminist psychotherapists from the front lines of the rape trauma and domestic violence movements. It might have been reasonable to assume that these socially conscious professionals, already deeply attuned to some forms of social injustice, would have looked next to issues of racism, classism, heterosexism, and other forms of oppressive inequality as they tried to enhance their comprehension of how trauma affected human lives; but that never occurred.

Why this next step did not happen has been a puzzle that writing this book has forced me to explore. As is true for most group phenomena, I believe that there are many reasons for this neglect of intentional multiculturalism, most of them benign and stemming from the same source as more general problems of modern aversive racism, classism, and heterosexism in progressive social movements as well as within the discipline of psychology (Bowes, 2007). Interrogating race, class, culture, and sexuality, by which I mean thinking critically and asking difficult questions about assumptions that are taken as truth in dominant culture, is threatening and induces shame in members of dominant groups, a category including the majority of psychotherapists. The critical analysis of systemic forms of oppression requires those in positions of dominance and privilege, such as psychologists and other psychotherapists, to acknowledge the social locations of greater power stemming from their professional training and status and to see themselves as benefiting from oppression through the privilege inherent in those roles, whether or not they actively oppress others.

This stance of admitting to privilege is not a comfortable position for any psychotherapist whose biases, such as they are, are mostly covert and well hidden from her- or himself, taking the form of what Gaertner and Dovidio (1977, 1986, 2005) have called "modern" or "aversive" bias, a form of bias that is denied by and invisible to its practitioners. Aversive bias has rarely been seen as the sort of very problematic countertransferential problem that it is because so much shame attaches to bias despite its nearly universal persistence. It is much easier for mental health professionals to be in the cultural role of supposedly neutral yet caring bystanders, to see themselves as good people who, because they are not intentionally perpetrating oppression, are thus not involved in it nor necessarily responsible for its alleviation through the mechanism of their work. To tell oneself the truth about how bias lurks in one's all-too-human nonconscious affective responses and one's personal symbologies can be a painful exercise in honesty and self-scrutiny.

Interrogating trauma and asking oneself to look closely at what its endemic nature means about the human condition are equally threatening. When people stare trauma in the face, it becomes impossible to engage in defenses against the reality that horrifying, unpredictable, disruptive things happen routinely in the lives of innocent human beings, and worse, that those things can happen to us, a phenomenon of painful awareness that Pearlman and Saakvitne (1995) have called "vicarious traumatization." Working with trauma requires psychotherapists to get up close and personal with stigma, which can and sometimes does rub off. Trauma therapy is not mainstream to training in any mental health discipline, even though some form of trauma is implicated as a psychosocial risk factor for most Axis I and many Axis II diagnoses (Briere & Scott, 2006). As Alpert (2006) noted in her comments in the inaugural issue of *The Trauma Psychologist*, scientists and clinicians in psychology do not generally familiarize themselves with the literature on trauma; those who do risk being seen as strange or suspect and are perhaps themselves secretly trauma survivors (which reads professionally as somehow less qualified to treat trauma because of bias or unhealed psychic wounds).

Each of these intellectual and clinical enterprises on the margins of society and psychology requires its practitioners to tell uncomfortable and often painful truths about aspects of the social status quo. Trauma and oppressive biases are close to the top of the list of what therapists generally do not like to talk about (Pope, Sonne, & Greene, 2006). If therapists do talk about trauma, they wish to speak of these painful and frightening topics from a safe intellectual distance, which is a stance antithetical to that necessary to work psychotherapeutically with traumatized people. From my professional location inside the circle of trauma psychotherapists and researchers who have taken the leadership in the field, most of whom appear to be of European descent whether living in North America, Australia, Israel, or Europe itself, it is apparent that many of us believed by that working with trauma survivors we were already doing social justice work and that trauma was sufficiently generic so as to not necessitate delving deeply into questions of cultural difference.

CULTURALLY COMPETENT TRAUMA THERAPISTS

It has also been true that for many well-intentioned Euro-American clinicians, diversity has been a topic reserved for those who work with special populations and for the clinicians who are themselves members of those very groups. Etic approaches to working with groups, which prescribed certain psychotherapeutic strategies for Asian Americans and certain others for African Americans and so on, although initially revolutionary because of simply raising consciousness about race and culture, eventually had the effect of ghettoizing discourse about ethnicity into the special populations class that was and still frequently is an optional course in the training of mental health professionals. Diversity came to be quite narrowly defined in mental health contexts; it was the study of the *other*, with each group placed in its own box. Race and culture were almost the only forms of human diversity addressed in the mental health realms for many years, and culture was defined in terms of those variables. Although feminist psychologists and other feminist psychotherapists have foregrounded gender, and lesbian, gay, and bisexual-affirmative practitioners began to make sexuality core to some components of the psychotherapy conversation, social class was and remains deeply neglected as a psychological topic (Lott & Bullock, 2007). Disability, immigration status, experiences of colonization, and other social locations have informed people's experiences of identity, and thus of trauma, and they have also largely gone unaddressed within the mental health discourse. Genocide perpetrated against Europeans has been of interest in the trauma field; genocide perpetrated by Europeans against indigenous people as colonial forces invaded the Western Hemisphere and the Global South has for the most part not been a subject of the field's attentions if one simply adds up the number of publications and conference presentations. The descendants and beneficiaries of the colonizers are among those controlling the professional discourse far more often than are the descendants of the colonized.

Trauma psychotherapists and specialists have not been an exception to this norm of disengagement from issues of human diversity within the context of U.S. culture. Ironically, the field of trauma studies has been international from its inception, owing largely to European and Middle Eastern heritages of war, the Holocaust, and ethnic strife of a longevity unknowable in a country as young as the United States. The journals and conferences of the traumatic stress studies field are well populated with materials about trauma from earthquakes in Armenia, wars in Kuwait or firestorms in Australia. Internationalism has been the trauma field's multiculturalism. In the largest published volume currently available on the topic of cultural diversity in trauma studies, the most frequent focus was on cultures outside of the United States or on individuals who refuged to the United States from other cultures. I can find more information about disaster survivors in the developing Spanish-speaking world than on the systemic trauma exposures experienced by persons of the many and diverse Spanish-speaking heritages living in the United States. This focus, although valuable in and of itself, has contributed to a neglect of multicultural competencies as regards issues of diversity in U.S. trauma survivors.

Whatever the causes, the dearth of formal commentary on what constitutes culturally competent trauma practice is not sustainable if trauma practice is to respond to the realities of trauma survivors who seek professional care. In this book I attempt to take one step in the direction of filling that lacuna by interweaving a paradigm for thinking about human diversity with knowledge from the field of trauma therapy to yield a framework for culturally competent practice with trauma survivors. The goal of this book is not to produce psychotherapists with etic knowledge, that is, specific knowledge about how to work with a specific population or their particular trauma histories. Instead, I invite my readers to an epistemology of diversity for understanding trauma and its intersections with humans' multiple and diverse identities.

EMIC VERSUS ETIC DISCOURSE OF CULTURAL COMPETENCE

There are numerous reasons for my decision to frame this volume within an emic discourse of cultural competence. First, etic models are themselves plagued by inattention to within-group diversities. To say "Here's how to work with a Bajoran trauma survivor" (Bajorans being a Star Trek ethnic group with a cultural history of trauma) ignores questions such as, is this a male, female, or intersexed Bajoran? Did this person live through the internment camps or is she or he the child of someone who did so? Did she or he participate in the resistance against the Cardassians (yet another Star Trek ethnic group who serve as a placeholder for perpetrators of oppression)? Did she or he see friends die? Spend time in prison? Refuge to another planet to seek physical safety? Is this Bajoran lesbian, gay, bisexual, or a transgendered person? Is she or he a strong adherent of the dominant Bajoran faith? As the list of questions grows, so does the complexity of issues facing psychotherapist and client. Yet these complexities are always present whether or not they are acknowledged, and the interplay and interaction between them and the trauma experience will have deep and lasting impact on how a person relates to what has happened and approaches the recovery process.

Etic models reduce people to one dimension of their identity and not always the dimension most strongly felt by trauma survivors themselves. My Bajoran client's trauma may have everything to do with being Bajoran or very little; her or his resources for responding to the trauma may also be affected or not by ethnicity and culture. If I only see the large dangling earring and the red clothing and immediately call up the "how to treat Bajorans" chapter from my inner database, I may miss what is important for me to know about this particular Bajoran's experiences of trauma. And I have not even begun to consider what it means that I am a human of this planet offering my services to this ethnically different human of another planet or to ask what we might represent to one another in symbolic nonconscious layers of our encounter. Representation, both individual and cultural/historical, constitutes two other vitally important dimensions of culturally competent practice.

Consequently, in this book I offer an epistemology of culturally aware and sensitive trauma competence of an emic variety. This strategy for addressing diversity teaches psychotherapists how to think about human difference, to develop algorithms for solving conundrums about diversity, and to consider themselves and their own diverse identities as they populate the social ecology of psychotherapy with trauma survivors. These models do attend to the various components of identity but with the goal of understanding how they merge within each person. The epistemology I use in this volume owes a large debt to the work of Pamela Hays (2001, 2008). Hays's model for understanding diversity in clinical context, which she calls ADDRESSING, is one that intentionally engages with multiple and intersecting identities in client and psychotherapist—age, acquired and developmental disability, religion, ethnicity, social class, sexual orientation, indigenous heritage, national origin, and gender. I draw on the ADDRESSING paradigm as an algorithm for thinking about human diversity and about how psychotherapists working with trauma survivors can understand their clients and themselves in terms of the intersection of trauma and multiple locations of social and personal identity.

TRAUMA IN THE LIVES OF PSYCHOTHERAPISTS

It is important to note that I refer to understanding diversity in both clients and psychotherapists. An assumption about what constitutes culturally competent practice, which recurs in this book, is that such practice involves knowledge of one's own multiple identities and their meanings. Along with one's sex; gender; and various ethnic, sexual orientation, cultural, and social class identities, there is also the question of how trauma is a part of one's identity. Some readers are trauma survivors. Research by Pope and Feldman-Summers (1992) has shown that approximately 30% of practicing psychologists admit to a history of childhood abuse. When I teach about trauma, I urge those in the audience to begin to speak of trauma survivors as *we* rather than *they*, given the ubiquity of this experience in psychotherapists' lives. Add in other common experiences of trauma such as combat, natural disaster, assault and sexual assault in adulthood, and traumatic loss, and the numbers of trauma survivors reading these lines grow.

Some readers will not have had a personal experience of trauma yet; yet because trauma is potential as well as actual. My colleagues living in New Orleans who reeled shell-shocked in the wake of Katrina, their homes, offices, and schools swept away by the floodwaters, were not trauma survivors (that I knew of, although there is a strong unspoken ban among psychotherapists and academicians about speaking of their own personal trauma histories) on the day that I agreed to write this book in early August 2005. When I saw them at APA's annual conference in New Orleans 1 year later they were trauma survivors, and for some of these people that change was visible and palpable. *Katrina survivor* had become an indelible component of their identities in that short timeframe.

Other readers are the children of trauma survivors, living with legacies of intergenerational transmission of trauma experiences (Danieli, 1998). Readers who are American Indian, African American, Jewish, Khmer, Native Hawaiian, or Armenian, to name but a few groups that have been on the receiving end of genocidal violence, are descendants of trauma survivors and of cultures marked by trauma. Readers who are South Asian may come from families that have been affected by the social upheaval and death attendant on the establishment of India and Pakistan. There is a plethora of additional examples; trauma has been pervasive in human experience.

They are we when speaking of trauma and its survivors. To work in a culturally competent manner with trauma each psychotherapist must be willing to understand her or his own participation, directly or historically, in the realities of trauma. Human beings evolved in terribly dangerous environments, surrounded by predators, and were likely to die before they reached age 40. The capacity for a response to trauma is built into the evolution of the species Homo sapiens; one's specific personal heritage is what creates the texture of one's trauma response.

Each individual is also diverse and possessed of multiple identities. Every person has a sex, a gender, a spiritual or meaning-making system (which need not include a divine being), and a culture with which she or he identifies, however loosely. If one's ancestors came from Europe or Asia to North

America, one is most likely a descendant of immigrants or refugees who arrived here to the chilly welcome that has greeted everyone from the Irish of the 1800s to the Eastern European Jews of the early 1900s to today's South Asian computer engineers and undocumented Guatemalans. Some came as indentured servants, sold into labor. If one's family came from South and Central America, one's ancestors may have crawled under the barbed wire fence at the border. Some ancestors came in steerage; others flew first class on a 747; but all experienced the loss of culture and language that is trauma for some.

Many individuals are also perpetrators. Some are the descendants of slaveholders, of soldiers who shot women and children in this country's genocidal wars against its indigenous people, or of those who imprisoned or tortured others in the countries from which they came. Many people have ancestors who suffered what Shay (1995) has called the "moral injury" of being trauma perpetrators, and in many cases that was traumatic to them and to the family cultures that they created and of which later generations are the inheritors. Some families served in the governments of Batista's Cuba, Stalin's Union of Soviet Socialist Republics, Hitler's Germany, or in South Africa under apartheid. Some individuals' ancestors have been beaten; some individuals' ancestors administered those beatings. Some people's ancestors include both; many African Americans carry the genes of a slaveholder great-great-grandfather who raped their enslaved great-great-grandmother. And people from positions of dominance and privilege can perpetrate oppression on others every day in their current lives without knowing or thinking of it (Vasquez, 2007). Perpetrator and victim consciousness live within people's cultures, families, and psychological realities. They are a component of our constructions of identity

If a psychotherapist does not understand her or his own diverse identities and the ways in which those identities include experiences of trauma, then no training in the application of eye-movement desensitization and reprocessing or prolonged exposure therapy or cognitive reprocessing will allow that psychotherapist to be culturally competent. The absence of cultural competence will detract from a psychotherapist's effectiveness as she or he applies these empirically supported modalities for reducing the distressing symptoms caused by trauma exposure because that lack will affect the quality of the therapy relationship. Research on common factors in psychotherapy has shown that for any intervention, a large percentage of the outcome variance is accounted for by the therapeutic alliance (Norcross & Lambert, 2006). Cultural competence enhances a psychotherapist's capacity to build alliances and enact the common factors of good psychotherapy even with those clients who appear to resemble their therapists in every way. I urge readers to think about trauma's meanings for psychotherapists as well as for the clients.

As noted previously, the field of trauma studies is a place in which it is disingenuous to speak of us, the psychotherapists, and them, the clients. We are they more often than psychotherapists like to think, and if psychotherapists tell themselves this truth, they come one step closer to cultural competence by acknowledging the ubiquity of trauma in human personal histories.

This is a difficult task with which to engage. At a large international meeting of trauma specialists that I attended in the midst of this writing, I never once heard trauma survivors referred to by other than the distancing third person, except for one distinguished presenter who, already full of gravitas and thus unassailable in his professional credentials, set aside his prepared remarks to speak about his own personal trauma history living in a country perpetually at war. Everyone who knows of this man and his work knows that he was born and raised in Jerusalem. As a Jewish Israeli, his trauma history is implicit in his citizenship. But for him to speak of it directly and explicitly was a violation of unspoken norms.

THE IMPORTANCE OF BEING IGNORANT

In her classic science fiction novel *The Left Hand of Darkness*, Ursula Kroeber LeGuin (1969) has taken her readers to the planet Gethen where all of the humans are intersexed and capable of being both male and female at different times in their lives and of being both and neither most of the time. Through the eyes of her protagonist Genly Ai, a middle-years adult male who is an apparently heterosexual, highly educated human of African descent from the reader's own third rock from a star, she has offered readers the opportunity to imagine how meanings are changed when variables that seem important and essential to their identities and understandings of one another become important and essential in entirely different and almost unfathomable ways.

On Gethen, sex is such a variable. Genly Ai cannot tolerate being unable to know which sex a person is, even though each Gethenian is usually neuter outside of a monthly estrous phase. Sex, and knowing a person's sex, is central to Genly's ways of relating; not trained as a psychotherapist, but rather as an anthropologist and diplomat, he is unable to set this strategy for organizing human experience aside. As a consequence of his insistence on putting Gethenians into boxes that do not reflect their lived realities, he makes continuous and dangerous errors of judgment, which form the themes of the book's drama and tragedy.

Psychotherapists are often like Genly Ai; they struggle with the ambiguity of their clients' identities and attempt to put them into the categories that they know and with which they are familiar. Trauma frequently has the effect of creating new and difficult-to-comprehend identities for clients, the identity of being broken, spoiled, dirty, and damaged. Sometimes those identities appear to make no sense to psychotherapists' preconceived notions of how humans organize identity, but they not only make sense for clients but also convey important information about the meaning of a trauma experience in someone's life. Culturally competent trauma practice requires that psychotherapists stretch their minds and let go of their categories so that they can open themselves to those parameters of identity experienced by the people with whom they work.

Another theme to be sounded here as I discuss how trauma intersects with identity is that no person has one identity. Drawing on models of identity development created by theorists observing the lives of people with multiple racial identities (Root, 2000, 2004a, 2004b), in this volume I encourage psychotherapists to understand trauma as it impacts each person's multiple identities, both additively and interactively. Each individual has a gender, and each individual has a gender as expressed through social class, age cohort, culture, and so on. When trauma intersects those multiple, overlapping, and sometimes apparently conflicting facets of selfhood, culturally competent practice requires psychotherapists to think not only of the easiest to see or most prominent aspect of identity but also about the intersection with the intersections, a sort of three-dimensional Venn diagram.

This leads me to another important point made by LeGuin. At one juncture in her narrative, LeGuin sends Genly Ai on a visit to a Gethenian religious sanctuary where practitioners of the art of Foretelling live. He approaches a member of the group and proclaims, "I am very ignorant." The Foreteller gently suggests to Ai that he is boasting, for in the philosophy of the Foretellers, ignorance is wisdom. So too with culturally competent trauma treatment; great ignorance, the stance of knowing that one does not know and thus openness to being informed, is a core capacity of the emotional competence informing culturally sensitive work. This is likely equally as difficult as being willing to interrogate one's own identities in relationship to trauma. The culture of modern mental health professions, with its reliance on a stance of empirical logical positivism, assumes that the psychotherapist is the expert who knows how to decode and explain a client's reality. Claiming ignorance is profoundly countercultural for people with doctorates, psychologists like me, or other professionals with advanced degrees and years of training.

Consequently another important goal of this book is to help each reader to become more ignorant, and thus wiser, about working with trauma survivors. After 3 decades of working intentionally with trauma I can say with utter certainty that I know that I have no idea of how any particular person will have experienced and made sense, or not, of her or his traumatic experiences. The clients I have worked with have taught me a great deal about what they have done to survive and thrive, and I have been able to amalgamate that knowledge into forms that function as useful heuristics, but no more than that. I have learned that my capacities as a psychotherapist and my ability to apply one or the other intervention effectively or to use my heuristics on behalf of any specific person are slightly less important than my willingness to stand in a position of ignorance in relationship to my client's suffering as well as her or his resilience, capacities, and struggles to make meaning in the wake of trauma. In that position of ignorance I am able both to join my client in intersubjective experience of ambiguity and noncontrol and also to relinquish my needs to act as if I, the psychotherapist, am immune to the vicissitudes of human existence of which trauma is only one.

AN OVERVIEW OF THIS VOLUME

This book's purpose is to generate in the reader the capacity to deliver culturally competent treatment to survivors of trauma. This book should not be read as a comprehensive text about trauma treatment or a comprehensive text about cultural competence. It is an introduction and an invitation. In attempting to adequately introduce readers to this topic in sufficient depth to be useful, I have chosen to omit large territories in both intellectual arenas. Everything written here presupposes that the reader has a basic familiarity with the diagnosis of PTSD and the ways in which the full range of posttraumatic symptoms can mimic a range of other diagnoses, including depressive disorders, anxiety disorders, and dissociative phenomena.

In chapters 1 and 2, I bring readers into the world of culturally competent models of psychotherapy. Here I go more deeply into Hays's (2001, 2007) ADDRESSING model and offer an extended version of that model that may be particularly useful in working with survivors of trauma. I explore how identity develops in the context of multiple, intersecting, and sometimes conflicting social locations and how trauma occurring at any point of identity development itself intersects with those other identity variables. In these chapters I invite readers to consider how the response to trauma emerges within the context of identity.

In chapter 3, I briefly review some common approaches to working with trauma in psychotherapy and discuss how cultural competence might inform their applications, emphasizing the process of therapy intake and transtheoretical paradigms of working with trauma survivors. I strongly encourage readers who wish to become more familiar with the topic of trauma treatment in general to delve further into sources referenced in chapter 3 regarding general paradigms and published guidelines for treatment of trauma sequelae. Working with trauma is a labor of both head and heart; specific, focused training in working with trauma within either a formal educational setting or through postgraduate continuing education is necessary for effective, ethical, and competent psychotherapy practice with trauma survivors. Ongoing consultation and supervision and copious applications of self-care, all of which are core to competent practice in the realities of trauma, cannot be acquired through reading. Doing culturally competent psychotherapy with any client is similarly not something acquired simply intellectually; this book should be a starting point, something that provokes the reader to think.

An additional goal of chapter 3 is to invite the reader to a competency-based view of trauma survivors. As I say to my clients who are castigating themselves for being symptomatic, "You arrived here alive." It can be difficult for psychotherapist and client alike to see a person who is profoundly impaired by flashbacks, numbness, and hyperreactivity as competent. Many survivors of interpersonal violence believe themselves to have been weak because they did not escape or they succumbed to posttrauma distress. Nonetheless, a competency-based viewpoint about clients constitutes a foundation of culturally competent trauma practice, in part because some of the apparent symptoms of posttrauma response are actually individually and/or culturally informed coping strategies. As psychotherapists know from the behavior change literature, people are more likely to feel hopeful about the possibility of their own transformation when they realize that what therapy is asking of them is not the acquisition of some new and entirely foreign skill but rather the expansion of a skill already in the behavioral repertoire.

In chapter 4, I expose readers to a diversity of paradigms for understanding what constitutes a trauma. I discuss trauma as a biopsychosocial/spiritual–existential phenomenon. I also look at multiple conceptual frameworks for understanding what might constitute a traumatic stressor and how experiences that appear to be normative or the background noise of daily life are potentially components of trauma. Feminist and multicultural models of trauma will be explored as additive to the *DSM–IV–TR* Criterion A definition of what constitutes a traumatic stressor. One of the many critiques of the *DSM–IV–TR* definition of trauma has been that it ignores the normative, quotidian aspects of trauma in the lives of many oppressed and disempowered persons (Brown, 2004), leading psychotherapists to an inability to grasp how a particular presentation of client distress is in fact posttraumatic. In chapter 4, I encourage readers to think beyond PTSD when they conceptualize the range of posttrauma responses, with particular attention to the ways in which various identity factors mediate how distress is experienced internally and expressed interpersonally.

In Part II of this book I look at particular social locations as they intersect with trauma. I examine age, gender, ethnicity, social class, sexual orientation, disability, displacement, health, and spirituality as factors in the experience of and recovery from trauma exposure. Each of these social location variables constitutes a source both of enhanced risk for exposure to trauma for some individuals and importantly a source of enhanced resources and resilience in the face of trauma. Each of these variables can also lend particular meanings to a trauma. I explore some of those meanings and ways to think about how social location can lend excess negative value to a trauma. Each of these variables can also influence how trauma is responded to, and thus in these chapters I explore in greater depth how to think in a diverse and complex manner diagnostically about the ways in which each survivor communicates about her or his distress. I also revisit the importance of looking at these variables as they intersect in the life of each trauma survivor.

In Part III of this book, I discuss interpersonal and psychotherapist variables. Working with the family, friends, and communities of trauma survivors is an important component of trauma therapy, but one that is frequently neglected in the focus on trauma survivors themselves. For many trauma survivors, these interpersonal contexts are the ones in which healing may occur if psychotherapists notice their importance and bring them, actually or symbolically, into the therapy room. Finally, the person of the psychotherapist working with trauma survivors requires attention. I discuss multicultural considerations arising from Pearlman and Saakvitne's (1995) construct of vicarious traumatization, with particular emphasis on how a psychotherapist's own social locations and multiple and intersecting identities affect the experience of working with survivors of trauma. I conclude with a discussion of future directions for deepening culturally competent trauma treatment, raising questions of where future research might be directed.

As always, my own social locations and identities form the standpoint from which I write. A component of that standpoint is the belief that ethics of authorship require a disclosure of those perspectives, because they create my biases and inform my understandings. I am an upper-middle-class Ashkenazic Jewish lesbian born in the last week of 1952, the granddaughter of immigrants who, arriving in the United States in the early 1920s as adolescents and young adults, never went beyond the seventh grade themselves but who sent all of their children to college. I am an inheritor of a rich intellectual tradition of critical thought; I am also an inheritor of a two-millennium-long history of cultural trauma, the descendant of those who survived. I was trained in the Boulder scientist–practitioner model of clinical psychology and have been a psychotherapist in independent practice since 1979. Most of the trauma survivors with whom I have worked have been individuals with histories of severe, repeated trauma exposure in childhood at the hands of parents and other caregivers, although I have also worked with persons who have survived combat and accidents. Most of the people with whom I have worked clinically are biologically female. In the mid 1990s I was deeply involved in the heated debate about trauma and memory, and some of my interests and allegiances in the field of trauma have been shaped by that experience.

As a long-time practitioner and theorist of feminist psychotherapy, I am deeply informed by that orientation and its emphasis on the role of power and powerlessness in the etiology of distress and dysfunction. I am also, because of that orientation, quite pragmatic about what I do in the office because I am mostly interested in the question of what helps and what works for the person sitting across the room from me. That pragmatism is reflected in my discussion of what works with trauma survivors and can also be seen in my general tendency toward a transtheoretical paradigm for good trauma treatment.

As a psychotherapist writing a book primarily for other psychotherapists I do not try to provide an in-depth review of every possible scholarly source on a topic. Rather, my interest is in inviting the reader to engage in a virtual conversation with me through these pages about how to become aware of opportunities for deepening cultural competence at all points in one's work with trauma survivors. I use clinical case examples as my primary instructional strategy because my own experience as both a learner and an instructor is that ideas stay with me when flesh and blood and emotion are hung on the bones of theory, something that I find is done best through clinical tales. This is a book about working with adult clients. I am not skilled or experienced in working with people younger than age 16. An entire separate book deserves to be written about cultural competence in work with children and younger adolescent trauma survivors.

The clinical case examples in this book represent, for the most part, disguised and merged stories derived from the lives of people who have sat across from me over the last 3 decades. Some examples also reflect and in some instances derive from the published biographical and autobiographical literatures on trauma and on human difference. My goal in including these examples is to give life and breath to the dry bones of theory and to illustrate how aspects of identity intersect, collide, and merge with the experience of trauma.

As McFarlane (2006) recently noted, the field of trauma studies began by attending to the literature created by trauma survivors from ancient times to the present to bear witness to their own lives. That literature, fictional and biographical, has been a source of knowledge for me and for the people with whom I have worked as a psychotherapist. In a few specific instances I have permission from a given individual to tell her or his story more fully. In those cases the client in question has read earlier versions of my discussion of our work together and agreed to my narrative of her or his life and the specific disguises given. However, most of the people discussed here are amalgams of two or more people I know. Having my clients read what I write about them has been another important stage in my process of learning about culturally competent trauma treatment, simply because their review of my manuscripts prior to publication afforded them opportunities to foreground aspects of their identities whose importance I had previously downplayed. These individuals have been my best teachers about trauma and its meanings, about what hurts, and what helps; they have also been my most powerful instructors about competence and resilience in the aftermath of trauma. This book would not exist without those lessons, and although none of them can be named, all of these people have my profound gratitude. They are the real authors of everything written by and about trauma by the "experts."

I

CULTURALLY COMPETENT MODELS OF TRAUMA TREATMENT

1

KNOWING DIFFERENCE
OR WE'RE ALL DIVERSE HERE

In this chapter, I explore some models for thinking about diversity and human difference, with particular attention to how those models inform psychotherapists' understanding of trauma. I also begin the process of looking closely at what it means that each psychotherapist represents something culturally meaningful to her or his clients as clients do to their psychotherapists, and these representations affect the process and outcome of psychotherapists' therapeutic work.

During my time on the faculty of a doctoral program in clinical psychology I took the lead in teaching a course with the well-meaning and benign-sounding name "Assessment and Treatment of Diverse Populations." When I took over the class on my arrival on campus and looked through the syllabus prepared by the prior instructor, I was unsurprised to find that this had been a class focused on rules for treating members of specific North American groups of people of color and other so-called minority groups; there was 1 week for African Americans; 1 week for Asian Americans; 1 week for lesbian, gay, and bisexual (LGB) people; and so on.

This model, referred to in the introduction to this volume as the etic strategy for understanding difference, has been so prevalent in psychology's discourse about cultural competence, difference, and diversity that I would be unsurprised if many psychotherapists picking up this book expected to find just that approach. The epistemologies of diversity in psychology have, until recently, been about deviance from an unspoken norm, the one in which "even the rat was White," to use Guthrie's (1976) not-quite-humorous words and in which a generic male human was seen to cover the experiences of all humans, including those who, unlike males, could and frequently did menstruate and give birth (Weisstein, 1970).

If one becomes deeply immersed in knowledge of a particular culture it may be possible to parlay the etic model into culturally competent trauma work in that culture alone. Psychotherapists who are intimately familiar with the norms, customs, languages, spiritual traditions, and histories of particular American Indian nations may be extremely well equipped to work with American Indians from those nations as clients. Trauma has been ubiquitous in the lives of this community, although there are large enough cultural and historical variations from nation to nation that deeply knowing Nez Pierce history does not mean deeply knowing Duwamish history or Dine history or Cherokee history, despite common themes of genocide and forced relocation. But even the most culturally steeped American Indian psychotherapist may not know what to do when the trauma for a particular client is one that happens outside the very broad parameters of the many and common traumas of this community. If, for instance, the client is a two-spirit person who has been gay bashed by other tribal members, the psychotherapist may not have all of the epistemic foundations necessary with which to assist the client in recovery with that particular form of within-group oppressive trauma.

What I have found useful in making sense of human diversity and people's multiple identities within that diversity is a model first proposed by psychologist Pamela Hays (2001, 2007). Hays invited her readers to see themselves and their clients through an intersecting web of what I refer to as "social locations" or "social identifiers." I define these as components of identity that are constructed in the context of social, interpersonal, and relational realities and that commonly inform the development of identity. Hays developed an acronym, ADDRESSING, for her epistemic system; this stands for age, disability (acquired and/or developmental), religion, ethnicity, social class, sexual orientation, indigenous heritage, national origin, and gender/sex.

Along with her acronym Hays proposed a series of strategies for developing culturally competent practice no matter whom psychotherapists are treating. A point that she made and that seems particularly germane to working with trauma survivors is that knowing the histories of cultures and societies, not simply the histories of the individuals with whom psychotherapists work, is a foundation of culturally competent practice. Understanding that social locations, the places in the social network where people are interpersonally situated, develop within a particular historical period and are also the helpful in understanding this discussion. I have come to eschew the use of the term *minority group* for a number of reasons having to do both with the message given to people by being called minority (e.g., perhaps less than) as well as the inaccuracy of the term (some minorities are now or are about to become numerical majorities).

Rather, I refer to *target* groups and *dominant* groups. Target groups are those social groups that have historically or continue currently to be targets of discrimination, bias, oppression, and maltreatment. Dominant groups constitute those social groups currently defined as the norm within a given culture. Thus, in the United States today, dominant groups include U.S.-born, English-speaking persons of European descent who are biologically male, heterosexual, affiliated however loosely or historically with some variety of Protestant Christian faith, married with children, middle-class, aged 25–49, with a college education or more, no current disabilities, not fat, normative in their gender expression, and adhering to conventional standards of attractiveness. Target groups constitute all others. Most persons have some mixture of target and dominant group status; even a person who today is entirely in the dominant group may move out of it as a result of aging beyond 49, acquiring a disability, losing his income and becoming poor, marrying a person of a target ethnicity, or converting to a non-Christian faith, to describe some very common trajectories for changes to social status. Movement among and between dominant and target social locations and finding ways to share both within one skin are other aspects of how identity develops. Understanding people's dominant and target statuses can emerge through exploration and examination of the most common categories of social location.

I also use the term *social location* as a broad concept that refers to a variety of different types of experience that can affect identity. The ADDRESSING model, for instance, lists many of the social locations that most commonly affect a person's sense of self as well as the ways in which others may respond to them. Even though some social locations have a biological component (e.g., gender, which is based in biological sex), all of them are to some degree or another socially constructed and variable from culture to culture. Although this terminology may be unfamiliar to some readers, my hope is that by using it I am inviting readers to reconfigure how they think about identity so that they eventually understand that it entails far more than a person's current or easily visible categories in the world.

ENTERING THE ADDRESSING MODEL

To understand how the ADDRESSING model can inform a psychotherapist's work, it is useful to explore in-depth each of the social locations identified by that model. This discussion will begin to interweave the topic of trauma into each ADDRESSING variable.

inheritors of other historical periods, allows for careful, critical examination of psychotherapists' assumptions about each of these potential components of identity. Many of these histories contain deeply embedded experience of trauma that go on to be the lens through which members of these cultures encode today's experiences. Inter- and transgenerational transmission of traumatic experiences cannot be well understood unless the histories that created those experiences are part of a psychotherapist's understandings of the world.

I often add to Hays's list, which she described as foundational but not all inclusive, such other social locations as vocational and recreational choices, being (or not) partnered, being (or not) a parent, attractiveness, body size and shape, state of physical health (different from disability), phenotype (similar to ethnicity in some instances, but not isomorphic with it), and experiences of colonization (which frequently but not always overlap with indigenous heritage in the Hays model). Readers are likely to have awareness of other social locations that neither Hays nor I have identified, and I encourage readers to consider including them in their understanding of themselves and their clients. ADDRESSING is useful because it invites psychotherapists to think broadly about the locations of diverse experience in each human.

Each person, client and psychotherapist alike, will have some relationship to most if not all of these social locations, and many of these locations will form core components of identity. Bias, oppression, and stereotype can be leveled at people on the basis of any one of these social locations; thus each person will have either been a target of such bias, will have practiced such a bias, and/or, as a result of being a target, will have internalized bias into identity. If a person has not her- or himself had such experiences, the experiences may have happened in the history of family and culture and may have left their psychological and relational traces. The presence of bias interwoven into the experience of social location in the context of social and cultural histories informs the meanings that those locations have for people's identities. This interweave of history, culture, trauma and identity also creates specific vulnerabilities as well as resistances to the experiences of trauma in the present day. It is important to explore each of these factors in greater depth and to begin the process of seeing where and how an enhanced comprehension of those factors can facilitate culturally competent, culturally sensitive, and culturally aware trauma treatment. The discussions in this chapter are introductory, and each topic explored here is addressed in great depth later in this volume.

A BRIEF WORD ABOUT TERMINOLOGY

A preliminary word about terminology to be used here and late volume to refer to groups of people who are usually referred to as mir

Age

Age is a social location with two components: one's actual age, which speaks to issues of developmental capacities, tasks, and needs, and one's age cohort, which informs the cultural contexts and norms surrounding one's life experiences. One's actual age is also a risk factor for certain kinds of bias; both children and older adults are targets of ageism, and because ageism is internalized, persons in adolescence and young adulthood frequently are affected by that internalized bias regarding their presumed future status as older people. To practice culturally competent trauma therapies, it is essential to understand the age (or ages, in the case of long-lasting trauma processes) at which trauma has happened and consequently to apprehend what developmental tools were available to the person for response to the trauma. The impact of trauma on succeeding developmental processes is also understood through the lens of age, because data suggest that traumagenic interference with one set of tasks affects, if not entirely inhibits, the successful accomplishment of other later developmental tasks. A very useful decision rule about age and severity of trauma impact is that younger persons are those most likely to experience longest term and most pervasive consequences of trauma exposure; this contradicts the common sense belief that the very young are very resilient and adaptable in the face of trauma and the very old are more vulnerable and reflects the reality that the foundational developmental tasks of childhood are more easily disrupted by trauma than are those of later life. I return to this topic and its ramifications for trauma therapy later in this volume.

Disability

As Olkin (1999) noted, it can be difficult to strictly define what constitutes a disability. She suggested that psychologists consider two continua, one of health and one of disability, which intersect in a variety of ways. Thus disability refers to changes and challenges to function at the level of the body that interfere with certain functions of life. Some conditions could disable an individual in some circumstances but not in others. Take severe myopia, for example. I am writing this sentence while looking through the lenses of my glasses. I am profoundly myopic and cannot see clearly much further than the end of my nose without those lenses; I have not been able to do so since about age 6. Living in a society that has developed corrective lenses means that I am not disabled from any function by my myopia, and I would not describe it as a disability. However, for an individual living in a pre-corrective-lens society this condition might be disabling and even life threatening, because my uncorrected eyes cannot tell what is lurking just down the road or looming beneath my feet.

Some disabilities come with few or no effects on general health. For example, a person may be deaf as a result of the failure of the auditory nerve to develop during gestation but may otherwise be in excellent health. A person might, however, be deaf because she or he had meningitis that damaged the auditory nerve and that has had various other long-lasting health consequences. A person might be born with spastic quadriplegia due to cerebral palsy and have quite severe disabilities of use of language and motor control arising from oxygen deprivation during the labor and delivery process; health problems that emerge for this person are not inherent in her or his condition but rather in the psychosocial consequences of having difficulty with voluntary movement and relying on others to move one's body so as to avoid decubitus sores from pressure.

Olkin (1999) has suggested looking to issues of function and the effects of a condition on a range of functions, noting that it is useful not to think of a "disabled person," but rather "a person disabled from" with the functions specified by a particular condition. A person might be disabled from reading by neurological difficulties, by visual difficulties, or by posttraumatic anxiety but not disabled from walking, speaking, hearing, or engaging in daily self-care functions, for example. Thus, an individual born without disabilities may as a result of cardiovascular disease become disabled from walking or cognitively impaired in later life. A person who suffers traumatic brain injury after adolescence or a war veteran who experiences traumatic limb amputation in combat has acquired a condition that can be disabling. Acquiring disability later in life can be traumagenic for some individuals.

Disability as a social location has both developmental and acquired components. Developmental disabilities as defined by Hays (2001, 2007) are those that develop in utero or very early in life so that they are long-lasting and core components of an individual's experience. Acquired disabilities can loosely be defined as those that occur or develop far enough into the life cycle that they are experienced or perceived as a change to the person. Thus, neuromuscular disorders that express themselves in childhood such as muscular dystrophy would be developmental, whereas a similar set of symptoms of muscular weakness arising in adulthood as the result of myasthenia gravis would be classified as acquired.

There is an important interaction of this social location with the previous one, age. The presence of a developmental disability informs a person's encounters with normative developmental tasks; the acquisition of a disability later in life informs the use of formerly acquired skills and may uncover the presence of tasks of emotional and cognitive development that were less than adequately accomplished. Because of the impact of both medical technologies and also the legal system on the lives of people who are on the high end of the continuum of disability, age cohort is also an extremely meaningful signifier in the lives of people with disabilities.

Disability is also a social construct. One can see this in the lives of people who identify as culturally Deaf (using the capital letter *D* to denote this cultural identification). Such persons do not see themselves as having a disability despite the fact that the inability to hear is so defined by the larger culture. Rather, they define themselves as an oppressed linguistic minority who, like other oppressed groups, have been forced until recently to learn the language of the majority culture rather than their own (Padden & Humphries, 1988). The spirited protests held by some students and faculty during the mid-1980s at Gallaudet University illustrate this defining process, with the protestors insisting that this unique university of Deaf culture have a president who was Deaf as well. Deafness is a physical condition defined as a disability in most laws, and persons who are deaf and those who are Deaf may request accommodations from schools and employers such as provision of sign language interpreter services under those laws.

However, many Deaf people do not personally identify as having a disability and define themselves as occupying a cultural location that must be defended from incursions by the larger dominant hearing world. This, too, is a function of social factors other than the ability or not to hear; age cohort as well as family history of deafness plays a large part in whether a person who does not hear self-defines as having a disability. A deaf child born to and raised by hearing parents is more likely to be defined by self and family as a person with a disability. A deaf child born to the deaf children of deaf parents, as a third generation "Deaf of Deaf" (to use the term from the Deaf community for those deaf by heritage as well as sensory capacities), is likely to see her- or himself as a person with a different language and culture, not a person with a disability.

I join with Olkin (1999) and Hays (2001, 2007) to suggest that culturally competent therapy with people with disabilities and their families requires what Olkin refers to as a "minority" rather than a "deficit" model. What is true is that people with disabilities have some (or several) aspects of their bodies that function differently than those of a majority of other humans. Frequently, however, the challenges for these individuals lie not in those physical differences but in the barriers created to fullest possible function by cultural institutions and practice. *Ableism*, bias against persons with disabilities, is pervasive, and because most people with disabilities do not come from families in which the parents are also people with disabilities, children with developmental disabilities almost always grow up in social environments distorted by ableist bias.

Trauma enters the issue of disability in a host of ways. Because of the risks inherent in applying a deficit versus a minority model, psychotherapists must be careful not to assume that the presence of the disability is itself traumatizing or stressful. This is especially true for people whose disabilities are developmental and for whom this way of being in their bodies is well-known and not associated with abrupt loss or change. Harriet McBryde Johnson (2005), an attorney, memoirist, and disabilities rights activist, exemplified this stance in her memoir *Too Late to Die Young: Nearly True Tales From a Life* (2005). Although her neuromuscular condition is progressive and has increasingly disabled her from using her legs and hands as she has grown older, her relationship with her body is one of deep familiarity. She knows that she is a person with a disability, but that is not a source of trauma to her; her stresses come from the barriers erected by others to her pursuit of her life.

Her story stands in contrast to those of individuals who are disabled by events or conditions that were inherently traumatic or a source of loss: accidents leading to paraplegia or quadriplegia or life-threatening illnesses such as cancer or multiple sclerosis. Such persons, prior to loss of their able-bodied status, may have held strong, even if not conscious, biases about the lives of people living with disabilities, and these biases now inform their understanding of the events that led to a change in function. Thus they may conflate being a person with a disability that made its appearance in the middle of their nondisabled life and life narrative and experience that entire change as traumatic.

Finally, as I discuss in further detail later in this volume, being a person with a disability can be a risk factor for some kinds of trauma exposure. The manner in which a particular trauma attacks a person at the location of disability and those aspects of identity affected by disability will both inform the experience of trauma. They will also shape that which may be useful in the healing process.

Religion and Spirituality

Religion and spirituality are the next social locations in the Hays (2001, 2007) model. Even atheists have a belief system; although they may balk at calling it a spiritual system, it will be one that allows for the making of meaning. All traumatic stressors are assaults on meaning-making systems, and most traumas will have lasting transformative impacts on the survivor's ways of making meaning. There is a pervasive interaction between trauma and issues of meaning making, with religion being equally a source of trauma, a location at which trauma is directed, and a source of coping in the aftermath of trauma.

Culturally competent practice necessitates inquiry into and comprehension of a survivor's religious, spiritual, and existential systems currently and prior to and during the trauma. Changes across time arising from trauma exposure and recovery are common, and the meanings ascribed to those changes by a trauma survivor will often become central to understanding some of that survivor's coping strategies in the face of trauma. It is also important for psychotherapists not to conflate religious identification with spirituality and existential meaning-making systems. Although for some people these are isomorphic, for many others they are completely separate, as is the case for the person who attends a Methodist church with his family on holidays and the occasional Sunday but describes his spirituality as being about his relationship to nature.

Some religious affiliations constitute target groups; which groups are targeted depends on history and context. For example, although the Mormon Church is currently a large, successful religious denomination, its founding history is full of stories of hate crimes perpetrated on the founders of the church by dominant culture Protestant Christians. In Utah today where Mormons constitute the dominant religious and cultural group and the numerical and political majority there continues to be a consciousness of target group status in the group's early history. Similarly, an individual raised in a cultural context in which her or his faith is dominant may develop religious target group status when she or he moves from that context into one in which her or his faith is no longer dominant; this is a common aspect of immigration to the United States from countries where Islam, Buddhism, or Hinduism are the dominant faiths, for example. The trauma of having one's faith marginalized can lead to distress that sometimes does not appear to be psychological but represents what happens when anxiety leads to rigidification of previously more fluid coping strategies.

Ethnicity and Culture

Ethnicity, the next factor in the Hays (2001, 2008) model, subsumes several factors. Ethnicity is commonly used in North American discourse to refer to persons of color, as in the phrase *ethnic minorities*. Hays asserts, and I concur, that ethnicity is not the same as phenotype. Phenotype refers to biology, the physical characteristics such as eye color and shape, hair color and texture, skin pigmentation, and so on, which are used as place markers for the construct of race, a concept that is then conflated with ethnicity. Ethnicity, however, is an intersection of a multiplicity of factors that include phenotype, culture, and language. Many Euro-American individuals are unaware that they have an ethnicity because they conflate that term with phenotype and may find a question about that topic confusing when coming from a psychotherapist. They may answer, "I'm White. I don't have an ethnicity." It can be helpful to give examples: One can be a "hyphenated" American of some sort (Armenian-American, Irish-American, or Norwegian-American); one can be of indigenous Euro-American ethnicity (Southerner or Northeasterner); or as one of my students phrased it, one can be "Heinz 57. A mutt," denoting a mixed and hybrid ethnicity of European descent whose distal origins have been lost in transmission over time.

A person's cultural identification, ethnicity, phenotype, and ancestry may not be isomorphic. Some fourth and fifth generation Americans of Japanese and Chinese descent are disidentified with their parents' and grandparents' cultures of origin. Statistics indicate that members of these groups are very likely to marry Euro-Americans rather than phenotypically similar persons and to identify culturally with Euro-American dominant culture. "I'm a White guy whose great-grandparents came from Japan" is the self-description of an acquaintance who although phenotypically Asian appearing and with a Japanese last name has no identification with any Asian culture, speaks no Japanese, and describes himself as fully assimilated into the Euro-American culture of which his spouse is a member.

Thus, ethnicity is a many faceted phenomenon containing a range of potentially traumagenic experiences that evolve out of family history and personal experience. Persons of non-European phenotypes and some of Eastern or Southern European phenotypes have been the targets of racist bias both historically and currently. Individuals who identify with ethnicities that are primarily defined by phenotype (e.g., race) may experience exposure to racism even when they are phenotypically more similar to the Euro-American dominant group. Consider, for example, Walter White, the famous African American activist who had fair skin and hair yet clearly was targeted by and affected by White racism.

Ethnicity has also been a source of other sorts of trauma exposures that may be unknown to the client because assimilation was a family response to trauma, but whose effects have been transmitted intergenerationally. Public figures such as former Secretary of State Madeline Albright and former U.S. Senator George Allen are two recent examples of offspring of Holocaust survivors who had no knowledge of their parents' Jewish origins until those histories were exposed to them in their middle adulthoods. In each case the family had used assimilation and religious conversion as self-protective strategies so that dynamics related to trauma in the family's history were buried and unavailable for understanding by either of these individuals.

Historical trauma, easier to identify in groups in which such trauma is relatively recent, is also present in the lives of most of the large immigrant groups who came to North America prior to the imposition of immigration quotas. Although the potato famine of Ireland that engendered the large immigration of Irish people to North America is 2 centuries past, the experiences of colonization and conquest by the English, the banning of indigenous Gaelic language, the disenfranchisement of the Roman Catholic religion, and other aspects of Irish historical trauma that preceded the famine are all components of Irish cultural identity that may be detectable in clients of Irish descent even when, at the point she or he enters therapy, that client's understanding of her or his ethnicity is consciously limited to her or his relationship to St. Patrick's day celebrations.

Social Class

Social class is the great invisible social location in the United States. Although national statistics increasingly point to growing income disparities between the richest Americans and all others and some social commentators speak of the disappearance of the middle class due to diminished availability of well-paying jobs outside of the learned professions, most Americans who are not abjectly poor are likely to describe themselves as being middle class. *Classism*, the bias against poor people as well as against those who work with their hands, is pervasive in American culture in which an analysis of class issues has rarely been a component of the public discourse.

Social class is also a complex variable. It may or may not reflect actual income level; some commentators on class have noted that middle-class status reflects the presence of social capital, defined in part by such factors as availability of literature in the home, parental or other close familial education, and a value placed on education for its own sake, even when financial means are absent or strained. A person of great wealth may have little or no social capital. Additionally, in North America barriers between classes are permeable, with social class not marked by accent, as is the case in Europe, or hereditary participation in a landed aristocracy (although informal aristocracies of wealthy visible families have long existed in the upper classes of U.S. society and now can be seen to form through families of celebrity). A person may live in many different social classes during her or his lifetime, with trauma sometimes being a factor contributing to loss of class status.

Social class is conflated with several other social locations. Persons with disabilities are more likely to be very poor, with some estimates being that 80% of people with disabilities are un- or underemployed as a result of systemic barriers to participation. For instance, a person with disabilities and a doctorate in psychology who requires multiple medications and the use of a wheelchair for mobility and also has a personal care attendant may be unable to find a job that both pays sufficiently to have a high quality of life and also provides adequate health insurance coverage; she or he can only afford access to necessary care if she or he remains on disability income payments, which then creates needs-based eligibility for that care. If she or he does find work that pays more than $700 monthly, she or he places all benefits in jeopardy (Panzarino, 1994). Additionally, if this person uses paratransit services to go to and from a job, she or he risks being terminated for repeated tardiness because a common complaint of persons who use paratransit systems is that they are rarely on time, sometimes being as many as several hours behind schedule. All of these factors can conspire in the life of a person with a disability to leave her or him impoverished no matter what her or his educational level, talents, or capacities. This person may thus be middle class in values and social capital but financially poverty stricken.

Age also interacts with social class. Very young children are more likely to live in poverty than any other group of Americans. In the past, older age was also associated with poverty, and this continues to be the case for many aging women and aging people of color. In those instances earlier discrimination in the workplace created a cascading effect from lack of financial resources earlier in life leading to reduced savings for retirement and smaller Social Security payments as a result of lower paying work. However, with the inception of so-called welfare reform in the 1990s, children in the United States are more likely to be living far below the poverty level than ever before.

Trauma interacts in a variety of ways with social class. Access to and expectations of care and safety are enhanced for middle-, upper-middle-, and upper-class persons. As I describe later, certain types of traumatic experiences, because they are more inconsistent with the lives and expectations of middle- and upper-class persons, are potentially more likely to be emotionally challenging for these individuals. Social class also directly affects the sorts of services and resources available to trauma survivors including insurance coverage for health and psychological services. Poverty creates risks for exposure to certain kinds of traumatic stressors including, given the all-volunteer nature of the U.S. military, combat trauma exposure.

Sexual Orientation

Sexual orientation describes the direction and expression of an individual's sexual and romantic desires. It is conceptualized on two continua, one of other-sex attraction and one of same-sex attraction (realizing, of course, that there are actually more than two sexes but that the other sexes generally sort into malelike and femalelike categories that allow the use of this continuum paradigm for sexual orientation). Each human being is to some degree high, medium, or low on each of these continua. Persons who self-identify as heterosexual are commonly higher on the other-sex attraction continuum; persons who self-identify as lesbian or gay are commonly higher on the same-sex attraction continuum; and self-identified bisexual individuals fall at roughly similar places on both continua. Persons' expressed sexual behavior is commonly, although not always, indicative of their desires; persons with strong same-sex and weak other-sex attraction may engage in sexual and romantic relationships with members of the other sex and not necessarily identify as lesbian or gay, for example. Not all of these relationships reflect some kind of suppression of true sexual self or self-hatred; they can also be about a strong relational connection with one particular other-sex individual.

Each person has a sexual orientation; for some individuals this is fixed throughout the lifetime, as appears to be true for most gay and heterosexual men. For others, including some lesbian and heterosexual women and some bisexual women and men, sexual orientation is experienced as more fluid. The best available data suggest that the origins of sexual orientation are poorly understood for persons of all orientations but that attempts to change orientation, the direction of desire, in individuals for whom this is not already to some degree fluid are generally unsuccessful and may be harmful to those persons. A discussion of the issue of sexual orientation conversion, or reparative therapies, is beyond the scope of this chapter but is addressed as a trauma risk factor in greater detail when sexual orientation issues in trauma are more fully discussed later in this book.

People who are lesbian, gay, or bisexual (LGB) are targeted by *heterosexism* (the systemic privileging of heterosexual ways of being and relating) and *homophobia* (fear and hatred of persons believed to be LGB) and are subject to a variety of forms of legal and attitudinal bias and discrimination. Currently most states in the United States ban marriages between members of the same sex; although same-sex sexual behavior is no longer criminalized in the United States, it was until quite recently. Persons who are LGB are forbidden to serve in the U.S. Armed Forces if their sexual orientation becomes known under the infamous "Don't ask don't tell" policy. (Readers might find it ironic that Israel, officially a theocracy, recognizes same-sex marriages from other countries, which the United States does not, and allows openly LGB people to serve in the military. Israel also makes survivor pensions available to the partners of those who serve, who are also likely to have been military veterans.) There are 17 U.S. states that have laws forbidding discrimination on the basis of sexual orientation in housing, employment, and public accommodations, but this means that the majority of states do not have such laws. Some states, most notably Virginia, do not even allow gay people to make nonmarital legal contracts such as medical powers of attorney for use in emergencies regarding their domestic partnerships.

Sexual orientation interacts with all other social location variables, both those already discussed and those to follow. Briefly, for purposes of this chapter, what is important in terms of beginning to approach culturally competent trauma treatment is for psychotherapists never to assume the sexual orientation of clients, regardless of such apparently obvious cues as the presence of an other-sex spouse or same-sex partner. Routine inquires into how a person self-identifies are an important part of conveying to clients that a psychotherapist is open to however they describe themselves. Psychotherapists who have personal difficulty with individuals of a given sexual orientation and have been unable to work through that aspect of countertransference should refer clients to other psychotherapists, as the risk of harm to clients from a psychotherapist's homophobia, biphobia, or negativity about heterosexuality can be great.

An aspect of sexual orientation that is rarely considered is that of what its practitioners refer to as *kinky* sex. This includes individuals who, along with attractions to persons of a particular sex or sexes, are aroused by such activities as bondage and discipline, the infliction or receipt of pain, various forms of role-playing involving dominance and submission, sexual behavior in relatively public settings known as *play parties*, or sex involving fetishistic elements such as clothing of particular fabrics (leather, rubber, vinyl, and velvet appearing to be among the most common). Sexually kinky individuals are gay, lesbian, bisexual, and heterosexual. Some have multiple partners for purposes of sexual activity; some will be monogamous with one partner;

and still others may be polyamorous (or *poly*), with committed relationships to more than one person that are not open to sexual activities with others outside the sexual partnership.

Although there are estimates available regarding the numbers of LGB persons in the U.S. adult population (generally ranging from 3% to 10% depending on how these counts are made), no data exist regarding sexually kinky individuals. Working with this group of persons requires a particular degree of cultural competence that includes a high level of open-mindedness about sexual activities of consenting adults. Again, as is true with a client of any sexual orientation, psychotherapists who have poorly contained countertransferences toward kinky sexuality should consider referring clients to other psychotherapists.

Trauma intersects with sexual orientation in a large number of ways, and not all of these are related to a client's membership in a sexual minority. For example, sexual assault of heterosexual women by male acquaintances and spouses is related to the risk factor of being heterosexual and female and thus in close relational proximity to the group of humans most likely to commit sexual assaults. For LGB people, however, trauma of some sort is a constant; working with LGB clients thus requires knowledge of both LGB issues and trauma in its many guises.

Indigenous Heritage and Colonization

Indigenous heritage refers to people first known to be dwelling in a location prior to its colonization. In the United States, this includes American Indians, Alaska Natives and Inuits, Native Hawaiians, and Samoans (this definition begs the question of whether these individuals were themselves colonizers of other now-vanished groups). World-wide indigenous people include Africans from formerly colonized countries, the indigenous dwellers of Taiwan who were colonized first by the Han Chinese and then by the Japanese, the Ainu of Japan, aboriginal peoples of Australia, and the Karen and Hmong peoples of Southeast Asia. Some settings also have semi-indigenous groups, originally European colonists who were then themselves secondarily colonized by ultimate conquerors such as Acadians in Louisiana, Spanish Americans and mixed-race Mexicans in the part of Spanish America that became California, Texas, New Mexico, and Arizona, all of whom experienced secondary colonization by English speakers.

What persons of indigenous heritage all have in common is a history of colonization by a group that invaded and stole land; imposed a different language, religion, customs, and ways of dress; often enslaved people for use in labor to produce trade goods; and frequently committed actual genocide. To say that trauma is an ever-present component of the lives and heritage of indigenous peoples is a great understatement. Historical, intergenerational, and present-day interpersonal trauma, called post-colonial trauma syndrome by some, are common in the lives of indigenous individuals (Duran, Duran, Brave Heart, & Yellow Horse-Davis, 1998). Poverty is commonly associated with indigenous status; the poorest place in the United States is the Pine Ridge reservation, the rural ghetto of the Lakota people. But most other social location variables cut across indigenous status as well.

National Origin, Immigration, and Refugee Status

National origin reflects the issue of immigration. Except for those people indigenous to North America, all Euro-Americans and Asian Americans and many African Americans living here are descendants of immigrants or themselves immigrants (differentiated from the experiences of people of African descent who if descended from slaves were not immigrants but rather victims of kidnap and enslavement). Each succeeding wave of immigrants has been greeted with hostility; the anti-Irish sign festooning New York City in the 1820s contained sentiments not unlike the anti-immigrant slogans being preached today by the vigilante groups who troll for undocumented people crossing the U.S. border with Mexico.

But the meaning of immigration has changed over time as well. When my Jewish grandparents fled their native Poland in the early 1900s they knew with certainty that they would never return, because Poland was an unsafe place for Jews. My partner's maternal great-grandfather who hid in a ship coming from Hamburg after running away from his home somewhere in the Austro-Hungarian Empire had a similar expectation of no return, although the issue was not as much one of safety. Immigration in the preairplane world was mostly a permanent phenomenon that had loss embedded deeply into its fabric.

Many of today's voluntary immigrants often come to the United States with the reasonable expectation of visiting home and extended family again once this is financially feasible. The losses of immigration still exist for voluntary and legal immigrants, but their configuration is different. More like the immigrants of the past are refugees fleeing unsafe places in their homelands; my dentist, a Baha'i born in Iran, cannot return home so long as the present government, which has criminalized her faith, is in power, despite Iran's being the place where the Baha'i faith was founded. Refugees thus have the usual losses of the immigration experience today but are also likely to carry with them specific experiences of trauma and danger that impelled their departure from their homeland. Persons who are undocumented also bear more resemblance in their experiences of immigration to those of earlier generations than to legal immigrants of today in terms of danger and risk associated with the immigration experience.

African Americans present a special experience of national origin. Persons of African descent whose ancestors came to the United States before the slave trade was banned in the early 1800s are all the descendants of those who survived the brutal Middle Passage of the slave trade. Although many also have Euro-American and American Indian ancestors as a result of sexual assaults and intermarriages and thus can be both indigenous and immigrant in their heritage as well, being transported to this continent in chains is a very different migration experience even than coming voluntarily as an indentured servant who shared phenotype and legal status with the master. Similar to the experiences of these persons are modern-day people who are trafficked into the United States and other industrialized nations for purposes of low-paid work or the sex trade. Trafficked people are in essence enslaved and come to the United States as a result of trickery or because they have been sold to pay a family debt. The meaning of migration for these individuals is not that of the voluntary immigrant, legal or otherwise.

Cultural competence around issues of national origin requires psychotherapists to consider carefully the various meanings of immigration and migration to their own and their clients' identities and then to explore how and where those experiences have engendered encounters with trauma. As is becoming clear, immigration intersects with every other social location; even persons of indigenous heritage in one place may become immigrants to another place, bringing with them their particular histories of living in their colonized countries of origin.

Gender and Sex

The final social location described by Hays (2001, 2008) is, ironically, the one that is generally primary in people's identities—gender. Gender is not sex. Sex is a term that describes the biological makeup of the body. As noted earlier, persons may be one of several sexes, with external genital morphology that matches or varies from chromosomal makeup or reproductive organs. One in 2,000 live births is of a person who is intersexed, meaning that the infant in question has genitals that are either ambiguous or inconsistent with reproductive and/or chromosomal sex. Generally, however, individuals in the United States regardless of actual sex are sorted into the two categories of male and female (the issue of intersex is addressed at greater length later in this volume).

Gender is the social construct built on the sex of the body. It is a series of schemata and roles that are both internalized and enacted and that begin to be imposed on children from almost the first moment at which the sex of a fetus is determined. Because of the very early imposition of rules regarding appropriate gender expression, gender is frequently phenomenologically experienced as isomorphic with sex and gender expressions as hardwired in the anatomy of the body. This position appears to be largely mythological, with careful meta-analysis of the sex difference literature determining that effect sizes for almost all sex differences are small and insignificant (Hyde, 2005).

Gender, no matter its origins, is quite a powerful determiner of identity and is generally the first identity that a person experiences, usually emerging with clarity for a child between ages 18 months and 3 years. Developmental capacities for greater and lesser flexibility of categories and less and more critical thought about rules frequently govern the gender expression of younger humans, particularly very young children. Younger individuals are thus quite rigid about gender roles and rules. Gender interacts with every other social location, because no matter what a person's social locations, that person has a gender.

Individuals whose preferred gender expression is at variance with that to which they have been assigned on the basis of sex are defined as *transgender*. Transgender itself operates on several continua, which may or may not include the desire to surgically or hormonally modify the body to bring it into line with gender expression. Overtly transgender individuals are frequently mistaken for being gay or lesbian, given stereotypes of cross-gender expression in sexual minority persons; however, transgender individuals come in the range of sexual orientations, which may or may not remain constant if and when a person has sexual reassignment surgeries.

Cultural competence in psychotherapy requires psychotherapists to have an awareness of their own gender schemata and the rules that they impose on the gender expressions of others. Gender nonconformity is a frequent risk factor for trauma exposure; however, what is less well understood is that particularly rigid forms of gender conformity also risk trauma exposure as well. Gender expression additionally appears to mediate response to trauma exposure, and posttraumatic symptoms are frequently expressed in manners reflecting an interaction with gendered ways of being in the world already utilized by a trauma survivor.

REPRESENTATION AND PRIVILEGE IN CULTURALLY COMPETENT PRACTICE

As noted previously, I have added several other possible social locations for consideration in the development of cultural competence for myself; each psychotherapist will, in deepening cultural competence, find social locations in her- or himself and her or his clients that enhance understanding of identity and its relationship to trauma. Culturally competent practice involves the psychotherapist's awareness of her or his own personal relationships to each of these variables of social location. Because of the manners in which trauma differentially impacts each of these social locations and their various intersections, a particular component of identity will have itself been a source of personal trauma or distress for many persons. Psychotherapists must also be aware that their various social locations, particularly those easily apparent to clients, will also have meanings that will color the therapy relationship. What psychotherapists represent to their clients and what clients represent to their psychotherapists through the lenses of their collective multiple identities affect therapy profoundly. The ability of psychotherapists to be aware of those issues of representation is core to cultural competence in practice.

The 19th century African American suffrage activist Anna Julia Cooper said, "When and where I enter, then and there the whole race enters with me" (quoted in Giddings, 1996, p. 13). Cooper's statement is true for each psychotherapist and each client. When and where psychotherapists enter the exchange of therapy, into the room with them marches their personal and cultural histories. They will represent things to their clients and their clients to them. This, I suggest, is more than simply issues of transference or countertransference, because the things psychotherapists represent are frequently alive and well in the social environments in which psychotherapists and their clients live and are not simply past experiences that are symbolically or unconsciously evoked or transferred into the therapeutic environment. These dynamics, even when symbolic, are not merely nonconscious representations of personal history; they are the interpersonal and political realities in which therapy takes place.

Culturally competent practice with trauma survivors or others requires a heightened awareness of what it is psychotherapists represent and what is represented to them. Culturally competent practice requires the sophisticated capacity to know when the dynamic in the room is about the psychotherapist's social locations, when it is about other representations, and when it is within the set of more usually considered dynamics of therapy as understood by the psychotherapist's particular theoretical orientation. This is especially the case when one or the other person represents a component of personal or historical trauma to the other.

A basic assumption of culturally competent practice is that psychotherapists can never and should not assume the trust of their clients. Trauma is itself destructive to trust; survivors of interpersonal trauma may take years to believe that psychotherapists will not become one of their perpetrators. Psychotherapists working with trauma survivors represent humans who were the source of trauma; psychotherapists' specific social locations and identities may enhance or decrease their overall role as a threat stimulus. As several of my clients have told me, it is only because my dog, who works with me, appeared to trust me that they then decided to accelerate their own process and view my actions as more likely to be truly benign rather than a trick designed to pull them closer to me so I could harm them further.

When certain kinds of difference are present, psychotherapists' clients will have even more reasons founded in experience and reality to view their psychotherapists with suspicion and uncertainty, not to believe that their psychotherapists' professional training trumps their life training as biased humans. In fact, for many members of target groups the mental health disciplines have been a source of pathologizing and disempowerment, making psychotherapists less worthy of trust than some other types of healers. When psychotherapists represent current or historical trauma to their clients and are aware of it, however, they increase the possibility of earning trust when they tell the truth about their acceptance of their role as representative of their culture. Acknowledging and validating the presence and stinky leavings of historical elephants in the therapy office can communicate to clients that psychotherapists are willing to tell truths that are uncomfortable for them as psychotherapists and not simply to invite their clients to experience their own discomfort. I return to this theme repeatedly throughout this volume as I explore the specific ways in which representation affects the therapy process in trauma treatment.

Cultural competence also requires attention to the phenomenon of dominant group privilege. Privilege is the collection of unearned advantages attendant on being a member of a dominant cultural group. There are usually corresponding undeserved disadvantages conferred on members of target groups. Some examples of how privilege manifests itself include the following:

- You can drive any car you want without worrying that you will be stopped so long as you are obeying traffic laws.
- You can marry the person you love and receive survivor benefits if they die first.
- You can walk into any store wearing anything you want pretty well assured that you will not be followed or harassed.
- You believe that if you are the victim of a crime that you can call the police and be helped by them.
- Your culture's holidays are always days off from work or school.
- You can be imperfect and few people will generalize from your imperfections to those of everyone in your group.
- You can swear or dress in second hand clothes or not answer letters without having people attribute these choices to the bad morals, the poverty, or the illiteracy of your group.
- If your day, week, or year is going badly, you need not ask in each negative episode or situation whether it has overtones of bias or whether you're being paranoid. (McIntosh, 1998)

Privilege lends power to one's biases; if I am a lesbian biased against heterosexual people, I may suffer from being prejudiced but I lack the social power to declare all marriage between other-sexed persons illegal. The heterosexual person biased against me has the privilege and power to legislate against me. Acknowledging one's privilege can be a trust-engendering and relationship-building action in therapy. Ignoring it or pretending that it does not matter will eventually undermine trust and endanger the working alliance of therapy.

When I sit across the room from persons of African descent, they cannot know that my ancestors arrived in this country in 1919, nor does it matter whether I personally benefited from slavery. What they know, and I must also know and be able to acknowledge, is that I have benefited from the unearned privilege associated with my phenotype of European-appearing skin and that they, in turn, have experienced undeserved social disadvantage associated with their phenotype of darker skin than mine. I know that my grandfather, who came off the boat in 1919 speaking no English, found work as a carpenter in Cleveland more easily because of the color of his skin than did a similarly experienced African American carpenter born and raised in the city to which my grandfather came.

I also know that when he built his home in a middle-class suburb in the 1950s no one questioned his right to be there. When the first two African American families tried to build their homes in that same suburb in the same time frame, their applications were held up for years by a zoning board raising one petty question after another. A carpenter with a seventh-grade education designed and built that first home; an architect with a master's degree in his subject designed, built, and finally was able to live in that second home with his daughter, who became the first African American girl in my scout troupe but not until the city did everything it could to make him and his family feel unwelcome. If I cannot find a way to convey to my African American client that I know this truth about the realities of phenotype privilege, she or he has no reason to go past a certain point of vulnerability with me because I will not have communicated an awareness of the power of my social location of privilege.

Other groups—heterosexual persons, middle- and upper-class persons, those not yet disabled, and so on—also benefit from unearned privilege and, when engaged in the intimate exchange of psychotherapy, will bring the effects of that privilege into the dynamics of the relationship. Privilege can protect against distress in the face of trauma, or it can be a factor leading to distress; disadvantage can instill resilience that is protective, or it can create vulnerabilities that spread the effects of a trauma exposure beyond their initial impact. The dynamics of power and powerlessness arising from privilege intertwine with trauma, and when they are treated as nonexistent, they will impinge on therapy for trauma survivors. Not yet being a survivor of trauma is, after all, very much a form of privilege that is unearned; being able to keep one's survivor status private and avoid the shame associated with disclosure, something that redounds to the role of the psychotherapist within the usual boundaries of the process, is also a form of privilege, associated as it is with the power of the psychotherapist's role.

Privilege is not a reason for guilt on the part of the dominant group psychotherapist. Individuals are not responsible for having inherited unearned privilege. I did not choose my phenotype or know the unearned advantages it would give me. In fact, guilt from privileged persons about their privilege invariably becomes an additional burden for the disadvantaged others, who then often feel compelled to do the work of reassuring dominant group members that they are not a bad, oppressive individuals, and become deflected from their own agendas. Rather, psychotherapists with some dominant group membership (and it is difficult to have none; the heterosexual Christian married-male African American has one set of privileges stemming from the first four social locations in his identity; I, a lesbian Jewish cannot-get-legally-married female Euro-American have a different set of privileges stemming from the last of my listed social locations) need to commit to personal work to become aware of their privilege and how it manifests in their worldviews and their work to achieve and maintain cultural competence.

A component of that work is leaving guilt and shame behind. I have privilege; my job is to know how to live responsibly with that reality, not to deny it or pretend that I can jettison it. Similarly, psychotherapists with social disadvantage must become aware of the effects of internalized oppression and exclusion on their psyches as they enter the relationship with clients who may have more access to privilege than they and notice how they or their clients may subtly disempower these psychotherapists as the dynamics of power and dominance from the larger society infiltrate the therapy office.

As McIntosh (1998) noted, any dominant group privilege, be it of gender, sexual orientation, ethnicity, social class, and so on, is generally operating at a nonconscious level. It is the nature of privilege to make itself invisible to those benefiting from it but very visible to those who do not have it. Internalized oppression may be similarly invisible because it has become a part of the consciousness and sense of self of the oppressed individual (Pheterson, 1986), a negative ascription about one's own group that feels true because it has been reinforced in oppressive social contexts for so long. In each instance, the psychosocial impact of culturally based hierarchies will have a residence in the therapy room and, if not brought into awareness and consciousness by the psychotherapist, may be detrimental to an effective healing process. Add trauma to the mixture and the potentials for problems may increase because trauma is itself a factor disadvantaging a person and frequently one that undermines power and privilege in ways that are confusing to all parties.

This perspective can be particularly important given that psychotherapists frequently constitute the privileged persons in the therapy room, with the power of the therapeutic role outweighing privilege or disadvantage that might operate in the social world outside of therapy. Because therapy is an elite profession requiring in most cases postgraduate study and thus the luxury of time and financial resources and the capacities to navigate educational systems designed by and for the privileged, few psychotherapists do not come from dominant groups holding social privilege. When the psychotherapist is not a trauma survivor and the client is addressing issues of trauma, then dynamics related to privilege will obtain even when all other aspects of social location are shared by client and psychotherapist. Ultimately, privilege is about unearned ease and the inequitable access to resources inherent in certain kinds of personal and structural power. Because trauma is about disempowerment and the loss of safety and ease, a psychotherapist's awareness of power dynamics will strengthen the work with trauma survivors no matter what a psychotherapist's general orientation to treatment might be. Awareness of privilege and disadvantage become important components of knowing what one represents because the social locations that enter the room with a psychotherapist generally carry messages about the privilege or disadvantage stemming from those markers of social realities.

The psychotherapist working from a culturally competent standpoint takes the position of an ally. Allies are not advocates, nor does an alliance stance require a deviation from the frame of one's theory of psychotherapy (Mio & Rhoades, 2003). Rather, alliance is the stance of externalizing the problem that has been placed on the client's shoulders and making it a collective problem; specifically as relates to the issue of privilege, an alliance perspective places the primary responsibility for responding to issues evoked by a psychotherapist's dominant group privileges in the hands of the psychotherapist. It is a stance of moral nonneutrality as regards the traumatic event, a stance that, as Ochberg (1988) pointed out long ago, is required in work with trauma survivors for whom moral neutrality is the functional equivalent of silently standing against the survivor. It is a stance of willingness to identify and validate the realities of systems of oppression that operate in the lives of target group people who are also survivors of trauma (Dass-Brailford, 2006).

This can be particularly crucial when working with trauma survivors who are a superordinate target group cutting across and through all other identities and social locations in part because of having been the targets of a traumatic event, rendering them members of a group stigmatized in Western cultures. Trauma is a feminizing event; trauma renders its targets weak, helpless, confused, and emotional, all characteristics that are associated with the target group of femininity. Many of the meaning-making systems of our cultures impute blame to the trauma survivor for what has happened; notice that even in the case of supposedly morally neutral natural disasters a discourse of "why did they live there in the path of the tornado/flood/hurricane/windstorm/earthquake fault" can be seen and heard in postdisaster public discourse. When the psychotherapist is her- or himself a trauma survivor, she or he is in the room not in that identity, holding the privilege of the psychotherapist position. As a therapeutic ally, the culturally competent trauma psychotherapist acknowledges the presence of stigma in the room, attends to her or his inner pulls to assume the privilege of *normalcy*, (which is a characteristic almost always ascribed to members of the dominant group, even in those contexts not officially dedicated, as is indeed true in the psychotherapeutic context, to defining people as normal or abnormal), and tells the truth to clients about the reality of their situations rather than attempting to minimize the experience of the trauma or failing to respect that the client has already made attempts to cope with its aftermaths. The culturally competent therapist contextualizes the experience of trauma in light of historical, systemic, and institutionalized dynamics of oppression and targeting, highlighting the interaction between trauma and those other phenomena in the client's experience of pain and of recovery.

It can be helpful to differentiate clearly between privilege or its lack and trauma. All trauma strips privilege from people; not all disadvantage is traumatizing. Oppression, as I discuss later at length, is a risk factor for becoming traumatized, with some writers arguing that all oppressive systems are inherently traumagenic. Nonetheless, oppressed people frequently also have available to them systems of resilience and coping that mitigate the traumagenic effects of oppression. Culturally competent therapists have the task of enlightening themselves and their clients about the complicated interrelationships between oppression, trauma, and resilience as well as between privilege, trauma, and resilience. As I discuss later in this volume, there are times when privilege increases a person's risk of experiencing an event as traumatic.

THE COMPETENT TRAUMA SURVIVOR

Alliance with a client and cultural competence also reflect a competency-based stance on clients (Bertolino & O'Hanlon, 2001). From this position a psychotherapist strives to see the people with whom she or he works as having already been making numerous biological, psychological, psychosocial, and spiritual attempts to solve the problems engendered by trauma exposure. Gilfus (1999) referred to this stance as a "survivor-centered epistemology," which she defined as "first and foremost the acknowledgment of the survivor as a complete human being with a cultural and historical context, capable of expert knowledge in her or his own right, to be viewed through the lens of a loving perception" (p. 1253).

Some of these strategies for responding to the unbearable pains of trauma will have succeeded magnificently for varying periods of time; some will have succeeded poorly if at all. But all of these strategies are evidence of the survivor's intentions and desires to deal with what trauma invited into her or his life. The Vietnam veteran nurse with whom I worked in the 1980s began drinking to silence her nightmares and flashbacks. In alcohol she had a strategy that worked very well for a decade or so, then began to break down as her dose increased and interfered with her other life functions, and worked even less well as even the increased dose no longer kept her intrusive symptoms at bay (Brown, 1986). It is important to note that because active alcoholism is more stigmatized in women than in men, her coping strategy led to more social isolation and rejection from her family than similar behaviors might have for a man. However, she was not helpless or a failure, although she believed herself to be both when she began to work with me. She had been actively trying to cope with her distress for almost 2 decades and was mostly in need of a method that worked better and lasted longer so that she could recover from the trauma and pick up the pieces of her life left by her initial coping strategy. Just as generally culturally competent practice rests on respect for the diversity of ways in which humans inhabit life and the world, so culturally competent trauma practice respects and honors the diversity of attempts that trauma survivors have made to solve the problems of distress and disruption that trauma has brought into their lives.

Some coping strategies will have worked not as well as wished for or lasted not very long. The heterosexual Euro-American man who was beaten in the parking garage at his office and then developed an unwillingness to leave home solved the problem of being in unsafe places by never leaving his safe home. However, he quickly replaced the problem of unsafe places with the problem of never being able to go to work. Because he was male in a culture that has no official social role for a man not working outside the home, his solution worked more poorly for him than it might have for a similarly traumatized woman, especially if she was heterosexual and married, two social locations that make it permissible for an adult not to work outside the home if she is female, but stigmatize that strategy for a man.

Nonetheless, both of these people and every single trauma survivor that psychotherapists encounter in their work will have created some sort of self-help strategy: avoidance, dissociation, overwork, abuse of substances or food or exercise, prayer, art, petting the dog, giving birth, or being celibate. They have arrived at psychotherapists' offices alive, if sometimes only barely so. Frequently the strategies that they have used reflect one or more of their social locations, both at and after trauma exposure; some of their strategies will have been learned from other people residing in a shared traumatized context, be it familial or cultural. Some of the reasons that they will have come into therapy also reflect their social locations and the capacities of their emotional and psychosocial environments to support their strategies or not. A stance of alliance is one that recognizes psychotherapists' client's desires to problem solve buried in what are now symptoms of distress and dysfunction and honors that problem-solving capacity in an overt and respectful manner as a component of the therapy process. Similar to Rogers's (1957) thesis that all humans are possessed of the drive to self-actualize, so I find useful the notion that humans have the will to solve the problems of their lives. As I discuss later, a component of culturally competent treatment for trauma involves exploring effective strategies developed not only by psychotherapists but by other similar survivors who are often the best experts on what works.

In summary, cultural competence in work with trauma involves two sets of knowledge and two sets of emotional skills that must then be skillfully combined into one set of strategies for understanding and interacting with those who seek psychotherapists' care. In the remainder of this volume I explore further how to think about diverse experiences and their relationship to trauma so as to deepen that combined set of skills in clinical practice.

2

LIVING IN MULTIPLE IDENTITIES
IN THE CONTEXT OF TRAUMA

I turn now to the question of identities and identity development as this interacts with the experience of trauma exposure and, in this chapter, look at models of identity development and their relevance to the understanding of trauma. *Identities* (the "who I am") emerge from the interaction of *social locations* (the "what other people think I am") and are different from social locations in their meaning to the individual by being more valued and more core. Some social locations become an important part of a person's sense of self, whereas others are more in the background of identity.

WHAT IS IDENTITY?

Specifically, an identity is defined for purposes of this volume as an enduring phenomenon that eventually comes to transcend social locations, to represent how the person knows her- or himself to be, and to reflect core values held by the individual. Although the social psychology literature on identity commonly refers to *public* identities (those I would consider social locations as well as potentially identities) and *private* identities (those known to the person but not necessarily visible or tied to social locations), my experience is that a culturally sensitive strategy for understanding identity is one in which this dichotomy is eschewed in favor of a more ecological model in which identity is interactive between public and private and in which everyone has multiple components of identity informing their experiences of self and interpersonal relationships (Brown, 2006a; Root, 2004a, 2004b). As such, each person's multiple identities interact with the experience of trauma.

How does one know if something is an identity? Jack had been a star on his college baseball team. He lost his throwing arm up to the shoulder when his car overturned on an icy road and crushed him. An important component of his rehabilitation process was finding athletic activities at which he could excel using his remaining arm and the rest of his body. Baseball player was not Jack's identity; it was the social location at which his identity of athlete had been lodged. When asked later in life about whether the accident had been traumatic for him, he told people, "Yeah, I guess so, until I got into paraskiing. You know, I just love it and would never have even put on skis if I hadn't lost my arm. So actually the accident was a good thing."

Identities as defined here commonly share certain characteristics. They are delineated by values and inform values in a recursive process. Threats to identity are experienced as challenges to those values. People's values predict their choices, the nature of their relationships, and the meanings that they make of life circumstances. Identities reflect what Comas-Diaz (2006) referred to as a worldview, an overarching strategy for understanding and lending meaning to all aspects of one's life. Identities commonly contain multiple social locations because those identifiers visible to others tend to evolve from the more core identities held by the person or to have informed the development of the core identities. Whether identity is experienced individualistically or collectively, which largely depends on the cultural contexts informing identity, it is the thing that the person describes as self. Although many writers have argued persuasively that the very construct of self is a Western, culturally insensitive creation, I suggest that the sense of *I*-ness experienced by a person, whether it is the singularity described by Europeanized cultures or the member of the family or tribe "I am because we are" version found in other contexts, is this thing I am calling identity; self is found in that emotional and cognitive location.

TRAUMA AND IDENTITY

Trauma has a role in shaping identity when it is a component of early life experiences and/or embedded in the context of early development. It challenges identity when it occurs later in life. Trauma is also a component of identity when it is an aspect of a person's familial and/or cultural heritage of oppression, intergenerational or historical trauma. This is because trauma often lands squarely in vital components of identity and can interfere with basic human expressions of self, particularly those aspects of being human contained in people's capacities for relationship. Internalized oppression, which constitutes the component of identity emerging from the introjection of external bias and stereotype about one's own group (Russell, 1996) functions as a variable creating vulnerability for target group members to be particularly affected by trauma. Because of trauma's emotional-shape-changing capacities, I have found that identity models that allow both for stability over time as well as recognition of transformation in context are useful for making sense of trauma's impact on identity. What such models propose is the notion of each person having multiple identities deriving from sometimes conflictual social locations that are integrated into a coherent whole by the individual. When that integration is problematic, trauma is frequently although not always a component of the difficulties being encountered by that individual.

Trauma can shatter that coherence and evoke conflict by undermining previously held values, blocking the use of capacities emerging from a person's prior sense of self, and changing the face of the world as known, thus altering the parameters of the social context in which self is understood. Feeling alienated from self and context is very common in the wake of trauma; the autobiographical literature by trauma survivors is replete with stories of "feeling not like myself." As Nancy Raine wrote about the anniversary of her rape, "It marked again the death of the person I had been for thirty-nine years. This woman had a history. . . . But on October 11, 1985 she died. Another person was born that day" (Raine, 1998, p. 2).

As Raine noted, her prerape self had a life, a career, relationships, interests, an identity; none of that lived through the day of her rape, although all of that history remained in place. Unlike Jack, who found a way to have his identity even after traumatic loss of a limb, for many survivors of trauma the trauma kills or sends into hiding the person they knew, and a new self composed of old identities as transformed by trauma comes to stand in that person's stead. When trauma survivors enter therapy they frequently come in the guise of that new person, who is seen as damaged goods by both the traumatized person and many in their emotional milieu. Their identities have been polluted by the trauma, particularly those traumas pointed directly at aspects of identity and social location. The presence of the pretrauma self may be known only by the grief over its apparent loss.

It is largely because of trauma's profound effect on identity and relationships with various social locations that Maria P. P. Root's (1998, 2000, 2004b) ecological model of identity development for persons of mixed racial heritage is one that I have found especially useful when thinking about the effects of trauma on identity and the reciprocal influence of identities on the experience of trauma. Root's model incorporates the possibility of a family or cultural heritage of trauma exposure into the process of identity development and is one of few identity development models of which I'm aware that takes trauma, both individual and historical, explicitly into account as a shaper of identity. The implications of this model are important for understanding how culturally competent trauma practice operates when approaching working with people from the perspectives of their multiple identities.

PARADIGMS FOR MULTIPLE IDENTITIES

Root argued that to develop an identity theory for persons of mixed social locations (which I would suggest includes almost all humans), several factors need to be present. First, this model needs to account for within-group bias and oppression, the sort of expression of internalized oppression or horizontal hostility that can occur when target group membership is present. In Root's original model, which refers to persons of mixed race, she pointed to discrimination and bias against persons of mixed race within the ethnic groups making up the various sides of their heritage.

Second, such a model must see as positive the experience of multiple identities. This is a striking deviation from prior models of mixed race, which saw having a unitary racial identity as the sine qua non of mental health; Root's model is a useful paradigm for understanding the identity experiences of trauma survivors by construing mixed identities as potentially mentally healthy. Her model next noted the importance of changes in social and political contexts and social reference groups available to an individual, thus informing individuals' understanding of identity and social location. Finally, the model must acknowledge the interaction of experiences in the person's social ecology, including family environment, history, and biological heritage. Root portrayed her model graphically as a series of nested, interactive, and overlapping boxes in which these various factors are in constant interplay and in which identity is in a continuous process of development rather than moving toward a fixed and apparently stable state.

Cultural competence in trauma practice is enhanced by this or similar models of identity formation because they allow the clinician to conceptualize the client's identity not only as a continuously transforming matrix of multiple social locations but also as not requiring a fixed and stable state to be functional. Because of trauma's potential to affect identity, work with trauma survivors requires psychotherapists to rethink their paradigms for mental health and good function; having a model of multiple identities with an embedded change process may assist both psychotherapist and client in finding strategies for creating a posttrauma life narrative that is healing for the client.

Many survivors of trauma exist in a liminal identity state, one in which transition is a constant. What is less obvious but equally important for the culturally competent trauma psychotherapist to take into account is the degree to which liminal identities are those emerging as a function of a post-traumatic healing process in which identity as a trauma survivor becomes integrated in a positive fashion into other aspects of identity.

Nancy Raine's narrative of transformation after her rape is an example of this experience of liminality. She is moving through a multiplicity of emotional and social positions, first appearing to lose then returning to and drawing on her pretrauma identities in her healing process. What is striking about Raine's memoir and what can be informed by Root's identity model is the manner in which interactions between various aspects of identity and the social ecologies available to her appear to have been core components of her healing process.

Five Identity Strategies

Root suggested that in attempting to develop an identity and self founded in multiple known social locations an individual has five possible strategies available. The first of these is to accept an identity as assigned by society. This implicitly includes accepting the social roles conflated with the identity because it involves internalizing and applying to oneself the rules created by the larger social context. She noted that this strategy is a passive rather than active one in which a person, by remaining congruent with societal expectations, is also disempowered in relationship to how realities are constructed by others (Root, 2004b). For those who have experienced trauma, having an identity constrained by an external construction of trauma survivors may be the position occupied by many people as they enter the therapy process.

This is not, it must be noted, a pathological or lesser strategy. It may reflect many of a person's social locations and the norms and values of components of identity in which not rocking boats or challenging authority are seen as central. It may also reflect a comfort with the identity that is assigned. However, when the assigned identity is one that is trauma related, it is likely that this identity strategy will be problematic in some manner because the identities that culture assigns to trauma survivors are commonly connected to the expressions of distress made by those individuals.

Marc, for example, was a survivor of sexual abuse by priests. He was a Polish-American grandson of immigrants who was brutally sexually abused by his parish priest for several years during his early adolescence. Although he had been an excellent student (and like many such men, an altar boy) and a star athlete, his behavior deteriorated sharply in the years after the abuse began. He kept the abuse secret from everyone; he felt deeply ashamed, betrayed by God, and guilty that he had had a homosexual encounter. Although he had a baseball scholarship to a small private Catholic college, he never completed his first semester; a terrifying flashback in the locker room during his first game of the season led to his dropping out and beginning to drink heavily. His life spiraled downward after that, with a series of dead-end jobs and failed relationships with women in which his attempts to prove his heterosexuality were undermined by the flashbacks that happened each time he attempted sexual intercourse. His family, not understanding that what they were observing was posttraumatic in nature, rejected him as a drunk and a loser. He came to take on this spoiled assigned identity, not himself understanding that his problems stemmed from the rapes and the degradation that accompanied them. It was only after the appearance of a series of articles in the local paper describing the first of many lawsuits against the priest who had abused him that he began to put together the possibility that any of his difficulties in life and the change of life trajectory from an A student and star forward to intermittently homeless and rarely sober had to do with the abuse he had suffered.

When he came in for a forensic evaluation a few months later at the request of his attorney, his identity was still firmly fixed in the one assigned to him by his family and society. He was just beginning to imagine, with help from his attorney and the psychotherapist that she had found for him, that this identity might be erroneous. It had come to trump every other aspect of self for him, an outcome not unusual for survivors of trauma. He told the evaluator that he was a "loser; I never fought back. I was 14; I could have beaten him up. So maybe I wanted it. I was weak." The constructions assigned by society to men who are raped had become Marc's identity.

Root's second strategy for identity creation in the context of multiple social locations is one of identification with one visible aspect of identity in which other aspects of identity are made peripheral. Her model suggests that this is a way in which people develop their identities in an active manner. The person's phenomenology of identity trumps social expectations and external variables, and the individual chooses how they will be known. This model still fits a person into social roles that are externally constructed as congruent for the identity chosen (in her original model, the role of the monorace, by which Root meant the one-race model). For a trauma survivor, choosing one aspect of identity might mean deciding to put the experience of trauma in the background because the attributes ascribed to the identity of trauma survivor are still unquestioned and experienced as stigmatizing and unacceptable.

Carla's story is an example of this strategy, which worked for a number of years (Brown, 1991b). A Euro-American lesbian from a blue-collar family, she had been repeatedly sexually abused by two older family members who were also her health care providers; her parents were emotionally absent, her mother deeply self-absorbed and critical. Bright and talented, she decided to put her past behind her, literally and geographically, moving 3,000 miles away from home as an adult. She came to therapy with the presenting issue of dealing with fertility challenges that had emerged as she attempted to become pregnant in her mid-30s. Her identity was that of an activist and a social services worker; trauma survivor was relegated to a distant corner of her self. While sharing her history with me, she mentioned in passing that she had been sexually abused and stated, "I've dealt with that," communicating her earlier decision to have this experience be peripheral to her identity.

Ironically, it was because the fertility treatments on which she was embarking, which were a component of pursuing the desired identity of mother, evoked aspects of the abuse that she had become symptomatic and sought therapy. The intrusive symptoms from which she was suffering interfered with the identity that she had constructed in which her trauma had no place, a common experience for those survivors of trauma who have made a conscious decision to make other social locations more important in their identity than the trauma. Until her encounters with medical care broke through this strategy, it had been an enormously effective one that had propelled her from a painful and problematic childhood and adolescence into an adult life in which her talents and competencies defined her to her social and emotional networks.

The problems in her life that she later came to see as associated with having been sexually abused had remained unexamined and unchallenged. Consequently, the emergence of posttraumatic symptoms brought with it a windstorm of self-hatred as the affects and cognitions associated with the trauma, which had been effectively dissociated, poured into her consciousness. She was faced with the challenge of working through and letting go of the toxic identities created by childhood trauma and integrating them into the nonsurvivor identities she had created for herself as an adult, integrating rather than having to choose one or the other as her true self.

Root's third alternative for identity development in the context of multiple identities suggests an active, creative strategy in which identity is core yet fluid and the social roles emerging from this identity may or may not be consistent with how the external social context defines the person. The identity that the person embraces will contain multiple components with each one informing the person's understanding of others. In this instance trauma may not take the foreground in identity, but its meaning has been interrogated sufficiently that social assignments of blame and stigma no longer predominate that social location. Trauma survivor will be a component of identity, although not a sole component.

This strategy embodies the feminist notion of resistance (Brown, 1994) in which a person finds voice by refusing, overtly or passively, to collude with oppressive social norms. With this strategy, the trauma survivor constructs identity freed from the constraints of social roles as defined by others and deconstructs identity to support multiple, apparently conflicting social roles that are experienced internally as consistent and supporting one another. Thus in the case of the racially and ethnically mixed people from whose lives Root derived her model, a person might decide that she is White and Filipina not either one alone and both in the ways not defined by others.

Selina, whose parents were highly educated Maronite Christian immigrants from Lebanon, had grown up encountering hostility in the larger community because she was Arab and in Arab communities because she was Christian. Her family of medical professionals had been decimated in Lebanon's civil war, with both of her parents having witnessed the deaths of family members during rocket attacks by hostile militias. The first American-born member of her family, she often felt pulled between her parents' more conservative norms for behavior and those of her friends at an urban public school. In her adolescence she engaged in increasingly risky behaviors as part of adolescent differentiation strivings, and while at a party where older men were present, she was raped by two other party goers while she was drunk and had nearly passed out.

In the aftermath of this assault Selina struggled with self-blame and the message from both her parents and herself that had she been more compliant with family norms she would have never been raped. It was only as she began to query her father more about what seemed to be his intractable distress at what had happened to her that she learned that one of the traumas he carried was overhearing his sister being raped by a gang of hostile militia men before she was killed. She felt confused; her parents' message to her while she was growing up had been that good Lebanese girls did not have such things happen to them, and because this had happened to her she was not a good Lebanese girl. Yet the aunt she had never known, who was held up to her as the model of this concept, had herself been raped.

Her parents' grief at having, in their own eyes, failed to protect this daughter, finally opened up a family discourse about the many losses that the parents had incurred, including loss of familiar country and language, in their hopes that the next generation could be kept safe. The family began to talk about the challenges of being a target group within a target group, and Selina became more aware of how her ambivalence about her culture had fueled her risky behaviors. As she moved through a healing process she decided that being a Lebanese-American, Christian Arab rape survivor was an identity that she could publicly claim "to honor my aunt's memory, to say out loud that this is not my shame or my family's shame." Her claimed identity included elements of many of her social locations and conveyed her refusal to submerge any of them in the service of others.

Root's fourth strategy is a level of identity creativity that can best be characterized as "grow your own." This strategy actively challenges the ways in which humans have been previously assigned identities by virtue of social locations (e.g., in her original model, by phenotype). This strategy engages resistance at a deeper level because not only does the person refuse to accept social prescriptions as to how identity should be developed but the person also refuses to legitimize the categories from which those prescriptions have arisen. These individuals will frequently be found saying that labels do not apply to them and will have an identity that is of their own making.

Eugenio was an artist whose collages of found objects were deeply symbolic stories about his experiences of torture and survival as a prisoner of the Chilean military junta. His parents, members of the Socialist party, had come to Chile from Germany to escape the Nazis, and the family had been active in leftist causes. Many of his friends from art school were among the *desaparacidos*, the disappeared ones murdered by the junta. He had moved to the United States after his unexpected and never explained sudden release from prison, where he had been tortured physically and mentally, and resumed his career as an artist, becoming a respected teacher as well as being sought after for his works.

When interviewed about his collages, he said that he had realized while in prison that nothing was more important to him than his artistic vision. "Yes, I was tortured. But that is not what defines me. It teaches me better how to be an artist, but the artist is first, always." He challenged anyone who suggested that he was in denial about the horrors of his experiences to "look at my work—there you will see the truth about horror." He told his physician that he indeed suffered from nightmares about his experiences and grief over the deaths of his friends and comrades and requested medication to help him with these symptoms. No stranger to therapy, given his mother's profession of psychoanalyst, he nonetheless chose not to use that modality because "I must grieve and heal in my own way."

Root's final strategy is what she described as the creation of a symbolic identity. In this strategy the person has never internalized social rules governing identity and decides that how they perceive themselves to be trumps how others perceive them and also trumps from where they came. This strategy can be controversial and can be incorrectly read as an endorsement of assimilation or passing by persons whose various social locations (such as phenotype, sexual orientation, social class, or gender) are not immediately apparent to an observer. This last strategy may figure heavily in the identity development of individuals with cultural histories of trauma, however, making it of particular interest for culturally competent trauma treatment.

Sokom's friends knew that she was Cambodian; her phenotypic heritage was easy for others to see, as was the fact that her mother, the only parent who had survived the Pol Pot regime, spoke mostly Khmer and relied heavily on her daughter to negotiate the English-speaking world. The family were poor, and Sokom, who came to the United States at the age of 5 as a refugee, grew up in a dangerous public housing development; her mother worked at home making traditional Cambodian embroidered clothing for a local shop, but the family's main source of income was inadequate social assistance funding from the state.

Sokom attended public schools where she was at first lost and bewildered by a language and customs not her own. She was intellectually very capable and was soon mentored by her teachers who encouraged her to spend time after school in their classrooms doing extra reading and learning about the skills necessary for living in America. She became a highly competent code switcher: At home she was a Khmer daughter, deferent to her mother; once outside the house she was an increasingly Americanized youngster, accent free and dressed in the latest fashions, which her teachers had helped her to procure by taking her on shopping trips to the local mall on weekends. She became a varsity athlete by high school, competing on an elite girl's volleyball team with promises of full scholarships to good colleges.

Sokom's college essay was an example of her creation of a symbolic identity:

> I know that I am Khmer. Nothing can change that, nor would I wish it changed. I am the descendant of a culture of decency, of art, a member of an ancient and lovely civilization. I refuse to have my understanding of my heritage shaped by its invaders and destroyers. So even though my residence in Tacoma owes everything to those invaders and destroyers, what they did is not a part of me because I am also an American. I am someone who sees opportunity and takes it. Because I am Khmer, I know that I will always share the fruits of my accomplishments first with my family. Because I am American I will pursue those accomplishments vigorously. My mothers, who include the mother who gave me birth and my teachers, are all expressed through me.

Sokom acknowledged that her social locations owed a debt to historical trauma, and she also located her identity outside of that trauma.

Root's various strategies demonstrate how it is possible to have a strong core identity containing apparently conflicting social roles or even an identity in which social locations recognized by the culture around a person are rejected in favor of a chosen identity. The conflicts, Root argued, are either externally imposed or reflect internalization of oppression. When persons become empowered to be the authors of their own identity or identities and to assert that any social role will be congruent in some way with those identities, some of the apparent conflicts diminish. Trauma, however, can evoke those conflicts anew or create fresh conflicts because of the manner in which it may emphasize some aspects of self and diminish or even delete others.

The chapters in this book separate components of identity to go into greater depth about how each one might contribute to the experience of trauma exposure and recovery. However, human beings can only be viewed as the intersection of those locations, the crossroads, as it were, of all of the various aspects of self. Most of the clinical examples that I use demonstrate how these multiple identities are experienced; although one aspect of identity might be in the foreground because it is related either to the trauma itself, the trauma's symbolic meaning, or the resources used for recovery, a person's multiple identities will always be the driving force informing her or his experience.

In culturally competent practice a psychotherapist is cognizant of the various components of a client's multiple identities, including those components contributed or influenced by personal or historical trauma. The foundation of culturally competent practice with trauma survivors begins with interrogating the meanings of those identities and their shaping of the experience of trauma and recovery

3

ENTERING THE HEALING PROCESS

Culturally competent psychotherapy begins at the first encounter. In this chapter, I look at how to integrate culturally competent practice into the intake and assessment phases of psychotherapy. I also examine specific treatments for trauma and the transtheoretical evidence base for culturally competent trauma treatment.

Some argument exists over precisely when Western medicine and psychology began to recognize posttrauma symptoms as such. This recognition of the relationship of trauma to psychological distress is a necessary first step in healing but one that mental health professions have only slowly and reluctantly taken. Apparently the writers of ancient texts of war and enslavement were able to identify such symptoms; the Biblical prophet Ezekiel, himself a survivor of the traumas of wartime conquest and captivity, spoke of having a "heart of stone" and of intrusive images of the Jerusalem he had last seen smoking in ruins as he was carried away to Babylon. "By the rivers of Babylon, we wept when we remembered Zion"; the Bible tells us of traumatic grief. Shay (1995) commented on the parallels between the stories of Achilles in the Trojan War and those of Vietnam combat veterans.

Yet aside from this sort of reference in sacred texts, trauma was rarely noted as a source of emotional difficulties until the middle of the 19th century when the concept of "railway spine," the symptoms now configured as posttraumatic stress disorder (PTSD), began to emerge in the medical literature. Pierre Janet, the great French psychiatrist, was one of the first modern commentators to both observe posttraumatic symptoms and name them as such. In the late 1800s he described the phenomena that are now called complex trauma and dissociation. He also proposed treatments, some of which resemble what psychotherapists now know empirically to be helpful for individuals who have suffered severe and repetitive interpersonal trauma (van der Hart, Nijenhuis, & Steele, 2006).

Freud considered, then rejected, a trauma model for understanding his patients' problems, a decision that had the effect of brushing trauma under the rug for another half century (cf. Herman, 1992). The British psychiatrists who treated "shell shock" in the soldiers of World War I similarly proposed treatment methods that appear to be precursors of current trauma therapies (Rivers, 1918), methods that were promptly forgotten once that conflict ended. Kardiner and Spiegel (1947) similarly revived awareness of war as a psychological trauma as a result of their work with World War II soldiers, but by the time of the Vietnam conflict it was as if their insights into the relationship of trauma to emotional distress had never been. When I interned in the Veteran's Administration in 1976 and 1977, veterans of the Vietnam conflict who suffered from what is now clearly known as PTSD were defined as characterologically disturbed, not traumatized.

As Herman (1992) famously noted, "The study of psychological trauma has a curious history—one of episodic amnesia" (p. 7). Trauma as a topic has gone in and out of favor in psychology and psychiatry, with treatment approaches being reinvented, sometimes with little or no reference to what has gone before. In the 1970s and 1980s when trauma was experiencing a resurgence of focus, a good deal of experimentation occurred in the trauma treatment field; some of these experiments were very helpful, whereas others taught psychotherapists about what trauma treatment should not be. Today a number of evidence-based practices for treating the symptoms specifically linked to trauma exposure are available. Additionally, outside of the framework of specific treatment techniques, consensus models have emerged as to how to work with survivors of trauma. Finally, there continue to be emerging paradigms for working with trauma survivors that still lack formal empirical foundation but that make intuitive sense in light of what is known about trauma as a biopsychosocial and spiritual phenomenon.

What is remarkable about all of these trauma treatment paradigms is that few of them were developed to take cultural competence or attention to human diversity into intentional account. Some of the transtheoretical conceptual models for working with survivors of interpersonal violence were designed by feminist psychotherapists and theorists and as such reflect an attention to gender and at times also to culture and social class. Research on specific treatment techniques for particular kinds of trauma that include such highly gendered stressors as sexual assault has also been conducted and constitutes an important portion of the empirical literature backing up some of those approaches. However, I have yet to find a major model of trauma treatment that begins with the question, "What does this trauma mean to these people, given their history, their cultures, and their identities?"

A challenge to any work with a survivor of trauma is that there is no universal human response to traumatic stress. Both PTSD and acute stress disorder (ASD) are enshrined in formal diagnostic nomenclature as the specific symptom clusters arising from trauma exposure. Yet trauma is a risk factor for a range of other conditions; although only about 20% of persons exposed to a *Diagnostic and Statistical Manual of Mental Disorders* (4th ed., text rev.; *DSM–IV–TR*; American Psychiatric Association, 2000) Criterion A stressor go on to develop PTSD, the remainder are not symptom free.

Rather, trauma exposure is implicated in a host of additional difficulties and expressions of distress, some of which will be shaped strongly by social location. Dissociative phenomena, including dissociative identity disorder, are very likely to be associated with a history of exposure to severe, repeated, and inescapable trauma (van der Hart et al., 2006). Interpersonal violence, one type of trauma, has been shown to be a risk factor for depression (Strickland, Russo, & Keita, 1989); depressive disorders are one of the two most common comorbid diagnoses made with PTSD (Briere & Scott, 2006), although some of this may reflect the overlap in symptoms between the two diagnoses. Many people exposed to trauma self-medicate through the use of alcohol, opiates, other central-nervous-system-depressant drugs, legal or otherwise, or nicotine, which calms the hyperarousal and anxiety resulting from trauma exposure in extremely effective ways. Others whose trauma exposure leads to problems of psychic numbing and loss of energy use stimulants to attempt to treat this posttraumatic depressive state. A history of trauma exposure is consequently common among persons seeking assistance to break an addiction (Briere & Scott, 2006). Specific phobias or other anxiety disorders can either be comorbid with PTSD or may emerge as distinct from PTSD, with a person manifesting only the anxious and fearful expressions of posttrauma response.

Finally, for many individuals trauma manifests in the body as well as the psyche. Somatoform problems, including in some cultures conversion disorders, are common in trauma survivors (van der Hart et al., 2006). Perhaps because of the pervasive systemic effects of the biological response to trauma (Mueller, 2005), persons with a trauma history also appear to suffer at higher rates than the general population from a host of organic health problems such as autoimmune disorders, chronic pain, and gastrointestinal difficulties (Walker et al., 1999). The difficulties in self-care with which many trauma survivors struggle, such as abuse of food, difficulties engaging in exercise, smoking, and use of self-inflicted violence to regulate emotions, may be the source of organic health problems such as cardiovascular disease or Type II diabetes, none of which are usually immediately linked to a history of trauma exposure but are endemic in the complex trauma population. Many trauma survivors manipulate food intake as a means of experiencing control (Root & Fallon, 1988) or use food to self-soothe, leading in turn to the range of medical problems associated both with disordered eating and, on occasion, very large body size. Finally, self-inflicted violence in the form of cutting, burning, hitting, or otherwise harming oneself physically is seen most often in persons surviving complex trauma (Brown & Bryan, 2007; Mazelis, 2003). Trauma has biological, psychological, psychosocial, and existential sequelae, and no one component of this multifaceted picture of distress can be understood in isolation from the rest.

CULTURAL COMPETENCE IN THE INTAKE PROCESS

All of this diversity of clinical presentation means that competent psychotherapy of any sort should likely consider the possibility of trauma as one of several variables informing the development of any client's symptoms, whether or not that client presents with either an expressed history of trauma exposure or the obvious symptoms of either PTSD or ASD. All intake histories should include questions about exposures to a range of traumatic stressors phrased in such a way as to increase the likelihood that clients will share these experiences if they are available as well as questions about the range of experience of distress not limited to those described by the PTSD diagnosis. Even when the presenting diagnosis is one now considered mostly biological (e.g., schizophrenia), a biopsychosocial and spiritual–existential conceptual framework should raise questions about the possible role of trauma as the stressor evoking a biological substrate or about trauma arising from a person's mental health status. I discuss later in this volume how trauma is a constant in the lives of many people who are persistently mentally ill; persistent mental illness in the United States frequently means a life spent in poverty, often on the streets, and consequently at the mercy of others' violent behaviors.

If specific questions about types of trauma are asked, the language should be such as to increase a client's ability to give the information the psychotherapist is seeking by being language that does not limit the sharing of life experience. For example, research on sexual assault trauma, particularly at the hands of known others, has shown that if women are asked if they were raped, many who are survivors of acquaintance rape will respond in the negative because the term rape is coded conceptually as representing a violent act perpetrated by a stranger, what Estrich (1988) calls "real rape." However, asking the same group of women if they have experienced sex that was unwanted, coerced, or occurred while they were asleep or drugged yields more accurate information about a type of trauma that may indeed have long-lasting psychological consequences (Koss, 1988).

Questions about trauma need to be phrased in neutral and behaviorally descriptive manners with verbal shorthand avoided. A disaster is not a disaster is not a disaster; what is disastrous to one person is a difficult but ultimately growth-producing experience to another. Asking about an experience in which one's life was disrupted by such events of nature as storms, earthquakes, fires, or mudslides will more likely evoke the narrative exposing what was traumatic as well as what was simply annoying. Cultural concerns that stand in the way of answering questions about certain kinds of experience also must be taken into account. If, for instance, one's family is shamed by one's experiences, then one may not tell of them unless and until the questioner has earned sufficient trust. Often, information about a trauma history can best be elicited by asking open-ended questions such as "I'm wondering if you can tell me about the life experiences you've had that *you* would consider painful, humiliating or frightening," which can then be followed up with clarifying questions as to specific experiences of trauma

At times people will be unsure if something qualifies for the label *traumatic*. Using such words as *painful*, *scary*, or *humiliating*, all affects commonly associated with trauma, or describing the types of responses people frequently have when traumatized, for example, "Sometimes people feel as if they're watching themselves in a movie or from a great distance during some kinds of confusing, painful, or scary events. Have you ever had experiences like that?" can be effective in both normalizing the experience of trauma and letting clients know that the psychotherapist is not unfamiliar with what they have suffered. This may, in turn, increase clients' abilities to narrate their traumas even very early in the therapy process. Because it is common for trauma survivors, particularly those afflicted with florid symptoms such as flashbacks or dissociative episodes, to wonder if they are crazy, this normalizing process in which common symptoms are identified by a psychotherapist as within the range of usual posttrauma response is basic to competent trauma treatment.

Issues of identity and cultural competence come immediately into play at this juncture in therapy and if attended to well can set a tone for the work to come. I discuss some important questions to consider for culturally competent history taking about trauma in the paragraphs that follow.

Does the psychotherapist potentially represent the source of the trauma? Representation becomes extremely salient at this early stage of therapy when the humanity of the therapist is less visible than phenotype, sex, and age. Examples of this include a male psychotherapist with a victim of sexual assault by a man, a Euro-American psychotherapist with a person of color who is a victim of workplace discrimination, or a native-born psychotherapist dealing with a client who is an undocumented immigrant awaiting asylum status. When psychotherapists are themselves reminders of a trauma, simply asking clients about painful or humiliating experiences may not be sufficient to elicit the information because clients may be unwilling to disclose their experiences to someone who is her- or himself unwittingly triggering their symptoms. Psychotherapists may need to take the time very early in therapy to contextualize what they represent in terms of the specific trauma and to consider how they and their clients represent members of one another's dominant or target groups.

A culturally competent psychotherapist might say,

> I realize that I'm a straight person who's going to be talking with you about being beaten up for being a gay man. I'm wondering how that set of circumstances is affecting your ability to tell me about your experience, and I'm also wondering what I can do to facilitate this process for you?

It is not always possible to find therapeutic resources for a trauma survivor that are not themselves somehow a trauma trigger; the strategy of "I'll refer this person to a gay male psychotherapist" may not be available, but the strategy of making power differentials and privilege transparent in the therapy session is always available and demonstrates cultural competence.

In culturally competent practice, these first steps of demonstrating cultural sensitivity, which frequently occur while the psychotherapist is taking a history, can be foundational for further therapeutic alliance building. When the psychotherapist begins the process by speaking out loud those variables that each person in the relationship brings to the table, then that psychotherapist has been culturally competent in a very basic yet quite powerful manner. Research on trust in therapy has found that in general the culturally aware psychotherapist, even when apparently culturally dissimilar, was deemed more trustworthy and empathic than an apparently culturally similar but not culturally aware psychotherapist. For effective and culturally competent therapy to occur, it matters more that the therapist demonstrates to a client that she or he actively considers who she or he is as a psychotherapist and what that might mean to the client than that the therapist appears to be a member of a particular group. Offering this sort of consideration to clients at the earliest possible opportunity is one simple strategy for demonstrating one's cultural awareness as a psychotherapist. As described in chapter 2, this awareness of what one represents in the transaction can be crucial to demonstrating one's worthiness of a client's trust particularly at this time in therapy when there is little else on which a client can base trust.

A second important question to consider in taking a history about trauma is the degree to which apparent shared group memberships may make it both easier and more difficult to tell the psychotherapist about a specific trauma if that trauma has culturally significant meanings. A woman who was genitally mutilated as a child in Africa may feel very uncomfortable talking about this as a trauma to another African woman. She may wonder if the psychotherapist was herself so mutilated. She cannot know if her psychotherapist did or did not experience it as traumatic or whether the psychotherapist has rationalized the experience in some way. This client may experience shame or humiliation about revealing, not what was done but the fact that it was traumatic to her because the frame put around female genital mutilation (FGM) is that it is a rite of passage for girls that protects their virtue and thus should be construed as a positive and valued experience. "Many women in our communities were cut when they were little," a culturally competent psychotherapist raised in Africa might say to her African woman client, "and many of those found it painful or frightening. My mother did. I'm wondering if that was true for you." Notice that here the psychotherapist does not directly disclose her own experience of FGM but does make it clear to the client that this is an issue about which she knows firsthand in an emotionally meaningful way.

Similarly some victims of domestic violence who hail from ethnic, religious, or other small communities may feel ashamed of being so victimized because of cultural mythologies that domestic violence does not occur in that community (Zimberoff & Brown, 2006); these clients may hesitate to tell the truth to a psychotherapist of their own group and be more comfortable speaking to a stranger or simply not be able to tell at all because of the taboo on revealing that domestic violence occurs in their community.

Irit was one such woman. An observant Jew with four small children, she was married to a man who had begun to beat her during her first pregnancy. He was prominent in their community, respected for his scholarly prowess, and a successful research scientist who created a financially comfortable life for his family. The regular beatings, which escalated with each successive pregnancy, had left Irit depressed and terrified, feeling trapped. Her faith discouraged her from speaking of his actions because speaking ill of someone else, even if true, is strongly frowned on in observant Jewish communities. She had once broached the subject of abuse in a roundabout way to her rabbi's wife and had received in return a lecture about how wonderful Jewish men were because they did not beat their wives. Irit left that discussion feeling even more silenced and alone. Her husband was also emotionally and verbally abusive of her in private.

She finally ended up in a psychotherapist's office after her obstetrician insisted that she seek psychological care for depression after the birth of her most recent child. The psychotherapist, who was a nonobservant Jewish woman, routinely asked about violence and trauma in her intake. Sensitive to the mythologies about abuse in her own culture and knowing that the strictures against discussing this could be particularly powerful in the social small towns of observant communities, she framed her questions to Irit by saying,

> I'm aware that there's a myth that there's no domestic violence in Jewish communities, which can make it hard to talk about it if that's been your experience. I just want you to know that I'm aware we say this to our-

selves and also that I know it's a myth because it happened in my Jewish family. So I'm wondering about whether there were people in your family who were ever violent with one another.

Both the acknowledgement of the belief system and the psychotherapist's self-disclosure allowed Irit to begin to consider disclosing what was happening in her home, although that disclosure came well into the 4th month of therapy.

Culturally competent trauma history taking proceeds by acknowledging this sort of dilemma that therapy can present for clients. Telling the truth about one's own culture, whether to an outsider or someone from within, can be a violation of strong proscriptions against speaking of such disowned ways of being. By normalizing the potential emotional barriers to sharing one's trauma story, the psychotherapist, in the intake process, makes visible and present the cultural issues that might serve as obstacles to initial disclosure by the client, taking into account those less visible but no less powerful barriers erected by shared culture as well as those more easily identifiable walls erected by difference.

This last topic points out an important side note to the discussion of taking a history, a side note that resurfaces throughout this text. Many psychotherapists, along with many of their clients, naively assume that when they share demographic characteristics this will ease the process of therapy and deepen empathy. When this comes to trauma I have found this not necessarily to be the case; sometimes this assumption has proven detrimental to the therapeutic process and outcome. Apparently shared experience can be a source of connection, but it can also be a source of distraction whereby either psychotherapist or client skips important components of a client's unique trauma narrative because of assumptions of similarities and shared understandings. My experience of being a lesbian is not any other lesbian's experience of being a lesbian; I cannot assume that the effects of heterosexism, sexism, and homophobia have affected her as they have affected me.

In culturally competent practice it is essential to consider the culturally tinged meanings of what it is psychotherapists are asking clients to reveal and what these revelations mean to psychotherapists as well as to clients. If psychotherapists are resistant to hearing about sexual abuse by a father from their own group or torture committed by a government that they support, if psychotherapists seek to rationalize failures to respond to a disaster by an agency they value or are unable to be present with the tale of a psychotherapist colleague who has sexually exploited, these and similar situations will often lead to a silencing of a client's trauma narrative; psychotherapists will use their power to ration the attention given, respond in a less than empathic manner, or otherwise push the client's experiences to the side. Psychotherapists can also have this sort of failure of empathy when their experiences appear to mirror those of their clients; if the psychotherapist is a cancer survivor she or he may find it more difficult to be fully open to another survivor's different cancer narrative if those differences evoke his own distress.

Although there are many circumstances in which similar experiences can assist in deepening empathy, the power of trauma itself to distort psychotherapists' emotional capacities as psychotherapists should never be underestimated. It is simply human to wish to distance oneself from the story of trauma. When that story brushes uncomfortably close to psychotherapists' own, they may engage all of their available resources for creating emotionally necessary distance. If the story is already too close in for comfort, psychotherapists' defenses against hearing that story may be even greater, with more problematic outcomes for not only the history-taking component of therapy but the entire process of treatment. Consequently, culturally competent practice, from the first moment of history taking, requires close and careful attention to the psychotherapist's own experiences as well as the psychotherapist's capacities to own and contain affects about their own personal or cultural histories of trauma and thus their capacities to create the emotional spaces into which clients can pour their stories.

USES OF PSYCHOMETRIC INSTRUMENTS IN TRAUMA TREATMENT: ISSUES OF CULTURAL COMPETENCE

Thorough assessment of any client is always a component of ethical practice. Not every psychotherapist will use formal psychometric instruments as part of assessment, but if a psychotherapist does, then choosing one that is reliable and valid for the assessment of posttrauma symptoms and sufficiently culturally sensitive to support culturally competent practice can be important to obtain accurate information that is not distorted by failures of cultural competence built into a particular test instrument. There are several excellent and relatively culturally sensitive psychometric instruments that assess a range of posttraumatic symptoms, including the Trauma Symptom Inventory (Briere, 1995), the Detailed Assessment of Posttraumatic States (Briere, 2001), the Trauma Attachment and Beliefs Scale (Pearlman, 2003), and the Inventory of Altered Self-Capacities (Briere, 2000). Each of these instruments has been well normed for use with the range of ethnicities within the United States, although data for use with persons from other cultures are not available as of this writing, and some clinicians have noticed that individuals who are not native speakers of English and who were raised outside of the United States or Canada have difficulty with comprehension of the items (B. Underwood, personal communication, January 14, 2007). Sensitivity to issues of gender and to cultural styles of reporting symptoms among African American and Latina or Latino respondents has been taken into account by Briere's tests, making them, in my experience, the formal assessment instruments of choice for culturally competent psychometric assessment of post-traumatic symptoms.

Because, as noted earlier in this chapter, posttraumatic difficulties are not limited to ASD and PTSD, some clinicians may wish to use a more general psychometric instrument. Of those available, I have found that the Personality Assessment Inventory (PAI; Morey, 1996) is the most culturally competent general objective instrument currently available. Test construction of this instrument, which makes available 11 clinical scales, each with independently interpretable subscales that include a trauma symptoms subscale as well as five treatment consideration scales and two interpersonal scales, was done in a highly culturally sensitive manner that included the use of community experts and focus groups who assisted Morey in eliminating test items that might pull for biased or culturally skewed responding. As such, the PAI is much less prone to the sort of Type I diagnostic errors committed by other commonly used general purpose objective assessment instruments, which frequently overpathologize trauma responses in general and those of people of color and women in particular.

A very small yet growing body of information exists regarding projective assessment of posttrauma manifestations. (Armstrong, 2002; Ephraim, 2002; Kamphuis, Kugeares, & Finn, 2000; Levin, 1993). Projective instruments are controversial, with some arguing that their use should be abandoned entirely because of problems of psychometric soundness, whereas others posit that the sensitivity of such instruments to individual differences makes them particularly valuable in assessment of subtle posttraumatic phenomena (see Hibbard, 2003, for a good description of this debate). Projective techniques have long been critiqued for being culturally insensitive, privileging Eurocentric ways of relating and pathologizing those of other cultures, particularly those valuing emotional expression and a fuzzy boundary between real and imaginal worlds (Dana, 2000). However, because they are idiopathic rather than nomothetic assessment tools, they may allow for culturally sensitive assessment of trauma by providing a strategy for the individual survivor's intrapsychic dynamics to emerge clearly. Some provocative work done by Sarlund-Heinrich (2007) supports this perspective, suggesting that changes to complex trauma symptoms resulting from treatment will manifest sooner on the Rorschach than on objective instruments such as the Trauma Symptom Inventory, although these findings require replication and extension. The culturally competent evaluator who is familiar with the use of projective instruments must also constantly assess her or his own bias in the interpretive process because it is at the point of interpretation that nonconscious bias is most likely to enter the process of projective assessment.

In choosing any formal psychometric instrument, psychotherapists must take care to read the manual to discover whether and how cultural diversity, as broadly defined, was a component of the test construction process. Many test instruments that are routinely used in mental health settings are poorly normed along those lines (Hays, 2008), and use of their findings may create a barrier to more culturally competent practice. Simply because a psychotherapist is familiar with a particular test is not a good rationale for its use, although such is common practice among North American psychologists. Finally, in using any formal psychometric instrument, it is important to be familiar with any research regarding trauma-specific information available from the test.

For instance, with the Minnesota Multiphasic Personality Inventory—2 (MMPI–2; Hathaway & McKinley, 1989), a validity scale called Fptsd, which assists in discriminating between the typical overresponse patterns of trauma survivors and malingered response patterns, is now available (Naifeh et al., 2003). Clinicians who use the MMPI–2 and are unfamiliar with the growing body of research demonstrating certain normative patterns of what would commonly be called overresponse on that test run the risk of making Type I errors in the evaluation of trauma survivors. Additionally, some research exists on MMPI (Hathaway & McKinley, 1942) and MMPI–2 response patterns of several different groups of trauma survivors (e.g., Rosewater's, 1985a, 1985b, or Dutton's, 1991, research on MMPI and MMPI–2 patterns of battered women), and those using this instrument in work with trauma survivors should become familiar with that research. Studies using the PAI with specific populations of trauma survivors are now also being published, allowing for greater specificity of its use with sexual abuse (Cherepon & Prinzhorn, 1994) and domestic violence (Swanson, 2007) survivors.

Finally, there is sadly little sensitivity to either culture or trauma in most computerized interpretations of psychological tests. Wherever one might stand in the debate regarding the reliability and validity of such materials (for the record, I tend to find them what Matarazzo has called "all mean and no sigma," i.e., utterly lacking in attention to contextual and cultural variables influencing response and interpretation; 1986, p. 14), culturally competent work with trauma survivors raises particular red flags with regard to the use of these instruments. Buchanan, Mazzeo, Grzegorek, Ramos, and Fitzgerald (1996) conducted an extremely interesting and relevant study in which multiple measures were used on sexually harassed women (a group of trauma survivors) and MMPI–2 answers were sent to six different prominent computer interpretation services. Their findings that the computerized interpretations were rarely in agreement with one another and even more rarely in agreement with the findings of other multiple measures used are indicative of the risks of computerized interpretations in culturally competent trauma practice.

Some clinicians find that structured clinical interviews can be an important part of their assessment process. Although these interviews are designed to be simply neutral information-gathering tools that organize the data shared by clients into diagnostic decision trees, clinicians choosing to use these in clinical practice versus in clinical research settings may wish to consider exploring how wording may need to be tweaked to reflect and respect cultural issues that are present for any given client.

What is most essential to cultural competence in the intake process, no matter how the clinician structures the gathering of that initial data, is that issues of culture, as broadly defined, be taken into account. Thus the intake process should also include questions not only about commonly identified traumatic stressors but also about direct or indirect encounters with unfair or discriminatory treatment as well as family histories of the same. As I discuss later in this volume, a number of commentators have argued that racism (and by extension other forms of bias) is traumatic by and of itself (Sanchez-Hucles, 1998) and need not come attached to overt violence to have some sort of posttraumatic impact. Inquiry should be conducted into people's ADDRESSING (Hays, 2001, 2008) and other social location experiences, and the clinician should be aware of those aspects of both target and dominant group status that might have informed the experience and aftermath of trauma.

MODELS OF TRAUMA TREATMENT—A BRIEF OVERVIEW

When the field of trauma therapy began to reinvent itself in the Western world within the past 3 decades there were no consensus models about how to work with trauma survivors. Early published works on the topic reflected the theoretical allegiances of their authors to particular therapeutic orientations rather than a specific paradigm for responding to posttrauma distress and dysfunction. This early literature also tended to generalize from the population of trauma survivors who were seen by the author to all trauma survivors, obscuring the important differences between exposures in adulthood and childhood, single-episode versus continuous exposures, and relational versus less relational trauma.

With time and experience, however, several broad consensus paradigms for working therapeutically with trauma survivors have emerged. These are variously known as *stage* or *phase* models of therapy because of the identification of somewhat distinct, although often recursive, stages of the therapy process. Although not formally researched quantitatively, these models are well based in the evidence of nearly 2 decades of application in clinical practice (see Norcross, Beutler, & Levant, 2006, for an in-depth exploration of the question of what constitutes adequate evidence basis for practice. I join with those authors in taking a very broad stance regarding the types of evidence acceptable to support trauma practice). These models address the overt symptoms of trauma that interfere with safety and functioning and then move on to the integration of the history of trauma into the individual's identity and personal narrative. I explore in depth five specific treatment models: Herman's (1992) ecological model; Gold's (2000) Trauma Resolution Integration Program (TRIP); Courtois's (1999) phase and stage model; Cloitre, Cohen, and Koenen's (2006) Skills Training in Affective and Interpersonal Regulation/Narrative Story Telling (STAIR/NST) model; and Linehan's (1993) Dialectical Behavior Therapy.

Herman's Ecological Model

Herman (1992) was one of the first recent trauma psychotherapists to propose one such model, an ecological model of trauma treatment (Harvey, 1996) used by Herman, Harvey, and their colleagues at the Cambridge Victims of Violence Program. As Herman noted, her concept of stages was not new but rather reflected much earlier recommendations made by the 19th century French psychiatrist Pierre Janet in regard to working with complex trauma or Kardiner and Spiegel's (1947) descriptions of effective treatment of soldiers with combat-related PTSD as well as more recent work by colleagues such as Putnam (1989). Herman's model, because of its broad dissemination in the field of trauma therapy, serves as paradigmatic for other transtheoretical treatments for trauma and has been integrated into the work of many psychotherapists working with trauma survivors.

An initial stage in Herman's model is that of establishing safety. Safety, like trauma, would appear at first glance to be a neutral, easily agreed on construct. However, there are many ways in which issues of culture and identity may inform what feels safe and what does not to a given trauma survivor. Some aspects of safety are basic and resemble the bottom layers of the Masolvian pyramid of needs: safe food, safe water, safe air to breathe, and safe housing.

Clearly, identity and culture affect these very basic safety needs. Safe housing in the United States as well as elsewhere in the world is commonly a function of access to financial resources. For my many clients with complex trauma who have lived in public low-income housing, safe housing was often a myth. Venturing outside into the hallway to the elevator could be an act of taking one's life in one's hands or at least be quite scary. One client came into her session shaking in fear after hearing through the apartment complex grapevine that her new next-door neighbor was a person with a history of sexually molesting children; she was herself a survivor of multiple sexual assaults in childhood. Moving was not an option because finding an apartment renting for under $100 per month required staying in the public housing system, which rarely allowed transfers from one building to another. Living in poverty often means increased risks of exposure to violence in one's immediate surroundings. Immigrants and refugees, who are also often poor, frequently deal with the intersection of unsafe neighborhoods and the lack of safety arising from biases expressed by neighbors who are hostile to the arrival of these newcomers.

Safe water and air are also not universally available. Environmental injustice situates toxic waste dumps in communities of poverty, dumps radioactive tailings on the lands of American Indian reservations, and builds garbage incinerators spewing smoke in communities of color; these are common aspects of unsafety in one's living environment for members of some target groups. Even though a person may not be consciously aware of the danger in which she or he lives, the presence of such threats to health and life resting omnipresent in the background may subtly undermine therapeutic attempts to work on creating safety for a trauma survivor.

Rico, a Chicano man in his early 40s, was a combat veteran of the first Iraq War who sought assistance from a storefront Vet Center for the nightmares that had increased in intensity after the second invasion of Iraq in 2003. Since his leaving military service in the middle 1990s with an other-than-honorable discharge conferred as a result of drug use and acting out in his final year in the service, he had had difficulty finding and then holding down a job. At the time he came into the Vet Center he was living with his mother in a two-room apartment in the barrio of his southern California town, subsisting on what she could share from her Social Security checks. The apartment was rat infested; the plumbing often did not work; and Rico and his mother lived on a diet heavy in fats, sugars, and starches, made up largely from the government surplus foods available at the local food pantry. Rico felt himself to be a failure on multiple dimensions: as a soldier, a man, and a son.

The psychotherapist at the Vet Center, himself an Iraq War veteran who had largely reduced his own PTSD symptoms during the course of his master's degree program, wondered out loud to Rico during one of their visits, which were marked by tension and silence on Rico's part, why Rico had such a hard time using the support that the center was offering to him to try to get him into different housing. Rico's response to this question was blurted out in a rage, "Man, why should I care about myself when The Man has been trying to kill me for so long anyhow?"

The psychotherapist, exploring this outburst from his usually taciturn client, uncovered Rico's family history of toxic exposures when working in fields picking vegetables. "Those government inspectors were no f—ing help at all, you know? And then what did I do, joined the Army because I didn't want to end up like my father," who, the psychotherapist now learned, had died when Rico was 15 from complications of chronic pulmonary disease that a clinic doctor had told them had been caused by years of pesticide exposures. "And then the sons of bitches, they sent me to Kuwait, and there they were again, blowing shit into my lungs." Rico had been exposed to the toxic fumes and smoke billowing out of Kuwait's oil wells; his drug use and disciplinary problems had occurred in the context of his feeling that the military health care professionals were ignoring his complaints about difficulties breathing. "They told me it was in my head, man. Like I was some sissy making it up." Rico's current neighborhood was downwind of a smelter. "They say they've got a scrubber on the smokestacks but why should I believe them?

So why the f— should I believe that the effing government wants me to be safe now, man? I mean, why? I'm no fool."

For Rico's psychotherapist to even approach issues of self-care in this stage of therapy, he had to be able to validate Rico's experiences of being a member of target groups whose health had been endangered through both direct actions and neglect and of then being invalidated for his fears and for his physical distress. He also had to consider how Rico's cultural context, in which a man's expression of fear was a loss of masculinity, affected his ability to identify fear as the root of his distress and problematic behaviors. Because Rico had rarely experienced safety, yet was constrained from admitting that he felt fearful and unsafe, attempts in therapy to engage him with this goal seemed laughable or enraging to him until the persistence of unsafe conditions in the air that he had breathed his whole life was acknowledged and a culturally acceptable manner for his expression of fear was made available.

Other forms of unsafety can be more subtle but equally pervasive. Glenda Russell (2004a, 2004b; Russell & Richards, 2003) has conducted extensive research on how antigay political campaigns can and do induce feelings of unsafety in lesbian, gay, bisexual, and transgender (LGBT) community members, which can lead to persistent symptoms of emotional distress. In the period following the September 11, 2001, attacks on New York and Washington, DC, the anti-Arab and anti-Muslim discourse present in all levels of society has led to a sense in many Arab and Muslim Americans that they are unsafe if their religious affiliation becomes suspected or known.

Iqbal (known to his friends and coworkers as "Ike") was a second-generation U.S.-born Pakistani American who was in a car accident in early 2002. The accident itself was a mild one; his car was rear-ended at low speed while he was alone in the driver's seat at a red light. However, when he got out of the car to initiate the usual exchange of driver's license and insurance information with the other driver, he found himself feeling unaccountably terrified of what that man might do. The other driver, who was Euro-American, was pleasant and apologetic, taking full responsibility for having not been paying attention. But as Iqbal told his primary care physician later that month,

> I haven't been able to sleep since. I kept having these images of some jerk leaping out of his car and rushing over to beat me up. Because I'm Muslim, because of how I look, you know. I mean, doc, I'm as American as the next guy. My parents would tell you that. It really bugs them how American I am. I'm Ike to everyone. Only my folks and my granny call me Iqbal. But that driver, he was a stranger. I couldn't know what he'd do when he saw me, saw my real name on my license. Strange White people scare me a lot these days—like maybe he saw me and my brown skin and thought I was a terrorist or something, rammed into me on purpose or something? I just can't keep the thoughts out of my mind. And I know I'm nuts, I mean, why am I acting like this?"

If the first stage of trauma therapy has to do with establishing safety, then culturally competent practice means extending the definitions of safety to include an understanding of how racism, classism, and other forms of systemic oppression and bias may be creating inherent and difficult-to-avoid unsafety for the client in her or his daily life. Iqbal, for example, was suffering from the effects of the post-September 11, 2001, outbursts of hatred against Muslims; he feared being targeted at any moment, although the fear had lain dormant and below conscious awareness until the accident. The presence of such systemic challenges to safety for members of target groups must be addressed and validated by the culturally competent psychotherapist working on issues of safety in therapy, given that some clients may be chronically responding to these embedded phenomena. A culturally competent psychotherapist working with the client on standard safety issues such as keeping away from overtly violent relationships with self and others needs to be willing to first name and address the persistent presence of systemic forms of absence of safety in the client's life.

Such a psychotherapist might say, for instance,

> I wonder how you feel discussing safety issues when we both know that there are so many that you can't yet figure out what to do with—like how you feel being the only person of color living in your neighborhood. I know that you've said that you like your house and feel safe inside of it, but that it's harder when you step out into this all-White environment. Can we talk about what we could do to assist you in creating a greater sense of safety? What would it take?

In this imaginary therapy encounter the psychotherapist acknowledges what is frequently true about issues of systemic unsafety, that is, that they represent the clichéd double-edged sword. As many residents of the Gulf Coast who fled Hurricanes Katrina and Rita have stated, their wish to return home, because home feels emotionally safe and familiar, is tinged with ambivalence and ambiguity by the experience of objective physical absence of safety in those same homes during the 2005 hurricane season. This has been worsened by ongoing threats to safety posed by flawed government responses to the hurricanes and the failure of those same governments for quite some time afterward to touch the surface of the worst devastation of people's homes and neighborhoods or to protect those who have returned from violent crime.

Issues of safety may also raise cultural dynamics when culture speaks directly to what constitutes safe ways of living and the means by which such safety is achieved. A traditional Navajo person may, for instance, feel safe only after going through a ceremony with a traditional healer. Had Rico been Navajo instead of Chicano, he might have sought an Enemy Way ceremony to rebalance his harmony with the world after having gone to war and felt unsafe in the world until he was able to perform such a healing ritual. The Muslim survivor of domestic violence who is in a physically safe shelter environment may feel unsafe if she is not able to eat halal food because the safety of her soul will feel in jeopardy; having to make herself visible as a Muslim by asking shelter staff about getting halal food will, in turn, add another layer of potential unsafety. Spiritual safety can often transcend physical safety in the meaning given to an experience, and its absence can undermine apparently safe settings; conversely, when there is spiritual safety, an individual may code an experience as less traumatic.

Safety in trauma therapy also addresses questions of strategies that people have adopted to soothe themselves and manage intolerable affects in the wake of trauma. Most of the symptoms associated with posttraumatic diagnostic pictures represent some component either of those intolerable affects or people's self-help strategies for trying to deal with them. Some of those strategies are problematic and risky, such as excessive consumption of mind-altering substances, cutting or burning oneself to evoke either heightened or numbed states of awareness, overexercise, overwork, eating less or more than nourishes the body, being sexual in unsafe ways or with unsafe partners, and so on. A major focus of many therapeutic interventions with trauma survivors during this phase of treatment has been on the replacement of these problematic and risky strategies with others that are nonharmful and may even be health inducing.

As I discuss in greater depth later in this volume in chapter 3, culturally sensitive, identity-driven, and culturally informed strategies for self-care and safety have the potential to be quite powerful when integrated with some of the empirically supported treatments for trauma. Conversely, prescribing a one-size-fits-all approach to self-care for clients may introduce culturally foreign or incompatible elements into the treatment process in ways that undermine the safety of therapy itself.

For example, Maryam was a modern Muslim woman who did not wear hijab but who did attempt to dress more modestly than the norms of her American-born friends in reflection of her cultural and religious beliefs. She was a survivor of politically motivated torture in her native Egypt and had refuged to the United States more than 20 years previously. She seemed superficially very assimilated into American culture, and her husband was a Muslim from a Bosnian family who was quite European in his attitudes and values. The family followed halal eating rules but rarely attended the local mosque, which both Maryam and her husband experienced as more conservative in its values than they were.

She came into therapy on the referral of her primary care physician who called the psychotherapist to say that Maryam had "fallen apart shrieking in my office" when the physician attempted to reason with her about joining a gym to manage her mounting blood pressure numbers. Maryam had been insistent that she could not join a gym; the physician had reminded her that there was a very nice 24-hour facility in her own office building, which had seemed to upset Maryam even further. When the physician pressed her and suggested buying some sort of home exercise machine, the conversation disintegrated completely.

The psychotherapist invited Maryam to use the session time however she might like, so as to avoid a trauma reenactment of Maryam's experience of feeling coerced and pressured by her physician. For several months their discussion was superficial, although Maryam was conscientious about attending her appointments. Finally, after yet another appointment with her physician where she was "berated like a child," to use Maryam's words, for her blood pressure numbers, she decided to experiment with telling her psychotherapist what was happening.

"I cannot exercise with men," said Maryam. "I know that I don't look especially modest, and I never did wear hijab, but something in me imagines feeling completely exposed to be sweating and straining and grunting in front of men." She then began to shake almost uncontrollably and, after her psychotherapist assisted her in becoming restabilized by using deep breathing, revealed that modesty was not the only issue evoked. Rather, one component of her torture had been being stripped and touched in front of male prisoners, including family members. The heat of the prison, the smell of her own and other prisoner's sweat, and the shameful experience of being physically exposed were all an unexplored part of her trauma history that she had avoided encountering for 2 decades by simply never being in the presence of any sensory triggers. She had moved to the Pacific Northwest in part because "it is almost always cool here and never humid when it is hot like at home." She did not exercise vigorously or do anything that she knew would make herself sweat. Her home had air conditioning, which was unusual for her part of the country.

As this narrative emerged, the psychotherapist was able to assist Maryam in asserting herself more directly with her primary care physician. Together, psychotherapist and client searched for and found a women's only swim session that was offered twice weekly. Although the swim session's primary audience was fat women (another group who often have difficulty entering gyms and swimming pools), the fact that it was in a cool swimming pool with only women in the room was soothing to Maryam's anxiety; no trauma triggers lurked unseen there, and there would be nothing that troubled her spiritually. She became a regular at the swim nights and after 6 months was off her blood pressure medication. She had also, importantly, begun to delve into and process her avoidance strategies for being safe and to develop new ones that had less risk to her health and well-being. She was able to claim her modesty as a Muslim woman in a manner not colored by the experience of violation. After 2 years she made an experimental trip to a mixed-sex swimming pool wearing her newly purchased triathalon swimming suit (which had legs down to midthigh and arms down to the elbow, thus meeting her cultural and spiritual modesty needs) and, although she experienced some increased anxiety at being in the presence of men, was able to use what she had by then learned in therapy to calm herself; she began to swim almost daily. Her health had improved dramatically during those 2 years.

Safety interventions such as the one described in the preceding case discussion also commonly involve health of the body, which is an important component of safety. Although few complementary and alternative medicine (CAM) treatments have been scientifically studied for their effectiveness, many of them are founded in long-standing non-Western systems of health care and have extensive clinical evidentiary support for their use. Specifically, CAM approaches have been studied with regard to certain ethnic groups within the United States; for example, studies of collaboration with traditional *curandero* in Hispanic communities (Comas-Diaz, 2006) or with traditional healers in American Indian communities (Robin, Chester, & Goldman, 1996) seem to indicate that integration of these CAM approaches into the psychological healing process can be extremely helpful. Culturally competent trauma practice invites psychotherapists to be open to methods of health management that are congruent with clients' beliefs, even when those beliefs run counter to those held by psychotherapists, many of whom are trained within Western models of medical care and standards of proof. Such clients are not always from the cultures in which these somatic interventions are most common.

An interesting example of this last issue can be seen in the case of Sylvie, a woman with complex trauma symptoms arising from childhood neglect and sexual abuse by older family members. During a stressful period at her workplace she had developed a symptom that she believed was caused by her having scratched herself too vigorously to alleviate stress. The symptoms appeared neurological in nature, and so her primary care physician referred her to a neurologist, who performed a series of diagnostic tests and, being unable to find anything organic, reported back that Sylvie's symptom was psychogenic in nature.

This might have been true, especially if one were to construct the concept of psychogenic very broadly so as to include those symptoms that are now organic but arise from posttraumatic changes to the body. However, Sylvie's physician did not have such a broad construct and told her that her symptom had nothing to do with the scratching but was, instead, anxiety related; she gave Sylvie a prescription for a mood-stabilizing medication. Sylvie took it and felt groggy and fatigued but experienced no remission of symptoms. Nor did her psychotherapist's attempts to offer nonmedical interventions for reducing anxiety seem to help. In fact, over time, the symptom persisted and worsened. Sylvie had long had difficulty trusting physicians because of some serious failures of care during her childhood; the medical response to her symptom seemed only to confirm that doctors would not or could not help her.

The psychotherapist, feeling desperate and willing to try anything that seemed semireasonable, referred Sylvie to a licensed acupuncturist of his acquaintance, because the acupuncturist had described having success with neurological-like problems that the psychotherapist thought of as conversion symptoms. The acupuncturist met Sylvie, started treatment, and called the referring psychotherapist to inform him that Sylvie's condition had a specific name in Chinese medicine along with fairly precise strategies for being treated with acupuncture, herbs, and other Chinese medicine interventions. Chinese medicine does not differentiate between psychogenic and organic causes but rather constructs all symptoms as problems of blockage, stagnation, or imbalance of the body's energy known as chi (ki, in Japanese, which has a similar medical system).

The acupuncturist, not yet knowing Sylvie's trauma history (as such history is of less diagnostic importance to an acupuncturist than the condition of the patient's tongue and the pulse as measured at several different places on the body), commented that many people with this condition were known in Chinese medicine to have had very painful experiences that led to this sort of profound imbalance and inquired of the psychotherapist if that might be the case here. Sylvie saw the acupuncturist twice weekly for several months and experienced a full remission of her symptom. More importantly, she came to see her psychotherapist as being allied with her because of his openness to the CAM treatment, which was the first somatic intervention she had experienced that did not require her to divide herself into psychological and organic boxes.

MOURNING AND REMEMBRANCE

The second stage of the Cambridge model is what Herman (1992) called "mourning and remembrance." This is the component of therapy in which a survivor tells the story of what happened and begins the process of integrating that narrative into the narrative of life, grieving for what was and what could not be as a result of the trauma so as to create the emotional space in which a life and a future can be constructed. As Herman and many other trauma psychotherapists have noted, this is actually a component of therapy that cycles through over and over as time goes on. I have suggested to clients the image of a Slinky toy or spiral in which issues are addressed repeatedly but in new ways as they work their way up along the coils of their trauma narratives and healing experiences and as new current life events intersect with old realities.

Cultural awareness and sensitivity and attention to issues of a survivor's identity are centrally important to the successful accomplishment of this component of therapy. As I discussed during the exploration of models of identity development, trauma frequently insinuates itself into multiple locations in an individual's identity and self. I return for a moment, to the hypothetical Bajoran trauma survivor who came into the psychotherapists' office.

For this discussion, she is a woman who was raped as an adolescent by a Cardassian soldier when she was part of the Bajoran resistance movement and captured during a raid on a Cardassian outpost.

This woman cannot tell her story without the psychotherapist realizing and acknowledging several things. First, what does rape represent in traditional Bajoran culture? Perhaps, because Bajorans have lived for a long time under oppressive Cardassian rule, a rape at the hands of a Cardassian is seen as not shameful nor as necessarily traumatic because this kind of experience "just happens" in the lives of Bajoran women. Herein lies the first dilemma; if the client cannot name this experience as trauma because of its commonality, yet it was terrifying and indeed traumatic for her, she must deal with her identity as a Bajoran woman to tell her own truth about this experience. Rape is violating, painful, and traumatic for most who experience it; simply because it is common in a given cultural context does not mean that it is any less of these.

Second, what does it mean that this rape was experienced in the midst of a heroic activity, being a member of the resistance attempting to attack the oppressor? But that the rape occurred because the attack, like many against the Cardassians, did not succeed? The failure of the attack and the capture by the Cardassians was another trauma; like many warriors in many cultures, however, this Bajoran client struggles against telling her story as one of fear and helplessness because as a resistance fighter she was supposed to be strong and to know that it was always possible to fall into Cardassian hands. A psychotherapist from another culture might see the failure of the raid as the trauma; for Bajorans, who rarely succeeded in their raids but continued in them because they would gradually weaken the enemy, permission to know this as traumatic might be culturally proscribed.

Inviting this client to tell her story, which means that she writes the narrative to reflect the intersections between her actual lived experiences, the identities that she brought to those experiences, and the meanings ascribed to those experiences by her cultural contexts, requires her psychotherapist to acknowledge the power of those cultural contexts in shaping the problematic posttrauma narratives. The culturally aware trauma psychotherapist might, consequently, assist this client in unpacking those cultural narratives as one component of uncovering and creating her own narrative. Such a process of disentangling oneself from the trauma narratives of a culture can be tricky and fraught with pitfalls. This Bajoran woman must be empowered to tell her own truth without feeling as if she has betrayed her culture's truths; her psychotherapist, to be culturally competent, cannot simply dismiss the official Bajoran lenses on these experiences as irrelevant to the client's realities but must invite this client to see how the truth of the cultural narratives was perhaps a necessary component of cultural survival but not a necessary component of her own recovery from the trauma. The psychotherapist must be an ally to the culture without being invested in the truth of its interpretations so as to fulfill her first responsibility to her client's need for healing.

At times cultural survival and safety of the group has led to suppression of individual narratives and experiences of trauma. In cultures in which certain kinds of trauma exposures are endemic, cultural and personal survival may have led to the development of a cultural narrative that minimized the importance of those apparently normative and usually inescapable events. "It's no big deal. This happens to all of us. It's the way of the world" are typical cultural descriptions of such endemic traumatic events. The survivors of those traumas have often suffered in silence or have enacted their distress in the absence of an aware connection between the trauma and their suffering. Many have, in turn expressed that suffering in ways that shaped their cultures and intergenerationally transmitted trauma.

This process of suppression of individual in favor of necessary collective narratives can be seen in many cultures in which colonization and or genocide have been prominent historical features. In these instances the problem is not the culture; rather, the culture allowed its members to survive in the face of danger. However, the presence of internalized oppression as a component of a person's trauma narrative cannot be overlooked.

I turn now to the traumas of combat, an endemic and highly valorized experience of U.S. culture. *Fortunate Son: The Healing of a Vietnam Vet* (Puller, 1991) is the autobiography of Lewis Puller Jr., the son (and namesake) of a hero of World War II, who enlisted in the military for service in Vietnam where he was gravely wounded, leading to the loss of both legs, most of one hand, and serious injuries to his internal organs. The book, which won the 1992 Pulitzer Prize for autobiography, purports to tell his story of trauma and healing. What is absent from the volume, which ends on an upbeat note, is that 3 years after its publication Lewis Puller, who had relapsed into active alcoholism soon after publication, shot himself to death.

Puller's tragic story is one of a trauma's cultural meanings overpowering the healing process and blocking the construction of a narrative in which all truths can be told. Puller's initial struggles with trauma in which he became a practicing alcoholic, are marked by his need to pay allegiance to the military culture in which he was raised, particularly the role of the war hero who is unfazed and uncomplaining about his horrific experiences. Alcohol and pain killers became necessary not only to deal with the physical pain of his wounds and their aftermath but also to deal with the psychic pain of having to uphold a public image of not being psychically traumatized by his experiences and with the spiritual and existential losses attendant on this ultimately impossible balancing act.

His book, which is a powerful and honest one, is nonetheless an example of the heroic narrative imposed by his culture on combat trauma survivors, especially men. This narrative proclaims that the pain and terror of that trauma can always somehow be overcome when those wounds are heroically incurred and that what is most important is being a man, a stereotypic gendered role (see Brooks, 2005, for an in-depth discussion of this phenomenon in male military veterans). On the day I read Lewis Puller's obituary in the *New York Times*, I wondered what pressure the publication of his book had created for him that had caused him to become rooted and perhaps trapped even more thoroughly and deeply in the hero role with which he had done battle his entire life as the namesake and son of an official hero.

Like the mythical Bajoran whose rape was a combat trauma as well as a sexual assault, the real human Lewis Puller was faced with a preexisting narrative about this particular sort of trauma that can and frequently does complicate the healing process of constructing a personal, experience-based narrative during the process of mourning and remembrance. The culturally aware enactment of this second stage of therapy is one in which trauma survivors are invited not to reject the narratives of their culture but rather to think critically yet compassionately about those narratives to develop their own healing stories about the trauma in their lives. Some of the grieving that occurs at this juncture is for the lost mythologies of trauma survivors' lives, the mythologies about "how it was supposed to be" woven into the dominant narratives of their cultures. At other times the process is about remembering and thus knowing of events banished from the original life narrative because of a cultural strategy of avoidance. Sometimes the grief is not simply for one's own losses but for historical losses sustained by one's ancestors and family members.

A clinical example of this last phenomenon can be seen in the story of Ruvein, who is the son of Holocaust survivors. His name is also that of his half brother on his father's side, who was murdered as a young child in a concentration camp. His parents, who each lost the children and spouse of their original marriages to the gas chambers, met and married in a displaced persons camp after the war; Ruvein was conceived and born there before the family emigrated to Canada in 1948.

As is common for many survivors of the Nazi camps, neither of Ruvein's parents spoke of their experience. Even though the Jewish community in Winnipeg was full of other adults with numbers tattooed into their arms, there was an unspoken rule about never bringing up the horrors of the Holocaust except to say that nothing that anyone who had not lived through the camps had experienced could be very bad. Epstein (1988) and Hass (1996), among others, have documented a similar common coping strategy of avoidance and silence used by survivors of the Nazi Holocaust and their communities in the first 3 decades after the liberation of the concentration camps.

Ruvein's mother was depressed during his entire childhood, grieving her terrible losses. His father, who likely was suffering both from depression and severe posttraumatic symptoms related to his having been forced to work cleaning out crematoria, was physically and verbally abusive to Ruvein on a regular basis, with several episodes in which he was injured severely enough to require hospitalization for broken bones. Ruvein, who was academically talented, told his psychotherapist that he "escaped" his parents as soon as he graduated from high school, moving to the United States for college and minimizing contact with them after that.

He entered therapy in his early 30s, depressed, struggling with emotional intimacy, and terrified by his own temper, which flared in the context of his important relationships. He did not identify himself as a survivor of trauma and for a very long time minimized what his father had done to him. He was professionally very successful, having earned an advanced degree; he was respected in his occupation into which he put very long hours and had an excellent income. His personal life was a shambles, marked by multiple failed relationships. He felt an urgency to get married and become a father but seemed unable to succeed at the first step of this goal because his over-work coping style drastically interfered with the establishment of intimacy, and any relationship that did take root was poisoned by his rage.

As Ruvein and his psychotherapist worked on issues of mourning and remembrance, she asked him about his parents' Holocaust experiences and was surprised to learn that this had never been discussed. He knew that he had been named after his dead half brother but dismissed that as simply part of a common Eastern European Jewish practice of naming children after a dead relative. She also began to press him on his minimizing response to the abuse he had suffered at the hands of his father. It was in the course of one such session that he blew up at her and began to rage verbally about the fact that he could "not make a big deal of this. It was not the Nazis, do you hear? Nothing is as bad as that. Nothing. How dare you, how dare I?" He then began to sob deeply.

Ruvein's family trauma narrative, although mostly full of holes, had one prominent and important feature that had been shared by members of the community of Holocaust survivors and their children in which he had been raised. That was the rule that nothing could be as bad as the experience of the concentration camps, and thus any other trauma, including the danger and emotional betrayal inherent in abuse at the hands of a parent, was not really traumatic. Ruvein could not name his own trauma within that narrative and, because of the ban on speaking of the losses of the Holocaust, could not participate in grieving for the siblings, grandparents, and cousins whom he had never known, or for the harms that had damaged his parents so terribly. He also felt constrained in his anger against his father, "How can I blame this man? He lost everything." For the psychotherapist to invite him to construct his narrative, to grieve his own experiences and know them fully, she also had to invite him to compassionately apprehend his parents' narrative, gaps and all, and the experiences that led them to be so impaired in their parenting of him.

She introduced him to the notion of *invidious comparison of harm*, a concept that describes how dominant cultural norms of scarcity of resources

lead to competition among individuals and groups for scarce emotional resources, with that scarcity expressed as a competition for "who had it worse"
(Siegel, 1990). This, she noted, was a perennially losing battle for him with
his parents because growing up a battered child in the relative safety of
Winnipeg in the 1950s was on a completely different continuum of terrible
from losing your parents, spouse, and children and nearly starving to death
yourself in a concentration camp. Nonetheless, she noted, no child should
be abused at the hands of her or his caregiver; such abuse is itself terrible and
terrifying to a child and cannot be compared and contrasted.

She thus invited him to sidestep that framework of invidious comparison and instead see his narrative as a survivor of physical and emotional
abuse by his father and emotional neglect by his mother, as existing both in
parallel and intersection with, but not in competition against, his parents'
narratives of extreme loss, near death, and enslavement, and his cultural
narrative of oppression due to anti-Semitism. She invited him, as well, to see
how he had also incurred losses at the hands of the Nazis; he had lost brothers and sisters, aunts, uncles, cousins, and grandparents as well as the opportunity to be raised by less traumatized parents, thus offering him a way to join
with his parents rather than have to distance from them emotionally.

She also suggested to Ruvein a strategy common to the grieving and
remembrance component of therapy, which was participation in a group of
similar individuals. In his case, she located and referred him to a group for
children of Holocaust survivors so that he would have support in his process
of differentiating from the family and cultural narrative, allowing him to
create space for his own story.

Culturally competent encounters with this stage of the therapy process
are those that are able to see such parallel, intersecting narratives in the
multiple social locations and complex identities of trauma survivor clients.
Such therapeutic exchanges can assist the survivor in deriving benefit from
the cultural narrative as it is available and letting go of its strictures as they
present barriers to personal healing without feeling as if the choice is between culture and self but rather that the choice is for self in the cultural
context. Psychotherapy has frequently been criticized for its overly individualist stance, focusing on the well-being of the one person in the therapy room.
Culturally sensitive trauma therapies cannot be individualistic, although they
entail a prizing of the suffering individual. An awareness of and attention to
cultural productions about trauma that influence the individual experiences
of mourning and remembrance are central to the recovery process from a
culturally competent stance.

Herman (1992) described the third stage of her model of trauma treatment as being about reconnection. In this stage, trauma survivors create active engagements with their interpersonal and relational worlds and come to
experience themselves as more empowered and fully alive. As I discuss later
in this volume, this is a phase of the healing process in which connections to

culture can become particularly valuable to the survivor. Briefly here, culturally sensitive trauma treatment invites survivors to deepen their own systems of meaning making and to integrate the discoveries of the healing process into the identities with which they initiated that process. This stage of therapy very much resembles the fourth and fifth components of Root's (2001, 2007) identity model described earlier in that the trauma survivor becomes able to make intentional choices about how to identify with components of social location in crafting an identity as a *thriver*, the person who has moved from surviving into a new identity of a person with an understood history of trauma.

Joann exemplified this stage of the recovery process. An African American woman in her middle 50s who had been raised in a loving middle-class family by college-educated parents, she had been among the first children of color to integrate her Midwestern elementary school and had been the target of enormous pressure in her family and church communities to be a perfect student and representative of her race as well as a daily target of biased and sometimes hateful behaviors from fellow students, their parents, and many of her teachers. "School was a living hell," she told her psychotherapist. "But I had to just keep soldiering on because everyone told me what an honor it was for me to be the first little colored girl at that school." She learned to keep her tears hidden and soothed herself with her mother's, grandmothers', and aunts' cooking. She weighed more than 300 pounds at the age of 30 and encountered a psychologist when referred for mandatory screening prior to receiving bariatric surgery for rapid weight loss.

Nothing about Joann had conveyed the message of trauma survivor. She was a respected public servant who had risen quickly into managerial positions; she was active in her church and in several community organizations mentoring younger African American women and girls. She had strong connections to her family, even though they lived in a different state. "I'm just someone who loves her mamma's home cooking," she told the psychologist, "nothing else wrong with me."

Because of concerns about some of Joann's answers on standardized testing, the psychologist had asked the "tell me about difficult or painful experiences you had growing up" question, which had evoked, reluctantly, Joann's story of being a child pioneer of the Civil Rights movement. Something about Joann's narrative led the evaluator to suggest that before undergoing surgery Joann might want to consider "a few visits with a colleague of mine, just to make sure you're completely comfortable with your decision to have the surgery." The word trauma was never spoken.

The psychotherapist was a visibly older Euro-American woman with a faint European accent and equally faint but visible concentration camp numbers tattooed on her forearm. Neither client nor psychotherapist ever spoke of the numbers, but as the evaluator had sensed, their presence conveyed to Joann that this woman knew something about hate and bigotry, which in turn made it a little safer for Joann to tell her story. Over the course of the therapy, which lasted several years more than a few visits, Joann moved with difficulty through the process of establishing safety, identifying that for her eating had become an entirely culturally and socially acceptable way to cope with the terror that had grown up in her during her childhood. "No one asks why a Black woman is fat," she said to her psychotherapist at one point.

> Fat was fine; I was a woman with meat on my bones, not some skinny White you-know-what. I didn't drink; I didn't use drugs; I didn't get pregnant; and I could sit in class in college and eat. My mom and aunties always loved how I appreciated their cooking.

She uncovered how her academic successes, which were many, had come at the price of good self-care, eating her way through school to cope with the anxiety of being in a classroom surrounded by White people in a historical and cultural context in which to acknowledge her emotional pain felt like a betrayal of her entire community and its strivings for equality.

Safety merged with the process of mourning and remembrance. Joann was able to be angry at her parents and her pastor for not being able to see how terrifying it was for her to go to the mostly White school every day and at the same time to come to a place of love, pride, and compassion for their striving to make her world a better and more just one. "They wanted that school for me so much, those good textbooks, all of those language classes and wonderful science labs, and I'm glad they wanted that for me. It wasn't their fault that it all came wrapped in hate." She explored her family's legacy of fat women, acknowledging as she did the many early deaths from diabetes and high blood pressure among the women of her family who had followed cultural and familial prescriptions to be strong and stoic in the face of endemic racism and had cooked and eaten themselves into early graves with fried and sweet comfort foods. She began to experiment with changing her relationship with food, which, as her body slowly diminished in size, evoked having to deal with developmental issues of sexuality and attractiveness that she had long ago shelved. She was able to name her experience as both brave and important and as traumatic and abusive.

Ultimately, Joann came to see herself as "a veteran of the war for social justice in America," to use her words. She never became as small in body as she might have had she undergone the stomach-stapling procedure, although her weight did drop by nearly 100 pounds during the course of the therapy. Her anxiety had become muted as she was able to tell the truth of her experience, and she had found a new self-soothing strategy in her study of African and Afro-Caribbean drumming; "I can drum anywhere, no drum needed, just a surface and my hands," which also gave her entrée to a community of artists and musicians where she could find a new framework for telling her story. The connection between the drumming rhythms, whose roots were in Africa, and her own African heritage felt spiritually meaningful to her.

She found that another way to self-soothe was to increase her sense of giving back. Already actively involved in her community, she developed a mentoring program for children of color in her city's gifted and talented classes, matching adults like herself with children like the girl she had been, poverty-class youngsters of African, Spanish-speaking, and indigenous ancestries who were frequently alone in classes full of Euro-American and Asian American peers with college-educated parents. Part of that program required mentors to introduce their mentees to self-care strategies such as meditation, exercise, and healthy uses of food "because it's scary out there. But we can give our children new ways to stop feeling scared so that they don't die early with their masters degrees like I almost did."

At each step of the therapy her psychotherapist honored Joann's multiple identities and cultural ties; she never asked her client to change how she ate, but rather offered Joann the chance to explore themes of food and cooking in African American cultures as rituals of celebration and healing as well as images of what it meant to be a strong woman and how that had been an important component of African American cultural survival (Greene, 2000). Joann was able to revise her personal narrative to include the reality of having been a trauma survivor, and to use that revised narrative as the springboard for connecting in new ways with self and community.

OTHER TREATMENT MODELS

Several other specific models for working with trauma survivors, all of which draw to some extent on the work of Herman and her colleagues, have been developed more recently. Each of them can inform the work of a culturally competent trauma therapist by offering a framework for generally understanding the challenges faced by survivors of complex trauma exposure.

Gold's Trauma Resolution Integration Program

Gold (2000) proposed a similar model for working with survivors of trauma within the family context, the TRIP model. He argued that trauma is not a sufficient conceptual framework for understanding the difficulties faced by these individuals, who also fall under the general rubric of complex trauma, and whose trauma exposures were usually the fabric of their early lives and thus central to their sense of self and coping strategies. Although he divided his model into more specific component parts, the directions taken by treatment in his paradigm are quite similar to those proposed by Herman (1992). Gold focused on the culturally competent task of assisting the survivor of intrafamilial abuse to identify the effects of the chaotic family context and to understand how those are both interactive with and distinct from specific abuse that may have occurred as a first step in developing a collaborative relationship with shared, clear treatment goals and priorities. He then iden-tified the importance of working with survivors to learn how to manage and modulate distress, reduce dissociative coping, engage in critical thinking, change problematic behaviors, and titrate exposure to the trauma narrative. Gold deemphasized the importance of thorough scrutiny of and exposure to the process of remembering trauma but emphasized the value of creating a postabuse narrative with clients that emphasizes the shift from postabuse functioning to liberation from the power of the abuse and abusers.

Gold argued that if clients wish to delve into their personal narrative of abuse, then the psychotherapist should support them in so doing. However, he noted that many of the clients treated by him and his copsychotherapists in their clinic found that once they had behaviorally and emotionally freed themselves from the problematic coping strategies used for dealing with the sequelae of trauma, they were no longer very interested in engaging in a narrative exploration of those experiences. He suggested that when a neces-sary component of solving the problems of life is understanding the roots of difficulties in the trauma experience, then specific exploration of that expe-rience can be useful because it is in the service of empowering a client into improved functioning. He further emphasized that this process needs to be client driven and initiated, a stance consistent with a culturally sensitive approach to trauma treatment. In Gold's model the mourning and remem-brance phase of therapy is set further in the background, with the greater emphasis placed on disruption of the family culture of chaos and neglect that enabled abuse to occur.

Cultural competence is necessary in working within this model to sepa-rate family culture from other cultural contexts. For persons raised in cul-tures in which genocide and colonization have been internalized, leading to pervasive and ubiquitous violence and posttraumatic manifestations, it can be difficult for survivors of family trauma not to blame the culture from which they come as a source of the problem. Culturally competent implementation of the TRIP model involves casting the cultural context in terms of the his-tory of a target group and then nesting the analysis of the family's own cha-otic and abusive culture in the framework of intergenerational impacts of larger cultural trauma.

Courtois's Guidelines for Working With Trauma Survivors

Similar to the work of Gold (2000) and Herman (1992) is Courtois's (1999) proposal of guidelines and principles for working specifically with trauma survivors who are experiencing delayed recall of childhood trauma. Although her focus is on individuals who report childhood sexual abuse memo-ries surfacing in adult life, her specific focus on phases of treatment and the value of putting containment and self-care at the top of the priority list ech-oes the recommendations made by other authors whose work has been largely with the complex trauma group of clients. Courtois's work is notable because of her careful attention to the question of memory for trauma and how she elucidates the impact of hyper- and hypoarousal in the consolidation and retrieval of trauma memories. Although this issue became controversial in the early 1990s as a result of accusations that psychotherapists were creating false beliefs about childhood abuse, the question of how a trauma survivor credits her or his recollections transcends the specific content of what is remembered or difficult to recall. Survivors of many kinds of trauma, including combat trauma and single-episode adult interpersonal violence trauma, frequently struggle with questions of accuracy of recall of events. Courtois's work offers a very solid and empirically founded framework for psychotherapists to use in approaching this aspect of trauma treatment.

Skills Training in Affective and Interpersonal Regulation/Narrative Story Telling Model

Cloitre, Cohen, and Koenen (2006) have proposed the STAIR/NST model aimed specifically at working with survivors of childhood trauma. This model, which is a technically integrative one, uses interventions from exposure therapies, attachment therapies, and narrative therapies, each configured to address specific components of the distress experienced by survivors of childhood sexual trauma. The STAIR/NST model exists as two modules. The STAIR module focuses on the reduction of specific posttraumatic symptoms and the development of healthy relationship patterns, whereas the NST Module targets the narratives developed by trauma survivors and aims at their transformation into narratives of recovery. Similar to the TRIP model, STAIR/NST prioritizes assisting clients in developing skills of affect regulation and life management before attempting exposure to the memories and narratives of the trauma itself.

The STAIR/NST model is a semimanualized treatment; although the authors give a specific framework for how it is to be used and steps that are to be followed, they also emphasize early in their work that flexibility and clinical responsiveness are important because the therapeutic alliance is core to work with survivors of trauma. A theme and curriculum for each session of a 12–16-session treatment are described with examples of how clients might respond to each theme and how psychotherapists can use the themes and curriculum in manners responsive to the particular clients with whom they are working.

Dialectical Behavior Therapy

Although not conceived of specifically as a treatment for trauma survivors, Linehan's (1993) Dialectical Behavior Therapy has emerged as one commonly used strategy for working with individuals who, like those described by Gold and Herman, have experienced repeated severe traumatic abuse and neglect in the context of early childhood development. Linehan's model focuses on the development of skills at affect regulation, self-soothing, and effective use of interpersonal relationships and support, very similar to the safety and skill-building phases of the Herman and Gold models.

EVIDENCE BASES FOR TRAUMA TREATMENT

The evidence base for trauma treatments locates in two dimensions. The first dimension is that of empirically supported treatments for specific posttraumatic symptoms. The second dimension focuses on empirically supported psychotherapy relationships (ESR; Norcross, 2000). The volume *Effective Treatments for PTSD: Practice Guidelines From the International Society for Traumatic Stress Studies* (ISTSS; Foa, Keane, & Friedman, 2000) constitutes an excellent resource regarding that dimension of evidence-based trauma practice. These guidelines, developed by task forces of the ISTSS, are founded in in-depth literature reviews of the trauma treatment literature; each treatment approach or modality described in this volume is rated in terms of the strength of empirical evidence for efficacy by using a standardized coding system. As the editors note, all of the studies reviewed and all of the treatment guidelines proposed reflect the challenges of studying trauma survivors and their treatment, including issues of single versus multiple traumas, the chronicity and complexity of the posttrauma picture presented, the presence of diagnoses other than PTSD, and so on. Psychotherapists wishing to be competent in their work with trauma survivors are well advised to familiarize themselves with these guidelines. Similar ISTSS guidelines for working with individuals with complex trauma are under study as of the writing of this volume, and information about them should eventually be available on the ISTSS Web site.

The International Society for the Study of Trauma and Dissociation (ISSTD) also has published guidelines for working with complex trauma in which dissociative features are a prominent component of the client's distress (ISSTD, 2005). These guidelines were developed through reviews of literature and consensus inputs from experts in the field of dissociative disorders treatment, generally regarded as a specific subspecialty of the trauma treatment field. The ISSTD has also developed similar guidelines for working with dissociative children. Both sets of guidelines can be downloaded at the ISSTD Web site (http://www.isstd.org/indexpage/treatguide1.htm). These guidelines can be quite useful for psychotherapists working with clients who have complex trauma presentations even in the absence of severe dissociative symptoms given the overlap of issues and problems of these groups of individuals.

Because these guidelines are available, I have not gone into detail as to specifics of any one approach to alleviating the overt symptoms of trauma exposure. Rather, what I wish to explore here is the issue of how ESRs are an essential evidence-based aspect of culturally competent trauma treatments. ESRs constitute the second empirically founded dimension of trauma treatment. Norcross (2000), a theorist of the transtheoretical common factors model of therapy, has been a proponent of establishing the empirical basis for certain well-studied aspects of the therapy relationship by commissioning multiple meta-analytic studies of those relationship variables while president of the American Psychological Association's Division of Psychotherapy.

When it comes to matters of cultural competence in therapy generally, the literature appears to indicate that the only empirically supported components of therapy with individuals from target groups are the ESRs (Fischer, Jome, & Atkinson, 1998). The absence of empirical support for psychotherapies with members of target groups is highlighted by reviews addressing the question of how and whether empirically researched therapies have been found useful for people of color (Sue & Zane, 2006), issues of gender in psychotherapy (Levant & Silverstein, 2006), LGBT people (Brown, 2003), or people with disabilities (Olkin & Taliaferro, 2006). All of these authors found an absence of data supporting applications of formally researched therapies with their respective target groups, and all noted that what has been empirically supported are issues of the therapeutic relationship such as empathy, collaboration, genuineness, positive regard and respect, and the nature and quality of the therapeutic alliance. Culturally competent practice, when it was possible, required attention to those relationship variables, which are estimated to account for 10% of the outcome variance of any approach to psychotherapy (Norcross & Lambert, 2006), but which may carry heavier weight when issues of cultural competence are present in the room. As Najavits and Strupp (1994) noted in their study of psychotherapy process variables contributing to good and bad therapy outcomes, "basic capacities of human relating—warmth, affirmation, and a minimum of attack and blame—may be at the center of effective psychotherapy intervention" (p. 121).

Integrating and synthesizing these disparate commentaries on the relationship in therapy, I would like to argue very strongly that taken together these findings underscore the empirically demonstrable necessity of the quality of the relationship for culturally competent trauma treatment. Individuals living in the emotional, biological, spiritual, and psychosocial aftermaths of trauma exposure can often challenge their psychotherapists with the complexity of their distress and with their apparent difficulties in making change. It can be exceptionally difficult for people to let go of coping strategies, even dangerous and deeply dysfunctional coping strategies that were developed as a response to the need to contain trauma-induced terror, helplessness, shame, and disgust. It is difficult in parallel for psychotherapists to be emotionally present with those coping strategies, and a psychotherapist may feel strong pulls, both internal and interpersonal, to overpower the client's process to more quickly produce a particular behavioral outcome. In this difficult emotional exchange, the relationship and its quality become paramount. Cultural competence improves relationship quality, which in turn is what the ESR research tells psychotherapists lies at the core of good psychotherapy outcome.

Countertransference

As Dalenberg (2000) cogently noted, "trauma victims figure prominently in virtually every well-known therapeutic dilemma or disaster associated with strong countertransference reactions" (p. 12). She went on to say that "psychotherapists often have countertransferential reactions to the *fact* of trauma . . . the psychotherapist's pre-existing thoughts and beliefs about the trauma may affect the course of therapy greatly" (p. 13). Many of these problematic psychotherapist responses to work with trauma survivors reflect the experiences of fear, terror, disgust, shame, and powerlessness felt by psychotherapists in the face of their clients' powerful feelings and apparently unreachably self-destructive behaviors.

It is beyond the scope of this volume to address general issues of trauma-related countertransference; readers are strongly encouraged to read Dalenberg's (2000) book, which contains a large body of important empirical research on countertransference in trauma treatment. Suffice it to say that issues of culture, privilege, and representation cannot but aggravate unexplored nonconscious dynamics on the part of the therapist working with trauma survivors and that a mindful awareness of all aspects of psychotherapists' responses to their clients enhances cultural competence and therapeutic effectiveness.

Competent work with trauma survivors, whether intentionally attending to cultural competence or not, thus requires careful attention to all aspects of the therapy relationship. When, as suggested by Najavits and Strupp (1994), psychotherapists avoid attack and blame, which many survivors of trauma have already experienced in the rest of their lives, and focus on warmth and empathy, two therapeutic conditions well supported by research as actual curative factors rather than placebos, therapy with trauma survivors is most likely to be effective. Cultural competence takes those capacities and deepens them by adding attention to issues of identity and culture in such a manner as is likely to render clients feeling more heard, seen, and known, in other words, more deeply empathized with because they are being dealt with not as some generic human but as a human with an identity shaped by a variety of social locations and experiences.

4

DIVERSIFYING THE DEFINITION OF TRAUMA

In this chapter, I explore the range of possible definitions of what constitutes a trauma, inviting the reader to consider going beyond the *Diagnostic and Statistical Manual of Mental Disorders* (4th ed., text rev.; *DSM–IV–TR*; American Psychiatric Association, 2000) definition. The importance of understanding how culture, context, and identity can render an experience traumatic for some individuals is examined, and several models for identifying trauma are presented.

The *DSM–IV–TR* defines a traumatic stressor, Criterion A of the diagnosis of posttraumatic stress disorder (PTSD), as

> an extreme traumatic stressor involving direct personal experience of an event that involves actual or threatened death or serious injury, or other threat to one's physical integrity; or witnessing an event that involves death, injury, or a threat to the physical integrity of another person; or learning about unexpected or violent death, serious harm, or threat of death or injury experienced by a family member or other close associate. The person's response to the event must involve intense fear, helplessness, or horror (or in children, the response must involve disorganized or agitated behavior). (American Psychiatric Association, 2000, p. 467)

This definition would seem, on its face, to be an adequate one and for many people an accurate one. Trauma is a wound to the psyche, one that spills over the dams of peoples' coping strategies, flooding them with intolerable affect.

Yet feminist and multicultural writers about trauma have long critiqued the *DSM–IV–TR* definition for its failures of inclusiveness (Brown, 1991a). In this chapter, I attempt both to deconstruct and to reanalyze this criterion through the lens of culturally aware models of practice and also to explore other ways of defining and understanding what might constitute a traumatic stressor for an individual. A genuinely culturally competent approach to working with trauma survivors requires this expanded understanding of what makes something a trauma, because Criterion A, although broad, is narrow enough to make some important sources of trauma invisible or unknowable as the traumas that they are. Because many of these invisible traumas are related to a survivor's multiple identities, ignoring or invalidating these experiences diminishes empathy in general and cultural competence in particular.

I begin with the end of the *DSM–IV–TR* definition, which speaks of trauma arising from learning of threats to the well-being of family or close associates. In dominant U.S. cultures, family is most often defined as those persons to whom one is related by biology or law. But for many persons, family is defined either in broader terms or in completely different ones. The common use in American sexual minority communities of the term *family* refers to any other lesbian, gay, bisexual, or transgender (LGBT) person, as in, "Is she family?" when inquiring as to another's sexual orientation. This language should not be taken lightly, because it represents linguistically a sense of connection and community that can have implications for how and whether an event is experienced as a traumatic stressor. Similarly, in many communities of individuals of color are thought of as family members because of their roles in people's lives, rather than their formal relationships. Hearing African American people referring to one another, even when strangers, as my brother and my sister conveys once again the sense of relatedness emerging from shared culture, heritage, and oppression. Strict constructions of the concept of family are consequently at risk to lead to a failure to understand how an event that happens apparently outside of the family or close associate circle might be perceived as equally threatening and meaningful as one occurring within those identifiable boundaries. "I am because we are" goes the African American saying; thus, if one of *we* is harmed, then harm to *I* may also be felt.

What constitutes a threat of death or injury or a threat to physical integrity is also not intuitively obvious. The happy bungee jumper who leaps out into space tethered by one foot to a long cord is objectively risking her or his life, but rarely does that jumper, or those witnessing the event, experience traumatic stress; those involved tend to describe the experience as fun and exhilarating. Similarly, the Formula One race car driver who spins out and crashes during a race is unlikely to see the experience as traumatic, but rather as part of the "living on the edge" draw of the sport. Farley (1991) has described persons who seek out such life-threatening yet pleasurable experiences as exhibiting "Type T" behavior. These are experiences that are purposefully sought and experienced as under the control of those partaking in them, no matter their danger. Contrast this with the same race car driver who walks away from a car accident on a city street in which her vehicle is crushed. Because this occurrence was neither chosen nor experienced as occurring in her control, the life-threatening aspects of that accident loom larger in the foreground than do those of the car crash occurring in the controlled environs of the race track. In dominant cultures that value the illusion of control over one's life, control over high-risk activities is a sine qua non of participation in that culture, and the illusion of having such control in life is common.

However, on the other side of the spectrum, it is possible for a person to experience threat to life and physical integrity simply from a word being spoken. Many African Americans report that when they hear the epithet commonly referred to as "the N word" they feel at such risk because of the resonances between that term and violence against their communities. Darrell was an African American man in his mid 50s who had served with distinction in the military in Operation Desert Storm, earning a medal for valor under fire. He had retired from the military after a career served largely in combat zones or preparing to enter them and was known by his friends and family to be a calming presence to all around him because of the equanimity with which he faced the risks of combat. Although exposed repeatedly to Criterion A traumatic stressors, he did not develop posttraumatic symptoms during his service or for several years afterward.

On retiring from the military, where he had been the sergeant major of a transportation organization, he took a similar job in civilian life in middle management at a trucking firm. However, unlike in the military, where he had found a mostly bias-free work environment, his new civilian job was rife with overt and covert racism. Although he had been hired into a management role in the company, he was frequently left out of meetings and decision making, and when subordinates were disrespectful to him, his boss refused to discipline them, telling him that he was "hypersensitive." When one subordinate used the N word, the boss laughed at Darrell's discomfort. Darrell was the only African American employee at the firm, which added to his sense of isolation. After 2 years in the job he began to suffer crushing headaches, which his physician determined to have no organic origin, and he was referred to a psychotherapist for stress management. He reluctantly followed his physician's advice because he was used to following orders, but came into the office angry, feeling dismissed and disrespected further by being told that "it's all in your head."

Several sessions into the therapy, which appeared to be going badly as a result of Darrell's apparent reluctance to participate, he mentioned, as if in passing, that he was having some difficulties sleeping. This led the psychotherapist to take a more careful history, at which point Darrell disclosed that he was having recurrent nightmares of the office in which his White employees surrounded him, jeering. Further exploration determined that he met full criteria for PTSD. However, the psychotherapist could not give the diagnosis because there was no apparent threat to life present; Criterion A was missing. Darrell worked in an office, not in a war zone, and his symptoms had nothing to do with his combat experience. The psychotherapist, puzzled, sought consultation from me, and I suggested that the client be asked about how he experienced the issue of safety or its absence in his workplace. The psychotherapist was shocked to hear Darrell tell him that he felt in danger of his life at work:

> No one's got my back. Everyone thinks they can do whatever they want with me; I'm just window dressing to them, someone to pimp out to the customers. I felt safer with those damn Iraqis lobbing Scuds at me than I do in that office, wondering when I'm going to come out and find my tires slashed or my brake lines cut.

For Darrell, constant daily exposure to racism was experienced as traumatic and as an indicator that things easy to identify as life threatening might happen. In his narrative it was the unpredictability and invisibility of potential perpetrators that was part of what felt threatening to him; in combat he knew who the enemy was and, more importantly, felt safe in the embrace of his comrades, who did have his back.

Similar stories are told by women who have been sexually harassed in the workplace; being referred to by crude names for female genitalia or as a species of female dog carries with it a deeply felt symbolic threat of violence for many women. Although some authors have argued that it is impossible for sexual harassment to rise to the level of a Criterion A stressor absent an actual sexual assault, Fitzgerald (1993) noted that it is what the gender hostility represents to its targets that leads to the phenomenology of feeling unsafe. Many sexually harassed women speak of developing a fear that their harasser, who seems not to be stopped by requests or threats, will escalate to more violent or physical forms of sexual assault; thus the crude jokes about a woman's breasts or the pictures of women's genitals taped into her locker are rape threats, not just words and pictures. Culturally competent trauma practice requires clinicians to think broadly as to what might constitute a trauma for the particular person in front of them, rather than having a fixed list of possible traumatic events that are simple to perceive as traumatic. I explore more specifics about how events can acquire a traumagenic meaning in the chapters about social locations and trauma. However, it's important to begin the thought experiment of deconstructing the narrow range of possible traumas in people's lives implied by Criterion A. A psychic wound need not occur in close proximity to a physical one to be very deep and terrifying.

It is not uncommon for individuals whose traumata are more difficult for others to see to be diagnosed, and stigmatized, as having some form of personality disorder. In fact, some of the most popular conceptualizations of personality disorder (Millon & Davis, 2001) would see just this kind of distress emerging in the absence of a clear Criterion A stressor as evidence of an underlying personality disorder whose symptoms are being evoked by stressors that the "normal" person would respond to asymptomatically. As discussed in chapter 1, having one invariant version of human normal is very likely to obscure the presence of multiple norms of human experience. The normal Bajoran spent time in a Cardassian internment camp and saw friends and family members tortured during the war of liberation; this is not the experience of, for example, a normal middle-class American of European ancestry (although it might easily have been the experience of one or some of those ancestors, depending on their specific origins).

Because of the narrowness of the *DSM–IV–TR* definition, several theorists and psychotherapists working from critical psychology standpoints have offered other ways of understanding what makes an experience traumatic. As Briere (2004) noted, experiences of degradation, humiliation, and coerced activities in which power was abused to induce unwanted behaviors even when an overt threat of violence was absent can all be experienced phenomenologically as traumatic for some persons. Additionally, empirical research on trauma offers alternative paradigms for comprehending traumatic stress, and when these paradigms are used as a lens through which to view clients, they give clinicians a model for trauma that better supports culturally competent practice.

THE JUST WORLD BLOWS UP

"Victims are threatening to non-victims, for they are manifestations of a malevolent universe rather than a benevolent one" (Janoff-Bulman, 1992, p. 148). Janoff-Bulman, a social psychologist, advanced a paradigm of trauma based on the social psychological construct known as the "just world hypothesis" (Lerner, 1980). Janoff-Bulman argued that most human beings possess three "fundamental assumptions" (p. 6) that reflect their working models of interpersonal and social reality. She argued that these three assumptions are as follows: (a) The world is benevolent; (b) the world is meaningful; and (c) the self is worthy. Although not all people hold all three assumptions, many, particularly dominant culture Americans, do, to the extent that they are likely to be optimistic about themselves and their lives even when they are able to see that the world is doing badly. Trauma, says Janoff-Bulman, happens when those assumptions about the goodness, meaningfulness, and safety of the world are shattered by life events.

Members of dominant U.S. and other Western cultures are particularly vulnerable to trauma arising from shattering of just world expectations. The assumptive systems of these cultures tend to be justice oriented, with the underlying belief being that people get what they deserve. Calvinist Protestantism, which is a dominant theology of American life, teaches that the elect of God, who are not sinners, are known in this life by their worldly success, whereas sinners can be seen because their lives are full of poverty and misery (see Weber's, 1930/2001, classic *The Protestant Ethic and the Spirit of Capitalism* for the source of this argument). The classic Jewish prayer of Yom Kippur, the Day of Atonement, *Unetaneh Tokef*, states that "Repentance, prayer, and good deeds" can stave off the possibility of death during the coming year by one of a long list of painful methods (fire, water, stoning, wild beasts, pestilence, etc.), again implying that bad things happen to the unrighteous. Catholicism similarly teaches the necessity of confession and repentance of sins to avoid an unpleasant afterlife in places other than heaven.

The philosophies of life and death most prominent in the shaping of Western cultures are those that make connections between good actions and good outcomes and that convey a spurious sense of control over one's life to those who unconsciously adopt them (Langer, 1975). In these contexts, the bad thing happening to the good person is more likely to constitute a trauma because it explodes the neat equation between good deeds and a safe, happy life and leaves the person with a frightening sense of life being out of control—witness the Biblical tale of Job, whose meaningless sufferings have become paradigmatic for the experience of unearned pain.

In contrast with this Western view of good deeds equaling good life, many other cultures make no such equation. Cultures informed by Buddhist philosophy assume that suffering will be a part of life and that such suffering occurs out of the control of present-day actions; rather it is likely to reflect a current-life working through of errors made in a prior incarnation by oneself and even by one's ancestors. Avoiding the attachments that can lead to suffering is seen as of greater value than pursuing behaviors that might forestall suffering, which is seen as an ultimately fruitless goal. Similarly, Hindu beliefs are that one is continuously attempting to become closer to the divine, and thus one's behaviors in this lifetime will redound to the next life, not this one. This is not to say that people living in Buddhist and Hindu cultures do not experience the psychological effects of trauma. Rather, it is to suggest that if one expects the world to be full of suffering one is less likely to have one's expectations shattered when suffering emerges; pain and suffering will ensue, but potentially the existential challenge and potential for an event to be traumagenic will be differently configured.

Janoff-Bulman (1992) pointed out that when one subscribes to the just world hypothesis, one's expectations of life reflect that hypothesis. People do not expect bad things to happen so long as they are behaving well. In fact, the lives of many people who are firmly rooted in dominant cultural identities are defined by the comfort with which they experience their fit with the world, and the assumption, founded in dominant group privilege, that they will be welcomed no matter where they are in the world. The original definition of Criterion A, that an event was "unusual and outside the range of human experience" reflects that model of reality; bad things should be uncommon, unusual, and not normative because life is good.

In Darrell's case a component of what was traumatic about his racist workplace was that it shattered assumptions he had about the world of work. Even though he was not a member of the dominant ethnic culture, he had lived most of his life in the military, his sole employer between high school and retirement, believing that a man who worked hard, did well, and related with respect to superiors and friendliness to peers and subordinates would have a good outcome in the workplace. He had repeatedly had this kind of experience in his more than 20 years of military service. In fact, as he later told his psychotherapist, he had scoffed at relatives, all civilians, who complained about racism in their workplaces, telling them that they just had to "suck it up and do the job," so little did he believe that there could be no relationship between hard work and a positive outcome in the workplace. When his assumptions were shattered the door was opened for him to make associations between what was happening to him at work and the possibility of actual physical threat.

To offer culturally competent trauma practice, a psychotherapist must inquire carefully into what the client's assumptions about reality were prior to the experience of trauma. Ironically, having had a life full of misery and difficulty does not necessarily reduce the possibility of having assumptions shattered; it is possible to be informed by some component of the just world hypothesis even when the empirical data of life do not conform to anyone's idea of justice. An excellent and very painful example of this can be seen in cases in which psychotherapists have become sexually involved with their clients, as this clinical example illustrates.

Renee sought psychotherapy with Dr. Jones in her early 30s after leaving an abusive relationship with her husband of 8 years. She had grown up in poverty, one of eight children of a Euro-American family whose marginal life was characterized by parental alcoholism, child abuse, and neglect. She herself struggled with chronic health problems, some of them arising from childhood malnutrition, and had barely been able to complete high school. She told Dr. Jones that she was relieved to finally be having a relationship with someone safe who would be good to her and help her.

Approximately 6 months into the therapy, Dr. Jones began to loosen the boundaries, inviting Renee out to coffee after their sessions and eventually spending many hours with her discussing his personal life. She was flattered to have an educated man express interest in her. When their apparent deepening intimacy led first to hugs, then kisses, and then a sexual encounter in his office after a session one evening, she initially felt even more special and loved. Dr. Jones told her that she was indeed special, "I don't do this with other clients." He also said that because many other people would not understand their relationship and because he was married and she was divorcing her abusive husband, they must keep the relationship a secret.

After 2 months and many such late evenings on the couch, she was shocked by an article in the local newspaper, "Psychotherapist Charged With Sexual Misconduct." Dr. Jones's license had been summarily suspended by the psychology board after two women had come forward to complain that he had sexualized their psychotherapy. At first Renee simply felt hurt and lied to. She was not special; when she complained about this to Dr. Jones, he told her that she was experiencing a "narcissistic wound" and that he should perhaps pull back from the romantic relationship if she could not handle being less than completely special. Over the next few weeks she became increasingly depressed and despondent, and Dr. Jones became decreasingly available to her as he became focused on his own legal and regulatory difficulties. Ultimately Renee admitted herself to the inpatient psychiatric unit of her local teaching hospital.

There, slowly finding her balance through a fog of new medications, she poured out her story to the resident assigned to her care. The resident assured her that she had done nothing wrong and added that Dr. Jones should have known that having a sexual relationship with her would harm her because there was so much research to that effect available. This was the tipping point for her; the resident's attempts to reassure her in fact opened up an abyss of terror. As Renee told me many months and several suicide attempts later, while being evaluated in her civil suit against Dr. Jones,

> What was so painful was not that he abandoned me, although that hurt. I'm used to being abandoned and can actually handle that pretty well. It was that he knew that having sex with me could harm me. That he knew there was research saying it was like rape. And that he knew that in advance! That scared me so much, made me feel like I was in free fall. I knew that the world was a bad place, but I always thought that psychotherapists were safe, that you could trust them. He blew that up. It's like he was trying to kill me.

She had all of the symptoms of PTSD. Although she had not assumed the world to be just and safe, she had reserved a tiny corner of it as safe, the corner where psychotherapists practiced. She had believed that safety lay there. The absence of the more general assumption about the world's safety did not protect her from the traumatic effects of the shattering of those assumptions that she had managed to hold on to.

Culturally competent trauma practice thus includes the possibility that the event, although not directly threatening to life or physical safety, was traumatic because it broke apart an existential system and worldview that had generated a sense of safety, even a minimal one. If a client is acting as if she or he is traumatized and there is no apparent Criterion A event to be found, it can be extremely clinically helpful to inquire into the ways in which assumptions have been shattered for this person. Cultural and contextual locations may be the factors informing both those assumptions and the ways in which they have been shattered.

DROPS OF ACID FALLING ON STONE— INSIDIOUS TRAUMATIZATION

Another conceptual framework for understanding trauma in a culturally competent manner is through the lens of insidious trauma (Root, 1992), also known as "microaggressions" (Sue, 2003). In the lives of many individuals who are members of target groups, daily existence is replete with reminders of the potential for traumatization and the absence of safety. These reminders can occur in apparently banal ways, for instance, when a member of one's group is made a target of ridicule in a public discourse or when media consistently portray one's group in a stereotypical manner. Some of these insidious traumata are very painful; as I was completing this book the talk-show host Don Imus dumped viciously racist and sexist verbal acid on the heads of a group of talented young woman athletes simply because they were women and African American. These experiences are not traumatic per se, but they can be traumatic in a subtle way. They are the almost daily reminders of the threat of violence that underlies bias. Everyday racism, sexism, homophobia, classism, ableism, and so on (Essed, 1991) are the small but ever-present pulls of energy toward a survival level of consciousness, the reminders that someone somewhere is trying to make you and people like you less welcome on the planet.

Microaggressions and insidious trauma can also be more directly threat evoking. For example, as noted earlier in this volume insidious trauma occurs for LGBT people during antigay discourse that occurs when attempts are made to roll back legal protections or deny efforts to obtain such protections for LGBT people. Such discourse, in which LGBT people are described in the media and from pulpits as less worthy of protection than others and often as sinful, dirty, or perverted, evokes memories of a time in the not-too-distant past when people were incarcerated for being members of a sexual minority. These experiences of hate speech come dangerously close to the emotional edge of more current events in which LGBT people were murdered in hate crimes such as that perpetrated against Matthew Shepard. Glenda Russell (2004a, 2004b) has documented the traumagenic impact on LGBT people of such public discourse in states where laws have been passed outlawing same-sex marriage or retracting protections against employment and housing discrimination. As one of my clients commented during the 2004 election cycle when laws against same-sex marriage were being proposed in many states, "All of this makes me wonder when they're going to outlaw being lesbian and gay. And then what do I do? Stop existing? Move to Canada?" The public discourse, although never calling for outright violence, is a potent reminder that violence occurs under the cover of seeing LGBT people as other than fully human.

Root (1992) argued that when a person is subjected to insidious traumatization, that individual experiences a gradual and often imperceptible erosion of the psyche. A useful metaphor is that of very small drops of acid falling on a stone. Each drop by itself does little damage and may in fact etch the stone in such as way as to make it more beautiful. Thus, in some ways the experience of daily microaggressions may evoke resilient coping responses. Yet each drop of emotional acid creates just enough damage to render the next drop more damaging. At times the dilution of the acid is such that the particular microaggression is barely perceived; at other times its sting is more apparent, as was the case for Darrell. Over time a fissure develops in the form of an emotional vulnerability that is invisible so long as certain aspects of the biopsychosocial and spiritual environment remain steady or supportive.

But at some point, said Root, the insidiously traumatized person may appear to crack and develop symptoms of full-blown posttraumatic stress when the apparent stressor seems small and not threatening at all. Root argued that it is in the nature of insidious traumatization that symptoms are the result of cumulative microaggressions; each one is not large enough to be a traumatic stressor but taken together they yield a traumagenic experience for the individual that manifests in posttraumatic distress when enough acid has fallen or when the environment shifts sufficiently to open wide the crack.

Sara's experience illustrates the impact of insidious trauma. Born with a congenital condition that created progressive muscular weakness, she required increasing amounts of assistance from others to engage in normal daily life. Sara was an optimistic, outgoing woman with great intellectual gifts that had propelled her to a career as a professor of mathematics. Her family of origin had been supportive of her from the start, defining her as "Sara, the brilliant mathematician," not as "Sara the disabled person," and had taught her how to fight for all of the accommodations to which she was legally entitled to be able to express those intellectual gifts. It was not that her family denied her disability, rather that for them it was not the foreground of their relationship with her. She seemed to many of her friends and colleagues to be the epitome of psychological well-being and so surprised all of them when she landed in an inpatient psychiatric unit after a fairly serious suicide attempt.

Sara started therapy when she left the hospital, a condition of her early release to which she agreed only because of her hatred of being "stuck in sick people prison." At first she seemed reluctant or unable to tell her psychotherapist what had precipitated the suicide attempt and was mildly hostile to the entire endeavor, stating that she was only in therapy to soothe her parents' worries and to make sure that she did not end up as an inpatient again. "Don't crips just naturally want to kill themselves?" she sarcastically queried her psychotherapist, who responded each time this theme emerged that no, crips did not just naturally want to kill themselves. After the sixth or seventh iteration of this line, however, the psychotherapist confronted Sara, asking her just who had suggested that she should be killing herself.

It was at this juncture that Sara was able to disclose the emotional toll taken by repeated stories to which she had been exposed for her entire life of people with disabilities who, unable to end their own lives because of quadriplegia, had petitioned courts for assistance in ending their lives. Sara explained to her psychotherapist,

> It's not that they wanted to kill themselves, although that bothered me and made me feel very sad for them, It's that perfectly rational people without disabilities, people I know, seemed to think that it was quite reasonable for someone to want to die because they couldn't wipe their own ass. I haven't been able to wipe my own ass since I was 19, you know? And I didn't think it was a good reason to kill myself. At least not at first.

She recounted tales of well-meaning acquaintances (who as a result never made it past superficial with her) telling her that they could not imagine living with a disability as severe as hers and commenting that she was brave to keep on living as her ability to care for herself physically continued to diminish. Sara had even joined a disabilities rights group called Not Dead Yet to become part of the movement protesting this apparently pervasive attitude in mainstream society about the worth of the lives of people whose physical disabilities lead to enhanced needs for personal care from others.

The net effect of this cultural discourse of the worthlessness of disabled life had, however, had the effect of being insidiously traumatizing to Sara. She noticed that each time such a story appeared in the news she would have sleepless nights and nightmares whose content she could not recall. The tipping point, though, did not come from another story of a suicidal person with an acquired disability. Rather, as Sara told it, once again the batteries powering her wheelchair had died unexpectedly; her spares were also inexplicably dead as well. It was a holiday weekend, and it would be impossible for her to get new ones until the following Tuesday when the university's disabilities services repair shop would reopen. In the past such events had been annoyances, but nothing more than that.

But this time it felt much worse than an annoyance; Sara recounted to her psychotherapist that she had realized this time how something essential to her life and well-being was perceived as so optional and incidental in able-bodied society that it could not be obtained over a holiday. She raged,

> If you need a battery for your car you can get one on July 4. For your fucking cell phone you can get a battery 24/7. But a wheelchair battery,

well, hell, let the crip stay in bed. What the hell, she doesn't have a life anyways, does she?

Her rage that weekend had met her feelings of helplessness and spiraled into depression and despair; she became sleepless for a week, during which time her mind replayed the story line of "better dead than disabled." The fight stopped feeling worth it to her; meaning exploded and blew away in a thousand tiny pieces. The following weekend she took an overdose of her muscle-relaxant medication, noting to her psychotherapist the irony that she could not toilet herself but had enough muscle control still to open her pill bottle and turn on the specially adapted water faucet.

Sara's story illustrates how insidious trauma can operate. For her, the emotional acid was a lifetime of being treated as if her life were not worth living; insidious trauma became internalized oppression, the internal representation in the self of oppressive and hostile messages about aspects of self associated with target group status. The early effects of this insidious trauma appeared in her activism against cultural ableism; she started with a highly adaptive meaning-making response to being devalued. But when the physical environment's supports became unavailable and that unavailability became invested with excess meaning by a lifetime of oppression, Sara's trauma broke through all of the protections she had erected against it and became intolerable for her.

Another component of culturally competent trauma practice requires psychotherapists to consider how insidious trauma and microaggression may have been present in a client's life even when the particular client does not identify this kind of experience. Everyday racism, sexism, heterosexism, ableism, and other forms of institutionalized oppressions may seem so familiar to people as the background noise of their lives that they may have no cognitive construct into which to place these encounters; they simply have the posttrauma distress and dysfunction arising from doing battle every day against an army of small toxic agents.

When psychotherapists invite clients to acknowledge these experiences as traumatic they do two very important things. First, they raise the client's consciousness, allowing them to make sense of their distress in a helpful manner that externalizes some important component of their difficulties; "It's not me; it's the social environment," is a stance that many persons find empowering because it allows them to become proactive in dealing with the daily acid drops (Brown, 1994). Second, and as important, a psychotherapist's offering this paradigm to a client may be a message about how that psychotherapist is an ally, someone who, although not necessarily sharing the client's target group status, is willing to tell the truth about the realities of life. That stance is a powerful component of creating a sense of therapeutic alliance, which is itself essential to the good outcome of the therapy. But psychotherapists must make this offer at a time when people are ready to hear it, when they are safe enough to know how they are and that they have been unsafe, so that this awareness does not disrupt their capacities to cope or their abilities to deal with the painful realities that they experience.

BETRAYAL OF TRUST AS TRAUMA

In the early 1990s a controversy arose regarding whether children who had been sexually violated by family caregivers could lose access to their knowledge of such terrifying experiences, only to have conscious knowledge return to them later in life. This debate over what were variously called repressed memories or recovered memories of childhood abuse yielded a great deal of heat and light but was also a source of a new scientific model of what constitutes trauma. Freyd (1996; Birrell & Freyd, 2006) proposed the concept of Betrayal Trauma (BT) as a paradigm for understanding both the phenomenon of delayed recall of childhood abuse and also for conceptualizing such experiences as traumatic.

The BT theory provides a cognitive science model of how interpersonal and psychosocial dynamics can make an event traumatic even when threat to life or physical safety is apparently absent, which is frequently the case when children are sexually abused by family caregivers such as parents or by other caregivers such as priests or teachers. Freyd, drawing on evolutionary psychology, suggested that humans are acutely attuned to the possibility of interpersonal betrayal so as to know how to choose with whom to closely associate. Children, however, have no choice in the matter of their close associates; because human children are highly dependent on their adult caregivers for safety and nurturance and because those adults control children's lives, children who are being abused in their families will be placed in the intolerable position of having to manage betrayal and the need for dependency.

Freyd argued that this intolerable situation leads abused children to store their knowledge of the abuse in separate neural networks that are unavailable cognitively until such time as the child is either no longer dependent on the abusive adult or cues in the interpersonal or physical environment retrieve the information and bring it to consciousness (e.g., an abused child, now an adult, has a child who reaches the age at which the parent's own abuse experiences began to occur). Freyd and her colleagues (Freyd, DePrince, & Zurbriggen, 2001) found that individuals with delayed recall of childhood trauma are significantly more likely to have been traumatized by family members than individuals who never forget the abuse experiences.

The BT model posits that betrayal traumas are traumatic emotionally for humans when the extent of the betrayal becomes knowable. This is similar to Koss's (1988) conceptualizations of acquaintance rape in which the experience becomes traumatic only when the victim reappraises the meaning of the experience from merely unpleasant to one of violation. The BT model explains not only why memories for childhood abuse can become elusive or unavailable for many years but also why experiences that are confusing and unpleasant but not an immediate cause of fear, horror, or a sense of danger to life can become traumagenic for people. The betrayals of trust that can occur in contexts in which people can reasonably assume that a powerful other is looking out for their interests and welfare are also a form of shattered assumptions; thus, a betrayal trauma does not require a family relationship of caregiving to occur. Ruth's story (Brown, 1986) illustrates how a betrayal trauma can join with a more obvious form of trauma to generate psychological distress that goes beyond the *DSM–IV–TR* diagnosis of PTSD.

Ruth joined the military after receiving her nursing degree and in 1968 was assigned to a military hospital in Vietnam, where her patients were gravely wounded young men flown directly from the battlefields on medevac helicopters. Her service was marked by many directly traumatizing events, including the repeated shelling of the hospital and constant exposure to wounded, dying, and dead soldiers, many of them younger than she was. When she returned from Vietnam she began to self-medicate with alcohol, a strategy that persisted for almost 2 decades until the nightmares and flashbacks became too powerful for drinking to push back.

Ruth came into therapy with me in 1983, a few months after she had been discharged from a Veterans Administration alcoholism treatment unit, overwhelmed by the symptoms of her PTSD. As we worked together to assist her recovery, we uncovered a number of other traumas that were not as evident as the constant exposures to the horror of war but were equally powerful in informing her distress, powerful enough that they kept her in despair for a number of years even after the flashbacks and nightmares had subsided.

These were traumas of betrayal. Ruth had volunteered for military service and to be sent to Vietnam in part because she had strongly believed what her government and her church had told her about the rightness of this war. Saving Vietnam from communism was, she had thought, a just cause. Her time there had taught her otherwise; as we discovered together, this was a first level of betrayal. In therapy she struggled with feeling alienated and lied to by the institutions of authority in whom she had always previously put her trust. A second betrayal occurred when she returned to the United States. There she found she had nowhere to turn with her knowledge and experiences. Her family and former friends, still seeing the war as just, wanted to hear nothing about what had happened. Robbed of support, she withdrew socially and became deeply distrustful of others, with alcohol being the only factor that made social interactions other than deeply painful. She came to realize that the onset of her most troubling psychological symptoms had paralleled her failed attempts to reconnect with her support networks and the experience of feeling silenced that had followed.

For Ruth, being lied to and betrayed by her country and her church turned out to be the existential crux of her despair. Her trauma arose when she came to believe that these betrayals had occurred, which in turn made the other traumagenic components of her wartime service more traumatic; the deaths of her patients and her own brushes with danger could no longer be seen as having occurred in a context that lent meaning to suffering. When meaning making is stripped from an experience, its potential to lead to distress is enhanced; so Ruth's loss of meaning derived from her sacrifices and those of the wounded and dead of the war became the pivot point on which her trauma turned.

In our work together, dealing with flashbacks and terrible nightmares gave way to the search for meaning, which occupied the second half of a 10-year therapy relationship. She rediscovered a creative capacity that had lain dormant for decades and turned it into poetry that spoke to the experience of being a woman in a war zone at a time when supposedly no women were present. She became able to address how she had been betrayed by faith and country by finding a public forum in which she could tell her truths and be listened to. As she became able to speak from a place of personal integrity the wounds of her betrayal began to heal as well. Today she has been out of therapy for longer than she was in it. We stay in loose touch through a mutual acquaintance who lets me know of Ruth's deep capacities to move through all of the vicissitudes of life—parents who died, her bout with cancer—with her sense of personal agency and meaning in place.

Culturally competent trauma treatment thus asks the question, How might this experience have been not only threatening or dangerous but also an encounter with betrayal? The evacuees of New Orleans are experiencing prolonged and continuous betrayal. For those who came through the floods with life and family intact, the ongoing realities of being lied to and left at risk by governments and insurance companies is becoming a second trauma that may be as likely to leave psychological damage as the hurricane itself or even more likely. These are persons who felt inconvenienced by the flood but are traumatized by having their trust and faith in the government betrayed repeatedly and for a period of many months. The woman whose former husband hit her once but before doing so conned her out of her life savings and left her isolated and destitute is suffering not from the pain of the assault on her body but rather from the psychological pain of having had trust badly betrayed.

BAD ICING ON THE POISON CAKE—
TRAUMA WITH SPECIAL MEANING

Rape is rape. The violation of one's body for the sexual pleasure of the assailant is universally acknowledged to be a humiliating, degrading experience. Large-population research on risk factors for PTSD identifies sexual assault as the trauma most likely to lead to PTSD and with the longest lasting incidence of posttrauma symptoms (Davidson & Foa, 1993). But some rapes are weighted with extra negative meaning for the victim. These are rapes in which the motives of the perpetrator or his (almost all perpetrators of sexual assault are men) role in relationship to the victim gives the assault a more potent toxic force. Although not the only sort of trauma that can become invested with excess meaning because of the ways in which it lands directly in important components of identity, sexual assault provides an excellent example of this sort of traumatic stressor.

In her novel *The Sparrow*, anthropologist Mary Doria Russell (1996) tells the story of one such victim of the added-negative-value sexual assault. That her protagonist is a Jesuit priest, a man, is only incidental to this phenomenon, although in real life men account for only approximately 10% of known victims of sexual assault. That the assailant in question is an alien on a planet that does not exist is also incidental. What matters and what leaves her protagonist Emilio Sandoz suicidal and wracked by nightmares is that he had believed that this man, whose music drew the priest and his traveling companions to visit the distant planet, was conveying a divine message through his work and that he, Sandoz, had been brought together with this man by God. He explains to another group of priests who are trying to get him to tell his story so that they may make sense of what became of the space mission,

> I was scared but I didn't understand what was going on. I never imagined—who could have imagined such a thing? I am in God's hand, I thought. I loved God and trusted in his love. Amusing, isn't it? I laid down all my defenses. I had nothing between me and what happened but the love of God. And I was raped. I was naked before God and I was raped. (Russell, 1996, p. 394)

Emilio Sandoz saw his rapist as the instrument of the divine, a role that held special meaning for him as a priest who had struggled with his faith and had come to believe more deeply in God because of the music made by the man who later raped him. Similar to today's real-life victims of sexual assault by Roman Catholic priests, Sandoz felt raped by God through his messenger. Sandoz's story also carries many elements of betrayal trauma; he asks, "Why did it all happen like that, unless God wanted it that way?"

Trauma with added negative meaning can occur for a myriad of different reasons: the person who is assaulted because she or he left a place of safety to do a good deed, the survivors whose assailants were charged with their protection, the victims of clergy sexual abuse, and the trauma that repeats historical patterns of oppression and victimization. All of these can heighten the pain and the distress experienced by clients. As I describe in detail in the following chapters, social location can lend special meaning to trauma. Culturally competent trauma treatment involves looking for these added meanings and weaving strategies for addressing those meanings into the process of healing and recovery. One of the goals of this approach to working with trauma survivors is to be able to consider how a trauma might carry added weight for a survivor; the question that a psychotherapist should be asking is, "How might this particular event or experience evoke other meanings that resonate with this individual's multiple identities?"

Trauma is not, for many individuals an event that happens once, a single blow that then fades away to leave behind the traumatized person in the safe and protective environment. It is, rather, a frequent component of social and emotional environments in which daily life can become a series of encounters with threat. Even when it is a one-time event, the social environment and realities in which the trauma survivor has lived prior to the time of the actual traumatic event and the milieus to which that person returns in the aftermath of the trauma can inform how and whether that experience will lead to distress and dysfunction. Humans almost never come away from trauma unscathed emotionally. Cultural competence in trauma treatment helps to make sense of those frequent occasions when the wounds seem deeper than would be expected given the size of the blows.

To do this, it is necessary to understand how specific components of social location and identity are implicated in the experience of trauma. Although the following chapters focus attention on one component of the ADDRESSING model (Hays 2001, 2007) at a time, readers are encouraged to remember that these identities are interactive and never experienced in isolation one from the other. Each person has multiple identities informing her or his experiences of reality; it is only for the purpose of focusing in-depth on each of several important social locations that I separate those parameters here. Because each social location has particular embedded qualities that inform experiences of trauma exposure I endeavor to highlight those in my discussion; this means that a lopsided picture of each social location emerges, given the focus on trauma. Readers are urged to consider how to guard against allowing their own biases to distort the information shared here into validation of stereotypic beliefs about target groups, which is one of the risks inherent in discussing social location as a risk factor for trauma exposure. Rather than following the order of the ADDRESSING acronym I look at social locations that are closely related to biological factors first, then move to those more fully socially constructed.

II

CONTEXTUAL PARADIGMS FOR UNDERSTANDING THE NATURE OF TRAUMA

5

TRAUMA, AGE, AND AGEISM

In this chapter, I introduce the reader to the ways in which age interacts with the experience of trauma. Trauma in childhood as a precursor to possible life-long challenges in the accomplishment of normative developmental tasks is examined as I look in detail at trauma's effects at the more vulnerable ends of the developmental spectrum, childhood and older adulthood. Age cohort as a factor informing the experience of trauma is also discussed.

Age is a fundamental fact of biology, the count of how many minutes someone has existed on the planet. Age is also psychology, the growth of the capacities, intellectual and emotional, that develop over the life span or diminish as life lengthens. Thus age is about the varieties of power that are attendant on access to capacities and the resources that can be obtained. Age is about changes in autonomy and dependency, which convey variations in vulnerability. Age is a social phenomenon; the meanings ascribed to a given point on the age span are socially constructed, creating opportunities for various sorts of privilege and exclusion. Age is also about cohort effects and the historical and social realities surrounding people and informing their consciousness of self when they are at a particular age. Trauma can occur at any point in the life span, and for many people trauma occurs repeatedly through their lives. When in the life span a trauma occurs has much to do with the resources available to an individual for responding and coping and thus differentially affects vulnerability to trauma and resilience in trauma response. Trauma appears to affect people in a recursive, mounting fashion, so that trauma at one point in the developmental process undermines and makes more complex the achievement of developmental tasks and milestones later in the developmental process even when trauma is not actively present. Myths about age-related resilience and vulnerabilities also affect how those surrounding trauma survivors respond to what has happened to them.

Age, real or perceived, can also evoke ageism, bias, and differential treatment. As noted earlier in this volume, ageism is a bimodal phenomenon. Western culture disempowers but also eroticizes the very young, stigmatizes and frequently ridicules the signs of aging, and communicates a barely hidden message that it may be better to take risks and die young than to become full of years, but also wrinkles and gray hairs. Western medical systems offer new and more avenues to prolong life as well as a variety of invasive procedures to make people appear younger than their years. Ageism is differentially distributed depending on culture and context, and the meaning of age varies on the basis of these factors as well.

Consequently, cultural competence regarding age and trauma requires a nuanced understanding of the interplay of biological and psychological capacities with their social interpretations and meanings in the interpersonal context. No 12-year-old child will have the emotional and moral development of a 30-year-old adult, but depending on time, place, culture, and context, some of these children will be asked to shoulder more difficult social responsibilities and burdens than some of those grown-ups. Age cohort and cohort within culture will convey information about the relational world in which individuals have deployed those age-related resources and capacities that were available to them at the time of a trauma.

The study of traumatized children has an even shorter history than that of psychological trauma in general, with some of the very first work that informs our current understandings of trauma's effects being done by Terr (1979, 1983) with the survivors of the Chowchilla mass kidnapping. In this event, a school bus full of children was taken, and the bus was buried underground for several days until the kidnappers were apprehended and the children were freed from captivity. These children are paradigmatic in many ways for the ability to comprehend the interaction of young age with trauma exposure. They were not harmed in their families or homes; they were successfully rescued; and their kidnappers were found, prosecuted, and imprisoned. As Terr (1990) noted, the child psychiatrist from the local mental health center made a public pronouncement that "only 1 in 26" children would have any lasting impact of being kidnapped. Yet Terr found that every one of those children, as well as some siblings and friends who had not been on the bus that day, suffered posttraumatic responses to this event, some of which persisted for a number of years.

An entire focus of the field of trauma studies, developmental traumatology, has emerged in the past decades out of the work of such researchers as Terr and Robert Pynoos to focus attention on the specifics of trauma as they affect young children. Because the effects of trauma appear to be greatest at young ages and because the effects of earlier trauma have continuing effects on survivors' capacities to navigate later developmental stages, any competent psychotherapist must familiarize her- or himself with developmental considerations in trauma response.

DEVELOPMENTAL CAPACITIES AND TRAUMA

Humans are unique among the species in that they are born with most of their survival capacities absent and undeveloped; more than any other species humans' survival depends on the kindness of the older members of the species, parents, caregivers, and other extended sources of support. A century of research on child and adolescent development indicates that humans become capable through somewhat predictable processes of cognitive, emotional, and biological maturation, with differing capacities at each point in the process. This notion of children and adolescents as uniquely different from adults in their capacities is a relatively new one in the history of most cultures in which children have generally been viewed as smaller, weaker, and less intelligent adults.

Unfortunately for traumatized children (and for the adults into whom they grow), many of emerging popular culture's narratives about children's uniqueness have to do with their alleged greater psychological resiliency. Varieties of childhood posttraumatic coping mechanisms, which frequently mask the damages done until later in life, have been mistaken for an absence of impact. The reality that children's bodies and brains are more biologically plastic and resilient than those of adults has become conflated with the equally potent reality that children do not have either the psychological or material resources necessary for coping with trauma exposure on their own. Because in many instances trauma occurring in childhood is perpetrated by those on whom a child depends for the development of self-capacities and the provision of safety, children's trauma responses reflect not only the direct effect of trauma but also the damages done to and in the context of relationship and attachment. The most common sources of psychological trauma for children are parents, parent surrogates, teachers, and others who are socially sanctioned to have access to and control over the lives of children. These are also the adults to whom children must turn for resources in dealing with trauma. The age-related double bind for the traumatized child is huge, and the effects of being effectively trapped with the source of the trauma and dependent on that source for soothing of its own maleficent effects can be destructive and long lasting.

Even in those circumstances in which the source of trauma is not a caregiver, a caregiver's capacities to support a child's development and offer necessary soothing and emotional resources to the child are themselves often compromised by other kinds of traumas in which both parent and child are affected. Natural disaster, war, genocide, and motor vehicle accidents can all harm both parents and child, with differential negative impact on the child's system of resources and care. Parents whose lives are disrupted by a natural disaster and who have become homeless, jobless, and preoccupied with dealing with their own posttraumatic responses and the destabilization of resources will have less time and attention available to give to the needs of their child, no matter how secure the predisaster attachment or how skillful the pretrauma parenting skills might have been. Being in acute emotional distress makes a parent less empathically available, less attuned, and less patient with a child; if the child is also in greater need because of the shared experience of trauma, there can be an exponential decrement of resources for the child both at the moment of trauma and during the later course of development. Because children, and to a lesser extent adolescents, are dependent on the adults in their emotional environments to function as external ego states for them, anything that impairs the capacities of the adults will have far-reaching implications for the development of the children. As Cloitre, Cohen, and Koenen (2006) wrote, the traumatized child experiences the "interrupted life," with interruptions in the development of self-capacities, relational capacities, and possibly brain development as well.

Hobfoll (2001) characterized psychological trauma as involving a loss of resources. Age dramatically affects the resources available to traumatized humans, and trauma dramatically affects the resources available to persons who have experienced it as they traverse their lifetime. The younger the child, the less she or he will have by way of intrapsychic or autonomously generated interpersonal resources. This is as true for the child of wealth as the child living in poverty; in fact, ironically, because social welfare resource systems are more likely to cast their gaze on the parenting behaviors of poor people, a child being traumatized in a wealthy home may be at greater risk than a child raised in a poor home because the systemic mechanisms of child protection are less likely to extend into the homes of those of the middle class and above. However, no young child has learned to self-soothe as effectively as any adult raised with good-enough caregivers.

What do we know about children's intrapsychic resources in the face of trauma, and how does trauma interfere with those resources? Much of the current understanding of the effects of age on trauma response arises from research on the psychology and biology of attachment. Humans are driven by evolutionary pressures to attach to caregivers at birth; infants who are biologically impaired from being able to attach face serious difficulties with all aspects of both emotional and cognitive development. Children with normative attachment capacities who are born into environments where caregivers are incapable of adequate reciprocation of infant attachment needs will also experience impairments in functioning that can include difficulties with cognitive efficiency and problem-solving capacities, decrements in affect regulation and impulse control, problems of reading interpersonal cues correctly and thus in the development of relationships, and impaired capacities to trust (Schore, 2003).

Trauma arising from abuse or neglect by a caregiver creates impairments that are core to a person's development and can be more difficult to address therapeutically because of their residence in what the traumatized person experiences as the real or inner self. Trauma occurring in the context of good-quality attachment between child and caregiver can be disruptive in other ways as the child seeks to make sense of the disruption in care using the cognitive schemata that are available at a particular stage of development. For very young children whose view of reality is developmentally and normatively egocentric, either type of trauma is likely to lead to experiences of self-blame; bad things happen in the world of the small child because of something she or he has or has not done. When the caregiver is malevolent, deep shame also attaches; the good person, the caregiver, is hurting me, which means that I, the child, must be bad and causing this good person to behave badly. Developmentally normative feelings of omnipotence in the small child translate into problematic posttraumatic behaviors later in life.

Trauma to a child increases the child's dependency needs; indeed, the descriptions of childhood posttraumatic stress disorder (PTSD) in the *Diagnostic and Statisical Manual of Mental Disorders* (4th ed., text rev.) indicate that one marker of trauma in children is behavioral regression to younger stages of functioning, and dependency is understandably greater the younger a child is. When the source of trauma is also the source of getting dependency needs met, a child's developmentally normative autonomy strivings are likely to be interfered with. An ironic negative vicious circle ensues; the child becomes more dependent on a caregiver who inflicts more psychic wounding, leading to more dependency, leading to even more opportunities for psychic wounding. This kind of trauma bonding is familiar to psychotherapists and others working with abused children, who comment on how these children cling to their perpetrators when attempts are made by child protection services to separate them for the child's own safety. Reactive attachment disorder, which is best conceptualized as complex trauma of childhood, has as one of its primary symptoms a child's extremely impaired expressions of autonomy and dependency.

When the source of the trauma lies outside the caregiving realm but affects the capacities of caregivers to respond adequately to the child's own trauma, then this same phenomenon of delayed autonomy may manifest. In these situations a child may appear to others to be pseudomature, offering care and soothing to the traumatized parent as a means of then obtaining some modicum of developmentally appropriate and necessary care from that parent when the latter is soothed by the child. Children traumatized by caregivers may also develop this self-care strategy as they become older and develop an awareness that calming the parent by whatever means available will lead to brief periods of greater calm, if not actual safety.

These age-related effects of trauma can be seen in adult trauma survivors with a complex trauma presentation. Nathan's mother was likely severely psychologically damaged herself; he remembers spending his childhood being screamed at, beaten, and sometimes deprived of food for days at a time. His father, who traveled on business, was largely absent and disengaged emotionally and when home refused to believe that his wife had done any of the things that Nathan tried to report. Because "telling tales out of school," as his mother called it, only led to harsher beatings when his father left for work, Nathan quickly gave up that strategy. He recalls spending his childhood trying to figure out how to keep his mother appeased, and protecting his younger brothers from her, with limited success on both accounts. His many bruises and broken bones were explained by his upper-middle-class, college-educated Euro-American mother to school and pediatrician as a result of clumsiness and hyperactivity; at one point she even had him tested for attention-deficit/hyperactivity disorder, with negative findings.

Nathan had indeed thrown himself into sports and school as a means of having sanctioned and legitimate reasons for being away from home because any other absence was used by his mother as an excuse for more abuse. Polite to the point of overcontrol, deferential to adults (whom he feared because no matter how nice they were, he was never certain that they would not find out what a terrible person he was and then hurt him), bright and talented, he was also very vulnerable to the predatory hockey coach on whose team he found himself in midadolescence. This man sexually abused him beginning at age 14, threatening to tell Nathan's parents if he was ever reported, knowing from Nathan's earlier self-disclosures that Nathan did not feel exactly safe or loved at home.

Nathan came into adulthood confused about his sexuality, self-loathing, and terrified of every other human being. This inner core was a stark contrast with how others saw him—friendly, helpful, capable, and respectful. He had many women friends but kept himself from sexual encounters because of his fear of losing control. He did well academically and then professionally as a radiologist but ran into a speed bump when he found himself repeatedly unable to pass his board exams.

Nathan's story represents a fairly good outcome of childhood trauma—good in that his temperament, social class privilege, and intellectual talent had all combined to allow him to develop posttraumatic coping strategies that were highly socially desirable. His extreme distress was invisible, but his vulnerabilities were large; the trauma of sexual abuse that he experienced had occurred in no small part because his perpetrator correctly identified Nathan as an adolescent whose ability to accurately assess which adults were safe and which were dangerous had already been entirely undermined by the abuse he experienced at home.

For persons who are parented as Nathan was, it is common to see far more disorganized and problematic life trajectories in which attempts to self-soothe and regulate emotions lead to substance abuse, self-inflicted violence, problematic adult relationships, and sabotaged academic and vocational strivings (Cloitre et al., 2006; Gold, 2000). In fact, although the literature on trauma and age largely ignores the middle of the age range, it appears clear that like Nathan, many survivors of childhood trauma have difficulties with some or all of the tasks of adulthood as their capacities are tested past the breaking point by the normative challenges inherent in adult developmental milestones.

Age-aware psychotherapy thus considers the possibility of childhood trauma even in apparently high-functioning individuals, not only in those persons whose clinical presentation is consistent with known patterns of complex trauma response. A growing literature addresses the needs and childhood realities of people who have overt manifestations of disruptions of childhood attachment patterns and exposure to sexual, physical, and/or emotional violence. However, when psychotherapists consider the potential interactive effects of such trauma with other factors such as temperament, skills and talents of the sort known to support relational resilience, access to resources due to social class or cultural heritage, psychotherapists must, to be culturally competent, develop a more nuanced and broader concept of possible outcomes of childhood complex trauma so as to include persons like Nathan.

As his psychotherapist said to him several years into their work at a point at which he had decided that the psychotherapist was probably not dangerous to him,

> Simply because your life looked like it worked didn't mean that you didn't have terrible PTSD. It did mean that you were too successful at accomplishing your goal of not telling on your mother—look, nothing about your life let anyone know what she had done.

For Nathan, hearing these words from his psychotherapist was an enormous relief; "You get it," he told him. "You get how much it was all about protecting her because that was the only thing that sort of protected me and the boys."

"And that's why I scared you so badly when I asked you about maltreatment, didn't I?" asked the psychotherapist. "I was asking you to tell on her, and you had no idea then that I wouldn't turn around and let her know that you told like your dad used to do."

Although the data from this literature are not unequivocal, considerable scholarship would suggest that even good parents who are themselves traumatized may have difficulties in parenting their children in such a manner as to offer sufficient support in the development of self-capacities. Parenting is an excellent example of a normative developmental milestone that can be compromised by earlier trauma exposures. Clinically, as adults these children may present with very different sets of concerns. When the traumatized parent has conveyed to the child her or his lovability and can assist the child to cognitively appraise that what is happening with the caregiver is not the child's fault, outcomes are best, and it may require careful history taking by a psychotherapist who is aware of age-related trauma dynamics to uncover the possible contribution of parental trauma to a now adult's difficulties with normative developmental strivings. This appears to be a more common result of situations in which a functional caregiver–child relationship is disrupted midway by a trauma such as a natural disaster or social upheaval that temporarily impairs the adult's caregiving capacities but does not affect her or his basic love for the child or awareness of the child's developmental needs.

Somewhat more problematic appears to be parenting in which the caregiver is affected by trauma in her or his own history that has not been adequately dealt with by the caregiver. The literature on children of Holocaust survivors is the exemplar of this phenomenon. Thus, age-aware trauma therapy includes an inquiry about possible parental trauma exposures during the client's caregivers' lives prior to becoming a parent.

None of this suggests that adults with trauma histories should refrain from parenting; in fact, trauma survivors can be highly attuned to the needs and vulnerabilities of children because of a deepened empathy with those vulnerabilities and may do well at this developmental task. Rather, this focuses attention on the need for psychotherapists to be attentive to the childhood experiences of their adult clients and to include in those queries information about the trauma histories of those intimately involved in caring for the client in her or his childhood. Just as depression in a caregiver poses risks to a child's experiences of attachment and the development of self-capacities, so too can the presence of posttraumatic distress in caregivers lead to complex traumalike experiences for their children.

Although adolescence significantly reduces dependence on caregivers, it is another point of developmental vulnerability to heightened emotional risk from trauma. One of the terrible paradoxes of adolescence, well documented in the scholarly literature as well as in popular culture representations of this period of life, is that adolescents both are and are not children, with the inherent contradictions growing ever greater as the adolescent moves toward legal adulthood. Recent research on adolescent brains indicates that the capacity to control impulses is not fully developed in humans until early to mid-20s, creating a biological substrate for age-related reactivity to trauma exposure that places the 19-year-old soldier at greater risk for PTSD from combat than the 30-year-old, all other variables being held constant.

Adolescents also struggle with the paradoxes of their capacities and privileges in the psychosocial realm. American culture increasingly controls the lives of adolescents; they may drive at 16 but in many states under restricted terms. They may work in certain jobs at certain hours but only with a permit; they must attend school and pass standardized tests. They may not consent to sex even with near-age peers; although fully capable of sexual functioning, they are given the message that they should abstain from acting sexually and frequently systemically denied information on the grounds of their age about how to protect themselves from sexually transmitted infections or pregnancies. They are capable of abstract thought but usually engage in less nuanced use of abstractions. Caught in this in-between land, adolescents exposed to trauma have particular psychological and psychosocial vulnerabilities.

For example, Tsai, Feldman-Summers, and Edgar (1979) found that when sexual abuse occurred during adolescence, survivors expressed significantly more self-blame than did those sexually abused earlier in life. Tsai et al. and scholars since that time have learned that the adolescent's perception of capacities and resources can lead to an inaccurate assessment that she or he should have been able to stop interpersonal violence of which she or he was a target. As one of my clients, a man sexually abused by a coach in high school, said to me, "I was a 16-year-old kid. I was big and strong, I was a linebacker, I could have fought the guy off. What was wrong with me?" The adolescent target of trauma decontextualizes the experience in a way similar to that found in the larger culture; in this instance, the perpetrator was an adult, an authority figure who was well liked by other adult authority figures, and the boy's mentor who had no small degree of control over access to a football scholarship much needed by this son of poor immigrants from Honduras. The process of identity development so central to adolescence was severely undermined for this man, with subsequent capacities to form intimate relationships badly affected by his worries about whether he was *man enough*, which in turn led him to the domestic violence episode that forced him into treatment.

Age-aware trauma treatment with adults who had adolescent stage trauma exposures must be informed by caution so that the psychotherapist does not fall into the trap of seeing the adolescent's experience through the eyes of ageist attitudes about adolescents. The adolescent stage of development is alternately fetishized (the best years of your life) and stigmatized (bad kids misbehaving) in American culture, and as with all age-related biases, psychotherapists are affected by these pervasive images of youth. Additionally, if the client is currently adolescent, she or he will present a psychotherapist with all of the usual challenges of a helping relationship with someone who developmentally wishes to demonstrate greater autonomy (the "I'm fine, I don't need to talk to anyone" response to trauma in adolescents) and also developmentally may still be honing skills at effective communication of her or his desires, thus leading to some rocky and emotion-laden passages with the therapist. Psychotherapists must guard against ageist negative countertransferences about adolescents when working with an adolescent trauma survivor to avoid overpathologizing developmentally normative styles of trauma response. Additionally, a therapist working with an adolescent traumatized at earlier stages of development must be prepared for the emergence of evidence of developmental tasks hindered or interfered with by that earlier trauma.

Age and Resistance Strategies

Earlier in this volume I discussed the concept of symptoms of distress as attempts by the traumatized person to resist the loss of power and voice associated with trauma and to solve the problems of loss of safety, dysregulation, and disruption of relationships that emerge from trauma exposure. This framework for understanding distress leans heavily on an understanding of the interplay of age-related developmental capacities with the tasks and challenges of responding to trauma.

As noted previously in this chapter, children's developmental capacities, both cognitive and emotional, play a central role in their ability (or not) to grasp and respond to trauma exposure. Age awareness on the part of the trauma psychotherapist means looking at the symptoms and resistance strategies and considering what kinds of developmental capacities might have informed the then child or adolescent's response to the trauma exposure. The nature and variety of external resources available to a child at different developmental stages is also important to consider; an adolescent can autonomously feed and care for her- or himself, can somewhat successfully run away if needed, can seek shelter at the home of friends or relatives, can usually read and write, and can sometimes earn a living in nondangerous ways. A 10-year-old can feed and clothe her- or himself and read and write but is less likely to be successful in becoming self-supporting or getting alternative shelter without the intervention of the state. Very young children, of course, can do none of these things.

These are treatment as well as diagnostic considerations. The adult trauma survivor who self-criticizes for having created a developmentally appropriate response to childhood or adolescent trauma with the inner and outer resources that were then available may be empowered by the psychotherapist's provision of accurate information about what children and adolescents reasonably can and cannot do. Introducing clients to introductory text materials about child and adolescent development in which information is available that counters either family or cultural mythologies about children's capacities can be a useful adjunct to psychotherapists' proffered information. Culturally competent treatment also contextualizes the issue of age in the light of the type and quality of information available in the milieu of adult caregivers. The issue of age cohort figures large here because the time of the world at which someone was 5 or 15 or 50 makes a large difference in how their trauma is constructed. Middle-class American parents in the 1950s who were told by the experts of the time that their sexually assaulted children would forget what happened or be minimally affected were not being neglectful when they acted on that advice and silenced their traumatized children.

TRAUMA AND OLDER ADULTS

In American culture today, old age is socially constructed as ever older. Age 55 at the time of this book's completion, I am now 3 years older than either of my grandmothers was on the day I was born. They were old women at 52; I am, aching joints and all, not particularly old; I spend my free time practicing the martial art that I took up at 50, riding my bike, and doing other activities guaranteed to make the joints keep aching.

This difference in the social construction of the absolute number of years in one's age has a great deal to do with age cohort effects, both biological and psychosocial. My grandmothers, born late in the first decade of the 20th century, survived a childhood without antibiotics or vaccines, and their middle adulthoods lacked someone testing their cholesterol at 40 to get them to stop putting sour cream in their borscht. I, born at the tail end of 1952, had enough penicillin pumped into me as a child to become allergic to it by age 20 and can recall my polio vaccine shots starting around age 3 and the oral vaccine when it became available. My lipids well and thoroughly tested, I banished butter fats from my diet long ago and down niacin nightly to keep my cholesterol low. Some of the difference between my 50s and their 50s has to do with the differential access to health resources occasioned by our placements in the course of the history of Western medicine.

But the psychosocial construction of age cohorts also has a strong impact. My grandmothers were socially constructed as old in their 50s because they were more than halfway through the life expectancy for their age cohort. It is interesting to note that they lived in a time when the premium placed on youth was present, but less. Today people in my age cohort are the targets of relentless advertising to whiten their aging teeth, inject antiwrinkle substances into their aging brows, dye their aging and graying hair, and take drugs so that their sexual organs will respond as they did in their teens. The normal biology of aging, what I jokingly refer to as "running out the evolutionary warranty on the parts" has become culturally anathema.

Thus, age and its visible symbols have become stigmatized, and ageist assumptions about trauma's effects on older adults abound. However, as with mythologies about children's invulnerability to trauma, myths about older adults' vulnerability appear to be just that—inaccurate stereotypes founded largely in negative bias about old age. Although trauma can affect people at any stage of life, currently available data suggest that the experiences and skills acquired during earlier stages of development as well as the knowledge of one's capacities to deal with prior adversity are likely to function as protective factors for adults exposed to trauma. For instance, studies of individuals who were displaced by the 2005 hurricane season found the lowest level of symptoms and highest levels of resilience in the oldest age cohorts, even though many of these people lost significant social and human resources through the storms. They told researchers that although they were sad and upset by what had happened, it was not a new experience for them, and they had faith in their capacities to respond to disaster and loss because of having tested those capacities repeatedly earlier in life (Cherry, 2006).

That said, some aspects of aging may lead to differential vulnerabilities to trauma, and the age-aware psychotherapist will increase cultural competence and effectiveness by integrating those dynamics into trauma treatment. Psychosocial cohort effects may function to mask posttrauma symptoms until later in life for some trauma survivors. This phenomenon can be seen in the upswing of reported symptoms of combat-related PTSD in World War II and Korean War male veterans in postretirement years. The availability of culturally valued externalizing coping strategies such as work appears to have allowed many of these men to deflect the intrusive symptoms related to combat trauma exposure until, in retirement, those distractions and meaning-making activities were no longer available. Auerbach, Mirvis, Stern, and Schwartz (n.d.) also reported this phenomenon occurring in high-functioning survivors of the Nazi Holocaust, with one participant stating, "Since I retired, it hit me like a ton of bricks. Because now you have time. Everything comes out, it never really left you" (p. 21).

It is also possible that childhood trauma may only come to light in older age. For some individuals whose childhood trauma occurred within the family unit there has been a cohort and cultural-based pressure to remain silent so as not to hurt others or disrupt family systems in which perpetrators of abuse were valued members. Difficulties in functioning and in accomplishing the developmental tasks of middle adulthood have been ascribed to sources other than earlier, unknown trauma. The death of perpetrators does not bring relief, as those inexperienced in working with the survivors of childhood trauma might imagine. But it does sometimes create the permission for the survivor to tell her or his story of what happened half a century or more ago today, at a time when there is finally no one left alive to be troubled by the story. Psychotherapists working with older adults should, consequently, be careful not to omit questions about childhood trauma from the intake process out of ageist assumptions that these issues would have been dealt with or forgotten long ago.

Very great age can bring losses of functional capacities and increased dependence on others for care and safety. As a result, this group of older adults is at risk for precisely the same types of trauma exposure as are young children. Abuse by caregivers occurs in the lives of older adults simply because of the need to depend on others. In families in which a parent had abused a child and is now, in older age, dependent on the now-adult child for care, the former target may become a perpetrator, completing the cycle of violence in the family. Little is known about the specific trauma responses of older adults with dementia or other cognitive changes that lead to increased dependency, but psychotherapists working with cognitively intact older adults who are dependent because of physical incapacities need to be alert to possible posttrauma responses in this group of individuals. A common ageist stereotype is that older age is normatively accompanied by depressed mood; this bias may lead to premature cognitive closure about the distress being expressed by an older adult client on the part of a younger adult psychotherapist, who may dismiss a client's complaints of abuse as depression-related distortions, missing the possibility that the abuse is the etiology of the depressed mood.

AGE COHORT EFFECTS

Members of specific age cohorts will have been at risk for types of trauma exposures that reflect interactions between aspects of multiple identities and larger social forces. Active discrimination and bias against various groups has waxed and waned historically, and the nature of vulnerability to bias-based trauma will have varied within a group as a result of cohort effects. Persons exposed to more direct bias and discrimination due to their age cohort will have different experiences of the identity components linked to bias than will persons whose age cohort experienced more aversive bias and discrimination. Because of the nature of insidious trauma and the difficulty that those so traumatized often have with knowing that this kind of exposure has had cumulative negative emotional impact, people within the latter groups are more likely than those in the former to question the strength of emotional response or to accuse themselves of overreaction; this risk also exists for those treating them. If "nothing happened" as a result of cohort effects, then the realities of unsafety as experienced in a given age cohort may become invisible.

Psychotherapists working with members of target groups will enhance their cultural competence by being aware of historical factors that might have informed the nature of trauma exposure for members of particular age cohorts. The total load of lifetime exposure to trauma for members of any given target group will be affected by the age cohort to which an individual belongs.

Such age cohort effects can be relatively easily identified for many U.S. target groups. For example, overt malignant racist bias against African Americans in the form of legalized disparate treatment and lynching is no longer a regular fact of life; being the target of covert bias and invalidation is definitely a regular fact of life. Older African Americans today will have experienced both forms of bias; the age cohort of African Americans who are currently in their 30s will have been more likely to have experienced mostly covert and aversive racism. Both groups will have been affected by historical trauma and its legacies, but the expressions of that heritage will also have been impacted by cohort effects.

Although culturally competent practice does not require specific etic knowledge about cohort effects on trauma exposure, a general awareness of and attention to ways in which members of a given age cohort will have been differentially affected by overt discrimination, insidious trauma, and other forms of risk will enhance a psychotherapist's capacities to grasp how an experience in the present may be evoking previous unmetabolized trauma exposures. Of course, individual experience will always be more central to understanding a given trauma survivor's distress than cohort effect per se. But if psychotherapists consider how cohort effects create expectations of the world, they may also see how the expectational context generated by cohort membership may render an experience more or less subjectively traumatizing.

Roger was a 28-year-old African American man with a master's degree in international finance who traveled frequently to Europe and Asia to do business. He had grown up in a middle-class home with college-educated parents and attended private schools and universities. Although he was aware of and proud of his ethnic heritage, it was of considerably less importance to his identity than it had been to his parents, who had been active in Black student movements, or his grandparents, who had been founding members of the local National Association for the Advancement of Colored People chapter. Until the day when he was stopped by the police, yanked out of his car and slammed to the ground to the accompaniment of vicious racist language accusing him of a crime he had never committed simply because he was a Black man driving an expensive car, his phenotype and ethnicity had been of minor consequence to him; he had frequently remonstrated friends and older family members about being "too hung up about being Black. It's the 21st century, get over it," as he reported later to a forensic evaluator who he was seeing as part of his lawsuit against that police department for false arrest and assault.

> You know, I think it was worse for me because I had been lulled into believing that that kind of racism was dead and gone and over. No one, and I mean no one, had ever acted that way towards me before. I knew people could be mean spirited and stupid, but actively violent and racist? That was in my parents' time, not mine. Or maybe that was what happened to people who weren't smart enough or well educated enough to know how to act right. What a shock.

Roger's trauma arising from the assault was heightened by an age cohort effect; his expectations of being treated fairly and not being targeted for racist violence had been informed by his growing up in a cohort in which social class and education appeared to be protective factors against racism.

The interaction of ageism with other forms of bias is also likely to be informed by age cohort. This, in turn, has impact on how a person ascribes meaning to and responds to trauma exposure. Ageism itself has been more or less malignant for different age cohorts and differentially interactive with such phenomena as sexism, ableism, classism, and so on.

AGEISM AND THE PSYCHOTHERAPIST

As with children and adolescents, younger and middle-adulthood psychotherapists are at risk for both ageism and internalized ageism in their work with older adults. Cultural competence requires attention to these biases and to psychotherapists' responses to larger cultural pulls to resist their personal aging process. Whether to dye one's hair or be injected with antiwrinkle serums is a personal choice; to be a psychotherapist who does so in a nonmindful way creates the risk of unexamined ageist bias being perpetrated against the self. If psychotherapists oppress themselves about their normal aging processes and apply ageist bias and stereotypes to their own developmental experiences, they are at heightened risk to do so with their clients.

Ageism also intersects and changes meaning in relationship to other social locations and forms of bias. In cultures and communities where value is placed on great age and where the culture is in the midst of struggles against acculturation and assimilation into a dominant culture that devalues great age, cultural identification may be assessed by the degree to which a person conforms to one or the other set of values about aging. In North American indigenous cultures that have been working to reclaim culture from genocide and forced assimilation, a new attention to and valuing of elders has occurred within the past several decades. In immigrant cultures arriving in the United States from locations where age is valued, elders may find themselves dealing not only with the loss of culture and familiarity of language but also with the migration-based loss of status in the eyes of younger family members who assimilate to the dominant youthcentric U.S. culture.

Age also interacts powerfully with sex and gender, another factor of social location that begins in the bodily experience. Culturally competent practice relies heavily on an understanding of the diversity and complexity of expression of the universal experience of being embodied as a sex and socially constructed as a gender, and much of the experience of trauma streams through that lens.

6

TRAUMA, SEX, AND GENDER

In this chapter, I explore in depth the relationship between sex, gender, and trauma. I discuss sex differences in the experience of trauma, the interaction of biology and social realities in the construction of gendered trauma, and the specific concerns of people who are either sex atypical or gender atypical.

Sex and gender are two of the more central components of most peoples' identities and the two most frequently confused for one another. One of the first things known about any human, irrespective of culture, phenotype, social class, disability, or family history, is that person's sex. Shortly upon receiving that information, the culture surrounding each human begins to construct the roles of gender on the scaffolding of biological sex. Gender, which is tightly linked to sex for most people, is commonly the first identity that anyone has; before people know that they are anything else, they figure out that they are male or female and learn what that implies for their particular interpersonal milieu. When a trauma is aimed at or affects aspects of a person's gendered self then issues of gender will become important considerations in the design of a culturally sensitive and competent treatment strategy.

Current research indicates that in Western cultures, women are twice as likely as men to develop posttraumatic stress disorder (PTSD) when exposed to a *Diagnostic and Statistical Manual of Mental Disorders* (4th ed., text rev.; *DSM–IV–TR*; American Psychiatric Association, 2000) Criterion A traumatic stressor (Kimerling, Ouimette, & Wolfe, 2002); women are also more likely to experience chronicity of posttrauma symptoms. This is despite the fact that in almost every study done looking at large population samples men report significantly more actual exposure to Criterion A stressors than do women. Gender and sex are clearly informing trauma in several different ways that lead to different outcomes. Sex is a risk factor for total trauma exposure even when only formal Criterion A experiences are counted. Gender, on the other hand, is a risk factor for the development of certain kinds of postexposure emotional difficulties. Sex and gender may also be interactive in the development of symptoms as biology and the body each respond to experiences of trauma, and then gender lends meaning to those experiences and to the expectations placed on traumatized persons by the culture around them. Understanding how these extremely core issues intersect with trauma exposure can lead to more culturally competent practice as a psychotherapist is able to unpack the meanings that sex and gender give to the traumatized person's experience.

There are a variety of ways in which trauma and gender can become interrelated. There are specifically gendered traumas such as sexual harassment or assault in which the perpetrator is targeting aspects of the person's body or gender. In these kinds of traumas the event is occurring in part because of the sex of the person and how that is responded to by a perpetrator. There are traumas whose specifics are not gendered but that engage scripts and schemata about gender roles by leaving a person impaired in their capacities to perform those roles. These are traumas in which sex was immaterial to what happened (e.g., a natural disaster), but gender roles were deeply disrupted by posttraumatic distress. There are also traumas arising from punitive cultural responses to sex and gender nonconformity. In these traumas sex and gender role norms are transgressed by an individual who then is targeted and punished for that transgression. Underlying and informing all of these kinds of trauma are sexism and misogyny.

SEXISM AND MISOGYNY: ENDEMIC INSIDIOUS TRAUMA

Every culture known to modern humans is a patriarchal one. What this means is that each culture, no matter how lineage is determined and no matter whether it is a Western individualistic culture or one of the collectivist cultures of the global South, is a culture in which all that is determined in that culture to be masculine is prized and privileged and all that is associated with femininity is devalued and degraded, both in individuals and in cultural institutions and systems (Lerner, 1987). As noted earlier in this volume, these assignments of characteristics to male and female categories are largely arbitrary, reflecting cultural constructs of a particular society and era. Witness the lacy, flowing clothing of men of 17th-century France, which would today be coded as extremely feminine. Or consider the ponytailed basketball players who star on today's professional women's teams and who only a few decades earlier would have been derided as unfeminine but can now be found modeling sleek fashions in the pages of popular magazines. As Weisstein (1970) noted almost 4 decades ago, psychology and the larger society have constructed the concepts of masculinity and femininity around male and female bodies on bulwarks of myth and pseudoscience.

Sexism and misogyny are natural outgrowths of patriarchal cultures. The first can be defined as bias and discrimination against women (and men who violate gender role norms); the second is direct hatred of women and those attributes associated with them. Sexism is seen as arising from misogyny, which provides the philosophical underpinnings and rationales for unequal treatment based on sex. Sexism is easiest to identify when it is overt, such as when it takes the form of active discrimination against women. When women are present in visible and powerful roles within a society some people, including psychologists, make the assumption that sexism has been banished, ignoring the reality that it is deeply embedded into many of the institutions and norms of most cultures. As an example, Title IX of the Education Amendments of 1972 may have outlawed discrimination against girls and women in sports in the United States, but it did not transform the masculinist culture and misogynist underpinnings of coaching cultures in which a common insult hurled at a faltering athlete of any sex is "you play like a girl."

Men are also affected by sexism and misogyny. Masculinity as a narrow social construct penalizes those men who stray from its boundaries by labeling them weak, nerdy, or negatively feminine (Englar-Carlson, 2006; Good & Brooks, 2005; Levant, 1996). Pressure on men to be manly, as defined by their particular cultural milieu, can create high risks for behaviors that lead to trauma exposure, such as abuse of substances, use of violence as a problem-solving strategy, and reckless sporting activities that raise the risk of serious injury or death. When posttrauma distress arises, masculine norms informed by misogyny can aggravate men's difficulties and hinder and inhibit their abilities to seek help.

What Levant (1996) described as "normative male alexithymia" frequently prevents men, particularly those from dominant cultures, from identifying and expressing emotions, which can in turn lead to misattributions about the nature of posttraumatic problems. As he noted,

> Males learn that aggression and violence are not only acceptable but that they should take pride in aggression and violence because that's how they prove themselves men. Males are taught to be tough, daring, fearless, assertive, to respond to threats with anger, and never back down from challenges—all of which conspire to propel males into life-threatening violent situations and prevent them from retreating or fleeing once they're in them. (1999, p. 1)

The presence of sexism and misogyny in the background of a culture are forms of insidious trauma rooted in sex and gender affecting women in one set of ways and men in another. One of the most potent and often-cited examples of insidious cultural misogyny is advertisements. Since its inception, MS. Magazine has run what might be described as the worst-of series of advertisements illustrating the prevalence of misogynist themes in American culture, a feature called "No Comment." An example published in a recent issue depicts a man holding the buttocks of a scantily clad woman taking a package of chewing gum out of her tight jeans pockets, captioned, "Everyone wants a piece," with the caption referring to the term "piece of ass," which is a form of demeaning slang about women. The ad for the popular chewing gum appeared in a mainstream magazine targeting an audience of young men but likely to be read by women as well. Lest the reader protest that the ad was appropriately targeted to the audience (and thus inadvertently communicate the sexist belief that real men objectify women sexually), the reader should look no further than another ad featured in that month's MS. Magazine hall of shame. The picture is of a man in a suit staring up the extremely short skirt of what the reader thinks may be a woman (only her miniscule skirt and legs are visible; she is beheaded and disembodied, a not infrequent representation of women in advertising). The caption reads, "Change your perspective, view the opportunity." The ad for a series of new condominiums appeared in the very mainstream Miami New Times.

Because Americans are exposed to somewhere between 15,000 and 30,000 bits of advertising daily (W. Heusler, personal communication, October 4, 2006), the stream of misogynist images to which Americans are exposed is not inconsiderable. As Cole and Daniel (2005) noted in their recent work on media representations of women, this kind of image in which women are objectified, portrayed as body parts, sexualized, or violated is not confined to advertising alone but is ubiquitous in every aspect of visual representations from video games (e.g., in the popular Grand Theft Auto the player murders a female prostitute) to high-concept cinema. Increasingly, popular network television shows portray women being sexually assaulted in the most violent and degrading of ways; violence against women as a norm is embedded in the plot so casually that only careful observation unpacks the rise in misogynist images. The experience of seeing other women beaten, raped, or simply demeaned is so usual for most women that the insidious effects of this stream of imagery are unknown and invisible until a final blow is struck. For men, the insidious impacts of seeing themselves portrayed as sexually aggressive, predatory, violent creatures of instinct are also difficult to detect unless and until the psyche reaches saturation.

Zak was a fourth-generation Chinese American heterosexual man in his late 20s whose trauma experiences were of insidious misogyny. Like many men of Asian descent in the United States, he had struggled with stereotypes that depicted men of his ancestry as effeminate as a result mostly of the tendency of men of this phenotype to an ectomorphic body type, which conforms poorly with Western images of mesomorphic masculinity. He was slight of build and stood just under 5 ft. 9 in., making him somewhat short in stature compared with his friends of Northern European ancestry. Raised in the Pacific Northwest by his college-educated parents, he was an avid outdoorsperson whose choice of a career as a wildlife biologist had been shaped with the opportunity to blend work and play in mind.

He entered therapy after his latest snowboarding accident, which had occurred when, as had become his custom, he had taken his buddies up on a dare to go outside the official ski areas. Careening down the mountain he hit rocks, fell, and shattered his leg. He walked into the office in a thigh-high cast and with a depressed demeanor. He explained to his psychotherapist that his orthopedic surgeon with whom he had a long-standing relationship for the care of his variously broken body parts had jokingly suggested that Zak needed to stop paying for her vacations and figure out why he was trying to kill himself.

> I laughed when she said it, but then I started thinking. I get completely freaked out and anxious when I can't do dangerous things. I mean, really dangerous things that if someone else did them I would think they were stupid. Free-climbing, snowboarding outside the areas, I'll take any dare. It sort of hit me when she said that to me; I don't think I want to die, but I kind of know I will if I don't cut this out. So meanwhile, I'm feeling freaked out and bummed out, so here I am.

As the psychotherapist explored with Zak what he experienced as a compulsion to engage in risky sports that had been hidden behind the veneer of outdoorsperson, the insidious trauma of racialized sexism and misogyny came to light. Zak became aware that he had become tired of being teased by the mostly Euro-American boys he played with in early adolescence. "So I guess I figured out how to be a real man, huh?"

His death-defying activities did in fact contain his anxiety about being insufficiently masculine, which had, he revealed, been complicated by his having a distinctly nonmacho approach to women.

> Like, I love my sister. She's really my best friend. And all of her friends, that's where I've mostly met women. And I like them too. I don't want to treat them like a piece of meat. If the guys I hung with ever knew what a wuss I was with women I would never hear the end of it.

Zak realized that he had somehow determined that he had to compensate for being "too nice" in his romantic relationships and too small and slight of body by being fearless to the point of injury.

Stopped from activities by this latest broken bone and with his surgeon's comment still ringing in his ears, he was being tormented by fears of being exposed as not a real man; his insidious trauma manifested itself not simply as risky acting out and anxiety but also in the form of nightmares in which he was being taunted and urinated on by a group of boys. "And even though I'm my age now in those dreams, I'm helpless." He became aware of the lifetime of exposure to messages in the popular culture that informed him about the devaluation of other-than-masculine men.

Zak's experience illustrates how sexism and misogyny can combine with other forms of oppressive norms, in this case racism, to create insidious trauma. It illustrates the realities of holding multiple identities; for Zak, as for many men of color, being a man was not a generic experience of masculinity but a racially informed experience. Because of his residence in the Pacific Northwest where there is a large and long-standing Chinese American community and because of his own experiences of being highly assimilated into the surrounding dominant culture, Zak's experiences of insidious trauma had gender as their primary component, with the racism that tinged sexism much more in his emotional background.

Sexism is more difficult to see when, as is often the case in 21st-century Western cultures, it takes its modern or aversive form and becomes subtle and embedded in the norms of a milieu. Because modern sexism violates the just-world expectations of many people from the below-40 age cohort in the United States who were raised in a period after legal sexism had been outlawed, it can function as a trauma.

Mallory's experience illustrates how aversive sexism can serve as a form of insidious trauma. A 35-year-old woman of mixed Chinese and German ancestries who came from a loving family, she worked as a firefighter–paramedic in a department in which she was one of very few women. She had always told people that as far as she was concerned there was no longer discrimination against women. "That was then; these guys aren't like that anymore," she would say of her coworkers. A life-long athlete and beneficiary of the abolishment of discrimination against girls and women in sports through Title IX, she was as tall as most men and had developed her upper body strength through years of daily workouts. She was well respected in her department and rose through its ranks.

Like most people in her profession, Mallory had coped with the frequent painful experiences of her work through strategies that are typical for firefighter–paramedics (Brasted, Cruz, & James, 2005); she used humor, emotional avoidance, and exercise to work through her feelings about seeing dead and injured people and did not experience her work as traumatic, partly because of successful coping and largely because she experienced herself as helping people and saving lives. This worked well for her until the day that she found herself attempting to sustain the life of a woman who was trapped in her car, slowly bleeding to death while Mallory's colleagues worked frantically to cut open her vehicle's wreckage.

> I was holding on to her hand, and I was talking to her, and she was looking at me, I kept telling her to hang on, and then I saw her die. I felt her die. She died holding on to me.

Something about this experience moved Mallory deeply in a way that her previous encounters with accidents and loss had not; as she posited later, being in close physical and eye-contact proximity with this woman at the moment of death made it more difficult to use her usual distancing strategies. "I couldn't joke at all about this one; I just felt sad."

However, Mallory's problem was not that she was upset by this death; she did not initially experience much except grief, which she saw as a normal response to an extraordinary experience even in the life of a firefighter–paramedic. The problem, rather, was that she began to allow her upset to be visible to her peers at the station house. Instead of joking it off or not talking about it at all, she found herself needing to verbally process her feelings with her workmates, who until then she had regarded as her friends and allies. To her surprise, rather than supporting her, they turned on her in subtle but noticeably gender-tinged ways. This was intolerable to Mallory, who had never been a target of conscious and overt sexism.

> All of a sudden I wasn't Mallory, their bud. I was a girl. They didn't say it, but I was feeling it. They weren't honest. They just started to avoid me and treat me weird. Like I didn't get included in going out after shift, or like when we were out on a call and something went wrong and I asked for assistance people stopped taking me seriously. Like, "Oh, it's just Mallory, she's a drama queen."

Because a large component of coping for frontline workers like Mallory can be found in the social support available from peers in the workplace, the withdrawal of that support just as she most perceived the need for it felt like a huge violation of her beliefs about the way the world should be. She had made the assumption that her competence, strength, and contributions to her team would trump gendered rules about emotional expressivity. She also had believed until then that women who complained about sex discrimination were "crybabies. It never happened to me, and I was around guys all the time, so what were they (e.g., other women) talking about," thus experiencing internalized sexism and misogyny; she had herself denigrated behaviors associated with femininity, including tearful expression of emotions.

The withdrawal and emotional disconnect emerging in her relationship with her coworkers were similar to what Dovidio, Gaertner, Kawakami, and Hodson (2002) described as occurring between aversive racists and people of color; although the former disavow racism consciously, their nonconscious racism leads to disconnections in their interactions with people of color. So with Mallory, her coworkers' aversive sexism led not to overt sexist remarks or behaviors but to their withdrawal from and avoidance of her.

The aversively sexist nature of the situation became more apparent to Mallory when she confronted her colleagues angrily one day. They in turn denied that gender issues had anything to do with their changed treatment of her.

> They just said that my needing to talk about it so much made them uncomfortable. When I told my buddy Sean that it sounded like how he talked about one of his girlfriends he got pissed at me and asked me if I was accusing him of being sexist, so I backed off.

Mallory's expectations that she would be given support by her coworkers to deal with her feelings about this work experience were violated. She began to notice herself becoming anxious when she had to go out on a call, no matter whether it was a fire or an accident. As she reported later to a psychotherapist, her intrusive thoughts were not of the possibility of encountering injured or dead people but instead of breaking into tears and being taunted by the men in her team. In her dreams she replayed stories of relationship loss and weakness. Because the sexism by which she was targeted was subtle and nonconscious and was being denied by its perpetrators, her capacity to grasp what had traumatized her was elusive.

Eventually she was able to realize that as her peers withdrew social support from her for violating the gendered-as-male norms for emotional expressivity of their shared occupation, she had come to experience not only the ending of her expectations of a just world but also a fear that her coworkers would inadvertently or intentionally endanger her during a fire. "What if I told someone on the radio that we were about to have a flashover and he blew me off because he thought I was too emotional? I could die; other guys could die."

Aversive sexism is present in many aspects of many U.S. cultural settings today. An awareness of the role that gender can play in trauma requires psychotherapists to be curious about the potential for both aversive and internalized sexism as components of emotional wounding for a client, particularly in instances in which overt discrimination or misogyny is not evident.

SEX AND THE BIOLOGY OF TRAUMA

It is now well established that there is a biological component to the posttrauma response experience (Mueller, 2005). Studies have found disruptions in the hypothalamic–pituitary–adrenal axis, which mediates the stress response system, as well as changes to brain structure and function after even one trauma exposure. Because one of the best known differences between the sexes is in the production of sex hormones, one hypothesis that has been explored to explain the differential response of women and men to traumatic stressors has been the influence of those hormones as a moderating or mediating variable. Indeed, because women's and men's biologies respond quite differently to a number of environmental and psychosocial factors, many clinicians believe that those differences are the most parsimonious account of differences in trauma response.

However, research to date has not found a clear biological difference in response to trauma exposure between women and men. Rasmussen and Friedman (2002) conducted an extensive review of studies available until that time that had explored potential sex differences between women's and men's posttrauma responses. They noted at the outset that conducting such a review was made more difficult by the paucity of research on women's neurobiology posttrauma and the even greater lack of research that compared neurobiological responses between the sexes. At the time of their review and despite clear evidence in other research that stage of menstrual cycle affects mood and behavior, they stated that "no published studies have investigated the effects of the menstrual cycle or reproductive status on stress responsive system in women with PTSD" (Rasmussen & Friedman, 2002, pp. 43–44). Thus, although it would seem intuitive that these meaningful differences between women's and men's biologies that lead to differential experience of other phenomena should play a role in posttrauma experiences, the data to support that are either missing entirely or poorly developed. Ironically, given that it is now more than 3 decades past Weisstein's (1970) call to stop attempting to understand human women through research on females of other mammalian species, the bulk of research that is available on sex hormones and stress response systems has been conducted on such nonhumans. Rasmussen and Friedman (2002) noted, "if we really are to understand the neurobiology of PTSD in women, we must study women with PTSD—not men, and not female animals" (p. 44).

What psychologists may know is provocative and does suggest that some component of differential response to trauma based on sex is rooted in hormonal factors. Most of these suggestions do not come from studies of traumatized individuals, but from nonclinical populations; however, it can reasonably be assumed to be possible to extrapolate from sex differences in the general population to those in traumatized populations, with careful cautions placed around broad overgeneralizations. Thus, for instance, Rasmussen and Friedman noted that there are sex differences in neurohormone levels, with those differences being marked by fluctuations during the menstrual cycle as well. The point in the cycle at which a menstruating female is exposed to trauma may have some impact on how her body responds to that trauma. Men's hormonal variations, which are less regular and less easily detected than those of menstruating women, and the within-person contributions of those variations to the stress response system, appear not to have been studied.

What difference do those vague data make for the culturally competent clinician? At the moment, it appears more important that all clinicians working with trauma survivors have a thorough grasp of the meaning of the biological component of trauma response (BCTR) for the distress and behavioral problems present in traumatized people, because offering clients the information that some important component of their distress is biologically based seems to be empowering for many people, particularly those blaming themselves for being unable to stop their distress through sheer willpower. What this information adds to cultural competence is the clinician's capacity to assist the client to explore how other experiences of their body's response to fluctuations in sex hormones might aid them in clarifying and understanding changes happening within their own symptom picture.

Christopher, an upper-middle-class Euro-American man in his 40s told his psychotherapist that he had started to realize that his flashbacks of the earthquake in which he had been buried alive in the rubble of his home for almost a day worsened, not at the time of day that the quake had occurred, which was just before day-break, but rather in midafternoon. He was puzzled because this was occurring in the absence of any knowable trigger. He also told him that even on the days that he did not have flashbacks he had been noticing himself being more irritable, jumpy, and "generally PTSDish. The people I work with are all starting to avoid me midafternoon, I'm turning into a real butthead."

The psychotherapist, who had already done some psychoeducation with Christopher about BCTR, had a hunch based on his own experiences of living in a male body and decided to check it out. "What's your beard growth like around then?" he asked. Christopher looked startled, then thoughtful, then grinned.

> Yeah, like I also usually go take my second shave of the day about then because it seems as if I get this burst of whiskers showing up after lunch. Been that way all my life. Do you think . . . ?

The psychotherapist reminded Christopher of something they both knew, that increased beard growth was usually evidence of a circadian fluctuation in testosterone output. The psychotherapist shared with Christopher that although there was no strong evidence available suggesting that testosterone levels were implicated in PTSD symptoms, it might be the case that surges in hormone levels, evident in beard growth patterns, were having something to do with his uptick of symptoms at that time of day.

Christopher came back into therapy the next week grinning, telling his psychotherapist that he had come up with a perfect coping strategy using the hypothesis of sex hormone fluctuation as a starting point.

> So I told myself that I have to shave off the irritation along with the whiskers. I go into the restroom and lock the door and do the breathing exercises before I shave, and then as I pull the razor over my face I visualize the trauma draining away. It's pretty cool. And I told my best friend at work, you know, Sheila, the one who's always warning me about her

PMS, that I've got PMS too, I just get it every day. Cracked us both up. Now she's coming by in the afternoons and joking with me about my PTSDMS, that's what we decided to call it. And like you were telling me when we started doing the relaxation exercises, it's impossible to be uptight when you're relaxed or laughing.

In this instance the psychotherapist's cultural competence allowed him to consider the contribution of biological sex to Christopher's posttraumatic symptoms, which in turn empowered the client to develop a coping strategy in which he used other body-based means to reduce the impact of possible sex hormone fluctuations. Christopher's trauma was not itself rife with gendered meanings; he had been in an earthquake; his apartment building had collapsed; and he had been trapped there. His rescue had been seen on local media outlets, and the actual presence of his PTSD symptoms had never been construed as an overreaction either by himself or by those around him, all of whom knew of his very public trauma experience. However, even with the absence of gendered risk factors, sexual biology may have played in part in how his PTSD expressed itself, which in turn affected his psychosocial coping strategies in the wake of those symptoms.

Sex of the body can also be a risk factor for certain kinds of traumatic stress, primarily those experienced by women. Sexual assaults are most frequently perpetrated on women, cruelly mimicking the actions of heterosexual intercourse. Sexual assaults on men do occur and are discussed in the context of gender; however, the sex of men's bodies is less of a risk factor for these assaults than the gender roles occupied or ascribed to such individuals. Women are also biologically at risk for traumas related to reproductive experiences.

These include female genital mutilation (FGM), in which parts of the external genitals ranging from the tip of the clitoris to the entire labia are excised and sometimes sewn together, with the stated goal of protecting a woman's chastity. Psychotherapists working with women from those parts of Africa where FGM remains common need to routinely inquire into whether a woman has been cut and, if so, what meanings and emotions have been associated with that experience. Because FGM is also being performed by physicians in some parts of Europe and the United States to which families from Africa have emigrated, inquiries should not be limited to women born in Africa but rather should include those from cultures in which FGM remains common. The issue of FGM may be implicated in some women's refugee status and asylum claims because fear of being subjected to FGM has been recognized by U.S. immigration courts as a form of a reasonable fear of persecution. Because these women often seek an evaluation from a mental health expert as part of an asylum claim, awareness of FGM can be crucial in offering a culturally competent evaluation of the woman's narrative.

Women can also experience trauma from painful or extremely extended childbirth in the absence of emotionally sufficient care. Injuries to the vagina due to childbirth are less common in the developed world today but are still not unknown.

INTERSEX AND SEX-LINKED TRAUMA EXPOSURE

An entire group of individuals whose existence is poorly recognized by society are at risk for trauma due to the sex of their bodies. These are intersexed individuals, who represent one in 2,000 live births. Intersex, even though common, is stigmatized in Western cultures, seen either as a curiosity to be exploited or a medical problem to be fixed in secrecy. Intersexed persons represent an extremely heterogeneous group; they can be genitally intersexed, as is the case with Swyer's syndrome in which the sex organs do not develop and are present in the body only as a smear of cells. They may be intersexed in their sexual morphology. This group of intersexed persons includes babies with an XX (typical female) chromosomal makeup who are fetally exposed to high levels of androgenic hormones and are born with very large clitorises that resemble a small penis, but with other vulva structures and all reproductive organs normative for human females, as well as babies born with micropenis. This last group of children have XY chromosomes (typical male) and very small penises; they also have fully functioning testes. There are also children born with full or partial androgen-insensitivity syndrome (AIS); these babies have XY chromosomes and testes; but because their bodies are nonresponsive to testosterone emitted by the testes, they are born with external genitals that appear female. In addition, there are a variety of forms of chromosomal intersex that commonly lead to typical external genitals but reproductive infertility such as XO (Turner's syndrome) or XXY (Klinefelter's syndrome). There are also types of intersex in which external genitals are incompletely formed, such as vaginal agenesis, a condition in which the vagina, uterus, and fallopian tubes may be absent but the external genitals appear female and the baby has XX chromosomes.

Aside from the medical issues that arise for some of these babies (e.g., some infants with micropenis also have hypospadias in which the urethra is exposed and may become infected, requiring reconstructive surgery to ensure the child's health), what about intersex makes it a biological risk factor for trauma? The answer lies in a culture that requires its members to belong to two and only two sexes and that rejects and stigmatizes physical sexual ambiguity. As a consequence of this stance, many infants and small children with intersex conditions, particularly those affecting external genital morphology, are subjected to cosmetic surgeries early in life to "correct" the appearance of their genitals to more typical sizes and shapes. Thus girls with very large clitorises may have those organs amputated or cut down to a more sexnormative size, which can lead to later life difficulties in sexual functioning. Boys with micropenis have also been subjected to amputation of their organs, castration of their functioning testes, and the creation of an artificial vagina, similar to that built for transsexuals undergoing sex reassignment surgery, which the child must learn to keep open through the use of dilating rods. All of this is done in the name of normalcy and reducing stigma.

However, many adults who were subjected to these cosmetic procedures in childhood have come forward in the past several decades to describe the multiple forms of trauma resulting from these surgical interventions (Chase, 2003), including increased stigmatization. These children are targeted for early and medically unnecessary cosmetic surgeries on their genitals because of the belief communicated by many neonatologists that these children would suffer from having atypical genitals; parents, who are usually in something of a state of shock and confusion after the birth of an intersexed child, have been a receptive audience for these suggestions. Additionally, because clinical wisdom until recently was to hide the fact of her or his intersexuality from the child, such children experience not only physical pain and loss of function due to how their sex is treated by the medical community but also shame and confusion arising from the secrecy surrounding their medical treatments.

Cultural competence thus leads psychotherapists to inquire of clients about early experiences of surgery and medical treatment. Although there are other early procedures that may have been traumagenic, intersexed individuals are more likely to have had the psychosocial stigma of their sex become interwoven into the experience of trauma that will not be the case for children whose early medical trauma was due to nonshamed conditions such as childhood cancer.

Arlene was an intersexed woman born in the early 1960s with AIS. Her parents, who were living at the poverty level when she was born, had a home birth and were unable to afford regular medical care for her until she was around 6 months of age, at which time the presence of her testes was found when the pediatrician palpated her belly, and the absence of a vagina was also noted. The physician was mostly unfamiliar with AIS but knew enough to leave her parents frightened; they were referred to a university clinic several hours drive away from home, where the physician's message was that their daughter had a serious problem requiring surgery and hormones. They also received the message that they could not tell their child what was wrong with her. At age 18 months Arlene was operated on to remove her testes (good medical care because if left in they are at risk of becoming cancerous in AIS girls and women) and to create a vagina, which first her mother and then as she became old enough Arlene herself had to keep open with dilators. At age 11 she had a second surgery to widen and deepen the vagina; this surgery she remembered very well.

> It was painful for days; back then they didn't believe in giving pain meds to kids because they were afraid we'd become addicts, which I find hilari-

ous (Arlene had entered treatment because of alcoholism). And I didn't understand what the surgery was about; I was just a kid, I wasn't having sexual feelings, I sure as heck wasn't having sex with anybody. My poor parents just got pushed around by the doctors, so it's not like I blame them, they barely had a high school education between them. And then those weird rods (the dilators). I felt embarrassed. I never got my period, but no one would ever tell me why. It was years before my mom told me that the special *vitamins* I had to take every day were hormones, so that I'd grow some breasts and look more like a girl.

Arlene's reflections on her medical treatment for AIS, which she was more able to discuss midway through therapy, conveyed the traumagenic nature not of the surgeries per se but of the psychosocial atmosphere surrounding them and the secrecy about her sex. She began to become sexually active in risky ways around age 14, seeking out sexual partners indiscriminately and often getting drunk and being subjected to sexual encounters to which she was unable to consent. Her alcoholism worsened when around the time she turned 18 her parents finally disclosed her intersexed condition to her. "I really went into a tailspin around then." She dropped out of college and followed a boyfriend to Alaska where she signed on to work on a fishing boat on which drinking was officially forbidden. She intended to use the months at sea to get sober.

As is common for many trauma survivors when they stop drinking, Arlene's sobriety was the gateway to the onset of her other posttraumatic distress. She became very depressed and was reprimanded repeatedly by the boat's captain for engaging in risky behaviors. This led to her finally being put off the boat midway through its cruise and forfeiting her share of the profits of the trip. Once on land again she went into a severe drinking binge that resulted in her being committed for detox and alcohol rehab. In the more protected environment of the rehab facility she began to once again confront the pain, shame, and stigma of her intersex condition, which in turn led her to seek therapy.

For Arlene, the psychotherapist's cultural competence lay in several areas. Initially, Arlene's distress had to do with the surgery and secrecy. As therapy progressed and her sobriety lengthened, her distress began to center on the issue of stigma and discrimination against intersexed persons. The psychotherapist to whom Arlene had gone for her expertise in substance abuse recovery realized that her own attitudes about intersex were unexplored and that her own knowledge base was lacking. However, her basic culturally competent stance was her ability to affirm to Arlene that what had happened to her was a result of discrimination against her sex and that her risky adolescent sexual activities and alcohol abuse had been attempts to cope with and master her unspoken and then still preverbal understanding of having been surgically violated because of her sex. Arlene's posttraumatic symptoms included an aversion to being vaginally touched or penetrated, although she enjoyed other forms of sexual touch and was orgasmic with her partner. She told her psychotherapist one day,

> There's the irony. They built me a vagina so I could have so-called normal sex, and that left me too traumatized to ever want that. If they'd just left me alone I would be having sex the same way I am now and not been traumatized.

Although the experience of persons born intersexed seems to be an extreme example of trauma based in sexual biology and morphology, it also underscores the effects of sexism and misogyny. When the penis of a boy born with micropenis, fully functional and capable of sexual arousal, is amputated, and he is then castrated and rendered infertile so that his entire body will be a feminine-appearing neuter, this entire process has often been medically rationalized on the grounds that as a male he will be embarrassed by his too-small penis. This narrative of masculinity being equated with penis size is usually a source of mild to moderate distress to adolescent boys going through puberty and to some adult men as well. However, when it becomes a rationale for mutilating and sterilizing children who, if left untouched, would become both fully functional sexually and capable of reproduction, then the contribution of sexism and misogyny to the trauma of intersexed persons becomes more transparent. Additionally, this sort of trauma based in sex illuminates how the sex of the body can become the risk factor for trauma exposure.

GENDER ROLE AND GENDER PRESCRIPTION AS RISK FACTORS

As noted earlier, gender, although built on sex, is not sex. Gender roles are powerful social constructs, and much of the trauma differentially experienced by women and men and by boys and girls seems to derive from gender roles and the gendering of experience rather than from sex per se.

The following discussion of gender roles is broad and general in nature. Because gender is simply one of a person's multiple identities and because gender is constructed and expressed differently through the lenses of culture, age cohort, ethnicity, social class, sexual orientation, disability, and the host of other social locations, some of these generalities will not apply to a person with a given combination of multiple identities. The culturally competent psychotherapist will be sensitive to these interactive effects and also to the ways in which culture and social context shape the meaning and experience of gender, which in turn inform the experience of trauma exposure.

What are gender roles? They constitute the set of norms and expectations both ascribed to people by a culture as well as internalized by most individuals in that culture about how one's sex should inform all of one's experiences. The rules range from the very serious, regarding what occupations women and men may enter or what topics boys or girls may study, to the absurd, such as what color a child of a given sex should wear. Hence the ubiquitous pink-for-a-girl, blue-for-a-boy nature of infant clothing and accessories as well as the assumptions made that boys will be interested in guns and violence, girls in playing with dolls and making friends. Bem (1989) has suggested that each person internalizes these rules through the formation of gender schemata, which are more or less flexible depending on a person's developmental capacities and which act to screen out information about gender that is contrary to the organizing principles of a particular gender schema. Because trauma usually evokes a rigidification of all of a person's coping strategies, it is quite common for gender schemata to rigidify as well in the wake of trauma exposure and thus for the loss of gender-normative behaviors to be experienced as particularly traumatic.

As discussed very early in this volume, trauma is a feminizing experience, particularly when posttraumatic distress is manifested. In the Euro-American culture dominant in the United States, expression of affect, except for angry affect, is coded as feminine; fear, sadness, and guilt, are seen as weak or wimpy, particularly when expressed by men and evidence of women's lesser capacities when expressed by women. Thus sexism places an additional burden on men who are trauma survivors by defining much of the range of response as evidence of loss of masculinity (Levant, 1996). Sexism also redoubles the burden placed on women. Although expression of affect is seen as gender normative, it is also constructed as evidence of a woman's weakness or lesser capacities, something that many women spend a lifetime attempting to avoid. In Mallory's story, told earlier in this chapter, her internalized sexism, which was part of her motivation to avoid affect expression, left her more vulnerable and less comfortable with herself when those previously disowned affects emerged.

Gender role norms also increase or decrease risks for certain kinds of trauma exposure. Masculine norms that overvalue physical risk taking and that prescribe acting out of uncomfortable affects or that permit or even praise abuse of substances (e.g., "he can hold his drink like a man") place men who ascribe to those norms at greater risk of such traumas as motor vehicle accidents, being victims or perpetrators of crimes of violence, and sporting accidents. In a provocative qualitative study of adolescent and young adult men who had committed murder or aggravated assaults, Jordan (2005) found that for many of these men their crimes stemmed from feeling a need to establish control and force respect from others, both expression of masculine norms that require men to be in control and respected.

Feminine role norms carry other risks. These norms prescribe compliance, acquiescence, and nonassertion for women. The onus of making social relationships work well is also embedded in norms of femininity. Women in domestically violent relationships often stay because of their beliefs and those of their families and social networks that they bear the responsibility for making those relationships peaceful and functional. In sexual harassment situations women describe trying hard to ward off their perpetrator without hurting his feelings. Acquaintance rapes, statistically the most common kind, are often perpetrated on women who feel unable to say no or forcefully resist.

Gender role norms extend to the body. To be feminine, women must be whatever the culture currently defines as not fat, a norm that has changed dramatically in the past half century. Men must be strong, muscular without being muscle-bound. Hair lengths, the presence or absence of facial hair, and the depth or sweetness of vocal tone, all of these are given a gendered meaning. A feminine woman is pretty; a masculine man is not pretty. If and when trauma affects people on these variables an individual may experience trauma as neutering or degendering. A man with facial scarring from an assault may be seen as having increased his perceived masculinity and attractiveness (note how often male heroes in certain types of romance fiction are depicted as having some sort of facial scarring), whereas a woman with facial scarring is disfigured, has lost her attractiveness.

In addition to general cultural gender schemata, there are variations on themes that are created by specific cultures, social class expectations, age cohort memberships, and other aspects of multiple identities. Thus, for instance, in some Latin American societies, the roles of machismo and *marianismo* are the culturally specific expressions of masculinity and femininity, respectively. Machismo is not only an expression of extreme (by Euro-American standards) masculinity but also requires bravery and *respeto*, acting in such a manner as to receive the respect of others. Honor and the defense of one's honor are more explicitly built into this version of masculinity than the versions experienced by some non-Hispanic men. *Marianismo* is a model of femininity based in adulation of the Virgin Mary, who is construed as the ultimate woman. Self-sacrifice, especially the sacrifice of self for children and family, meekness, chastity, and humility are consequently more strongly coded into some versions of Latina femininity than into Euro versions.

Because of the history of slavery and racism in the heritage of Americans of African descent, masculinity and femininity also have particular culturally derived flavors. Being respected, being able to provide for one's family, and being able to protect that family, all characteristics stolen from African American men by slavery, have become extremely central to this version of masculinity. Because racism denoted African American women as objects of sexual use and gratification for slave owners, femininity for African American women has had a conflicted relationship with sexuality. The "strong Black woman" stereotype, which calls on these women to repress affect and shoulder the burden of suffering for the good of the family, is a distant echo of a time when a woman could suffer the loss of family through legally sanctioned murder or sale of her children.

The intent of this book is not to be etic and go deeply into each variation on the theme of a particular social location. The examples provided previously are to alert the reader once again to the importance for culturally competent practice of not assuming the particular meanings and schemata of gender for a given person. Instead, culturally competent practice starts with an awareness that each person has gender schemata and that an important component of understanding the meaning of an individual's trauma exposure will be knowing how those gender schemata have informed the meaning of the trauma and of posttrauma symptoms and distress.

These gendered schemata also lead to differences in coping styles, which are in turn related to norms of allowable emotional expressivity. In general the feminine role allows for more expression of negative and inward focused affect, including grief, guilt, shame, and sadness, and more overall expression of emotion than does the masculine gender role (Peirce, Newton, Buckley, & Keane, 2002). This is despite the fact that woman are apparently less physiologically reactive than men; thus men following prescribed gender norms may be more required to suppress awareness or expression of affect, leading to Levant's (1999) construct of "normative male alexithymia." Alexithymia was long ago identified as one of the common sequelae of severe and persistent trauma exposure (Krystal, 1969), which suggests that for men deeply influenced by and compliant with gender role norms, already present difficulties with affect awareness and expression may be complicated and worsened by trauma exposure. Ironically, becoming more emotionally aware and expressive will, for such men, require a violation of gender norms, which in turn can complicate a recovery process. Similarly, since feminine norms allow, and to some degree expect, women to be emotionally expressive and weak, the woman who does not express affect when exposed to trauma may be perceived as cold or unfeminine in some manner.

Gender also intersects with and complicates trauma recovery when trauma interferes with the expression of valued, gendered activities. Lisa, an upper-middle-class married heterosexual African American woman had been a full-time parent and homemaker, actively engaged in the lives of her two elementary age children when she was severely beaten during the course of a robbery in the parking garage of a mall by a man who was on work release. The beating left her with partial paralysis of her right side, persistent fatigue, and a fear of leaving the house. She had received treatment for her PTSD symptoms after the trauma, successfully completing a course of prolonged exposure and reporting a remission of her nightmares and flashbacks.

However, when she came to me for her evaluation during her lawsuit against the state, her ongoing distress had little or nothing to do with overt PTSD symptoms. She said, with tears streaming down her cheeks,

> I'm not a mom anymore. I'm not a wife. I can't drive; I can't take care of the house; I'm tired and overwhelmed all the time. My face droops. I know I shouldn't be so petty, but I really liked how I looked, I worked at it. I'm not good for anything or anyone anymore. I might as well be dead.

Lisa's trauma also included a strong loss-of-just-world component. She had learned through the discovery phase of her lawsuit that her assailant, who had beaten several other women before he was re-arrested, had in fact violated the terms of his early release and should have been put back in prison several weeks before his attack on her.

> They knew he was using drugs again, he had three dirty UAs [urine analyses]. Their own rules said that two violations was an automatic revocation of parole, and they didn't do anything. He was free to beat me up, and those other women, too.

Lisa, who had grown up and always lived in the upper-middle-class, had a reasonable belief that her government would follow its own rules much of the time, although she was aware, as a woman of color, that equal protections did not always extend to people like herself. But she had internalized a schema of womanhood that included carefully following of the rules, which she came later to realize had held an implicit promise of protection from danger.

Lisa's just world had collapsed and robbed her of her sense of self as a woman. Her persistent emotional injury from the assault was not PTSD, which had been well treated using an empirically supported method that works very well for single-episode adult trauma like the one she experienced. Instead, the lasting emotional consequences of this trauma were bound up in how she was no longer able to be a woman as she understood herself to be one.

Lisa's trauma also had to do with issues of within-group betrayal, as she revealed toward the end of the evaluation process, when she had become more comfortable self-disclosing to the Euro-American evaluator, that another complication of this trauma had to do with her assailant's ethnicity and phenotype.

> He was a Black man, and my husband's a Black man. There was a period after the assault when just seeing my husband made me scared. I felt like I was betraying the race, me, afraid of Black men. And then I thought, no, I was the one who was betrayed. That brother's job was to protect sisters, not beat them up. Can you see how confusing this was for me?

She reported that with her psychotherapist, who was also African American, she had been able to explore her guilt for feeling afraid of her husband and her guilt for testifying against her assailant. She told me,

> There's already too many brothers behind bars, you know. But the man had no right to beat me. He almost robbed my children of their mother, my husband of his wife. He had to pay a price for what he did. I had to remember that he put himself there, I didn't put him there.

Psychotherapists working with trauma survivors need to be alert to this sort of gendered and culturally flavored loss embedded in other aspects of the trauma and to invite clients to interrogate their narratives of gender. Notice that for Lisa these gendered losses were compounded and heightened by cultural themes and meanings. She commented at one point in her evaluation that she was the first woman in her family to be able not to work outside the home for pay and "stay home and raise my own children, not work raising someone else's children" as her grandmothers had both done. The loss of her capacities in her roles of parent and homemaker had a special significance for her as woman in a culture in which few women have not worked outside the home.

GENDER NONCONFORMITY AND TRAUMA

Gender conformity is enforced in a variety of overt and covert manners. Consequences ranging from shaming and humiliation to hate crimes that are often fatal attend on the lives of those who are gender atypical in some manner, particularly those whose gender atypicality extends to a clear disconnect between their biological sex and their lived gender role expression.

Transgendered individuals, whose gender atypicality may or may not include seeking the use of hormones or sexual reassignment surgery so as to conform their biological sex with their experienced gender, have been welcomed in some cultures and contexts. In traditional Lakota societies there were the roles of winkte (biologically male) and berdache (biologically female) transgendered people; certain healing rituals and chants could only be performed by these individuals, who were seen as having two spirits. Although these persons engaged in same-sex relationships they were socially constructed as transgendered rather than homosexual. Similarly, the hijra of India constitute a transgendered, sometimes transsexual, social group possessing a ritual function in Hindu societies.

In dominant U.S. cultures, however, and indeed in most cultures in the United States that have been colonized by dominant values, gender nonconformity is risky and can be a factor leading to trauma. Mike was a biologically female Euro-American transman (female to male transsexual person) who came into therapy after learning of the death of Brandon Teena, a transman whose biological femaleness was discovered by male acquaintances who then brutally raped and murdered him (his story is told in the film *Boys Don't Cry*). Mike's transition had not been easy; he had identified as a lesbian prior to having a mastectomy (top surgery) and taking daily testosterone injections, and many of his friends had deserted him as he transitioned from a lesbian woman to a man. His family had struggled to accept his becoming male, and his employer had asked him to take an unpaid leave of absence from his teaching job at a local community college until his transition was complete; because the state where he lived had no legal protections for people based on gender expression, he had no legal recourse to prevent this happening. He was working as a security guard, the only job he had been able to find in which his status as a transitioning person seemed to make no difference, "since I'm alone at night with buildings, right?"

Learning of Brandon Teena's death evoked Mike's own fears of being assaulted or killed were his transsexuality to become known to strangers. "Every time I go into a public bathroom now I have a panic attack," he told his psychotherapist. He reported that he would deny himself liquids during his work hours so as to avoid bathrooms at all costs. He began to have nightmares of being beaten up and being taken to a hospital where the staff yelled *freak* at him and refused to treat him for his injuries.

In therapy he disclosed a lifetime of being punished for his gender nonconformity.

> When I was a little kid and I already knew that I was a boy, I got into trouble big time with my parents. They believed that girls should be girls, and here I was, really a little boy. The kids in school called me freak a lot. It's probably why I got into drama, because there I could put on disguise and be a boy and a man and it was fine. But you know, none of that was traumatic.

Mike's exposure to insidious gender-based trauma was invisible to him; internalized sexism and transphobia had left him feeling as if his torments growing up were normal and to be expected. His strong posttraumatic reaction to learning of another transman's death through the media was an example of insidious trauma hitting a tipping point and exploding into full PTSD symptoms.

Gender is a starting place in cultural competence. Each person takes her or his biology of sex and roles of gender into her or his other social locations. A next social location likely to inform people's experiences is one also founded in biology–phenotype, which is culturally transcribed as race and ethnicity and which in turn forms culture.

7

TRAUMA, CULTURE, PHENOTYPE, AND ETHNICITY

Anyone interested in posttraumatic stress disorder must eventually confront the role of ethnocultural factors in the etiology, distribution, expression, course, outcome, and treatment.

(Marsella, Friedman, Gerrity, & Scurfield, 1996, p.1)

In this chapter, I look at the topic of biological phenotype, commonly thought of as race, culture, and trauma. The interactive nature of trauma and culture and the realities of racism and ethnocentrism as sources of trauma exposure are analyzed and explored.

Culture is a shared, acquired pattern of values, attitudes, beliefs, and schemata that consciously and nonconsciously shapes peoples' identities and behaviors. Cultures can be observed at very macro levels, such as the culture of a country, or very micro levels, such as the culture of an organization or even a neighborhood. My neighbors and I proudly proclaim ourselves "Fremonsters," people living in a part of Seattle characterized by odd public art, many Thai restaurants, and a summer solstice parade featuring people riding bicycles while wearing little more than body paint and feathers. But among Fremonsters are our other more enduring cultural identifications, which have had lasting effects on identity and well-being: my neighbor who is second-generation Latvian American and proudly informs me when someone in the news is of her heritage, the elder South Asian couple who take their exercise every day walking up and down our steep hills, the original resident of our block who talks about being raised by her Norwegian immigrant father in Montana in the 1920s, and the 60-something Navy vet who is our lone neighborhood Republican. If trauma were to strike, it is those enduring cultural values and experiences that are likely to be evoked no matter where these people live and work today.

Ethnicity is one way in which people code their cultural identification. In the United States, ethnicity has been ascribed to members of some cultures and not others; dominant Northern-European-influenced cultures are usually not defined as ethnic cultures, whereas cultures of color, Southern-European cultures, and Eastern-European cultures frequently are identified as ethnic cultures. The term *ethnic minority* has been commonplace to refer to Americans of African, Spanish-speaking, Asian, and American Indian descent, whereas the term *White ethnics* has been applied to Americans of Irish, Eastern European, Jewish, and Italian heritages among others. I use the terms *ethnic cultures of color* and *Euro-American ethnic cultures* to refer to these two different groups, including among the latter the Northern European Euro-American ethnicities.

From the standpoint of cultural competence in therapy each person, whether conscious of it or not, has a culture and an ethnicity. A psychotherapist working with trauma survivors needs to become aware of what that culture and ethnicity are because of the importance of those factors for understanding trauma's meaning; that psychotherapist must also be able to differentiate between phenotype and ethnicity, which are often but not always so deeply intertwined as to appear isomorphic. Some of those cultures and ethnicities have been targets of long-standing oppression, discrimination, colonization and sometimes genocide, meaning that members of these cultures often have distress that is tied to historical trauma, internalized oppression, current discrimination, and insidious traumatization. Other cultures have been those of colonizers and oppressors.

Racism, an expression of cultural domination founded in the erroneous belief that humans can be divided meaningfully by shared phenotypic characteristics and that some sets of phenotypes are less worthy than others, is a commonplace in every culture; it is an enduring and persistent source of distress for its targets and an ongoing potential source of trauma. Some would argue that racism is, in fact, a trauma by and of itself (Bryant-Davis & Ocampo, 2006; Sanchez-Hucles, 1998; Sue, 2003; Walters & Simoni, 2002). In the United States and other places colonized by Europeans, the possession of a phenotype that includes fair skin, light-colored hair and/or eyes, and hair that is silky rather than coarse in texture as well as being associated with descent from Celtic, Germanic, Viking, and Anglo-Saxon distal ancestry is defined as White and is the dominant and valued phenotype. White people who have darker skins tones and darker and less silky hair and who descend from Mediterranean, Magyar, or Slavic distal ancestries are generally considered less White, as can be seen by the coding of such individuals in terms of standards of attractiveness, perceived intelligence, or exoticism, which is a version of devaluation. In the United States, racism is an ideology of White domination, although it takes other forms in other parts of the world (e.g., in India racism is perpetuated through a caste system in which darker skinned Dalit people are devalued by people considered brown skinned and targeted for racism in the United States). In this volume I use the term *racism* to refer to White racism, which is most common in this country, and its dominant culture rather than other forms of racism. Members of ethnic cultures of color can perpetuate White racism on themselves and members of other, different ethnic cultures of color through application of racist norms and standards; however, the meaning and impact of these expressions of racism will be different from those deriving from racism at the hands of Euro-Americans.

All ethnic cultures of color in the United States and each member of those cultures have been affected to some greater or lesser degree by White racism, both current and historical. It is a source of insidious trauma, historical trauma, and systemic exclusion for anyone who is part of these cultures. For some individuals racism has been experienced directly and painfully in ways resembling *Diagnostic and Statistical Manual of Mental Disorders* (4th ed., text rev.; *DSM–IV–TR*; American Psychiatric Association, 2000) Criterion A trauma through hate crimes and active episodes of discrimination. For others it is manifested more consistently as insidious trauma or as a risk for traumas of betrayal or loss of just world. Racist trauma is also about the ways in which people of color are rendered invisible as individuals and subsumed into stereotypes (Franklin, Boyd-Franklin, & Kelly, 2006).

Racism functions to devalue persons and groups defined as racially inferior and to create negative associations between characteristics ascribed to those persons and groups. Well-known examples of this societal discourse can be seen in discussions in the sport world about the alleged ability or lack thereof of African American athletes to occupy positions that are coded as more cerebral (quarterback in football) as versus more physical (running back in football). It is interesting to revisit the iterations of this discussion over time, including those rationalizing the exclusion of African American players from baseball during the 1930s and 1940s because they were alleged to be insufficiently physical.

There are also invidious forms of racism that manifest as pseudo-idealization or envy. The stereotyping of persons of Asian descent as a so-called model minority, who are seen as dangerous competitors for the social positions in professions once held largely by Euro-Americans is one of the better examples of this phenomenon in American society today. The model minority construct also denies the reality of racism, implying that persons of Asian descent do not face discrimination but rather have some sort of culturally based social advantage, a narrative denying the extensive history and current reality of racist violence and exclusion faced by persons of Asian descent in the United States. This sort of racism also sets up a competition between ethnic cultures of color in which one group is encouraged to adopt White racist attitudes and values about the other.

Persons of mixed phenotype who have one Euro-American parent and dominant culture persons who have become family members or allies of people of color are also exposed to a variation of these forms of systemic trauma. Persons of mixed phenotype and ethnicity are subject to the rules of hypodescent, in which any visible non-White ancestry codes persons as being of color and makes them a target of racism, sometimes from within the Euro-American side of their own family. These individuals suffer from another and uniquely painful form of racism in that they are also often subject to within-group tensions, sometimes being insufficiently supported or included within one of their heritages because of accusations that they are not sufficiently a member of that group (cf. Root, 2004b).

Euro-American (White) people are affected by racism in its various forms as well, because perpetration has the potential to be traumatic. The shame experienced by perpetrators of racism and the ego-dystonic nature of racist values in the lives of otherwise well-meaning White people have been identified by Dovidio, Gaertner, Kawakami, and Hodson (2002) as the sources of modern aversive racism in which overtly racist values are denied but nonconscious racist values pervade interactions with people of color.

INDIGENOUS PEOPLES: THE ETHNICITY OF COLONIZATION

Persons of indigenous heritage, which in the United States most commonly include American Indians, Alaska Natives, Native Hawaiians, and Native Samoans, all share the historical trauma of colonization that informs culture more powerfully than phenotype, even though all of these groups are sufficiently phenotypically similar to the eyes of Euro-Americans that members of one group are often misidentified as being of the other. Colonization is an especially pernicious form of trauma in that one's historical home is invaded by technologically and/or numerically advantaged people who systematically strip out the value of language, spiritual practices, cultural norms, land ownership, and the humans themselves. Wholesale killings, rape of women, enslavement, and physical dislocation are common in the histories of colonized peoples and often occurred within the lifetimes of psychotherapists' clients or their family members, not only historically.

Not surprisingly, these are all cultures that suffer from endemic sequelae of historical trauma, including extremely high rates of interpersonal violence, which can be seen as a form of helpless horizontal hostility expressed within group, because the option of expressing it against one's oppressors is not available; high rates of substance abuse; and high rates of suicide as well as persistent poverty and educational and occupational disenfranchisement (Duran, Duran, Brave Heart, & Yellow Horse-Davis, 1998). Colonization histories, which weaken cultural coping strategies and create distress and vulnerability for all members of a society, can aggravate present-day trauma, as Paula's story illustrates.

Paula was in her early 30s, an enrolled member of a Pacific Northwest nation. Her father was Euro-American, but her mother's family had lived in and around the same area for many generations back. The family had suffered many traumas, and Paula had been sexually abused by her father, maternal grandfather, and some uncles; physically abused by her mother and some older cousins; and neglected. She was pregnant for the first time at 16 and addicted to alcohol by the time of her second pregnancy when she was 18; all told she had five children with two different fathers, both of whom beat her, before her 25th birthday. She told her psychotherapist it was a miracle that none of them suffered from fetal alcohol syndrome; she had stopped drinking with her last pregnancy and, with the arrival in sobriety of intrusive images of her childhood sexual abuse experience, entered therapy. She was in and out of a psychiatric hospital for 2 years and then stabilized. She returned to school, got her general equivalency diploma, and had started college when her Euro-American Indian Health Service psychotherapist began to sexualize their relationship.

To protect the secrecy that he required, he convinced her to leave the nation's lands (i.e., the reservation) and move into the nearest large city, using the excuse that it would be easier for her to attend college in Seattle now that she was nearing the end of her community college program. Her extended family felt distanced and somewhat betrayed; to the degree that they offered some support in the past they withdrew it now. Therapy ended. About 1 year after the move, the psychotherapist abruptly ended the sexual relationship, blaming it on Paula's sexual difficulties, which stemmed in large part from the history of sexual abuse for which she had sought treatment from him initially.

Paula's mental health took a sharp downward turn; she readmitted herself to the psychiatric hospital, where the nursing staff, on learning her story, urged her to bring charges against the offending psychotherapist, which she did. As she told the story to her psychotherapist later, there were multiple levels of traumatization and betrayal. The Indian Health Service, an agency of the federal government, was the direct target of her lawsuit against her first psychotherapist. She told her new psychotherapist that she realized that what her former psychotherapist did was yet another example of "Indians being screwed by the Feds. Only this time they were way more direct about it." She had noticed that one of her former psychotherapist's tactics was to isolate her from her community.

> He moved me off my land, off my spiritual source. He told me it was because he didn't want my aunties prying into our relationship, and you know that he knew how persuasive that would be to me because I'd complained about it more than a few times in therapy. But if they'd been

around they would have known there was something wrong and helped me and the kids.

Instead, isolated and alienated from her extended family, she struggled on alone in the middle of a Euro-American setting where anti-Indian racism, taking the form of bumper stickers about fishing rights and casinos, was ever present.

Things became more difficult when, in the midst of her lawsuit, the Federal Bureau of Investigation sent agents to the nation's land with the stated objective of "interviewing witnesses for the case." Paula received a barrage of angry hostile phone calls from relatives (as she commented with a combination of fatigue and humor in session that day, "Everyone on the rez is my relative somehow or another") for having exposed them to an agency perceived as very dangerous in Indian Country. "No one in Indian Country forgets what the Feds did to our cousins at Pine Ridge," she told her current psychotherapist, referring to an infamous recent episode of occupation of Indian land by federal agents, "And here I am causing trouble, bringing the Feds onto our land." Her pain at this, although slightly balanced with her rage that the government would first be the agent of her sexual exploitation, then use the excuse of her fighting back to terrorize her relatives, seemed for a long time to be more traumatizing to her than the actual sexual abuse itself. The entire experience was evocative of multiple layers of historical trauma for Paula; displacement, alienation from family and traditional culture, endangerment of her family, and oppression of indigenous people by the Euro-American U.S. government. Although she ultimately prevailed in her lawsuit, she reported that her victory felt hollow, as the costs to her relationships with her nation and her family remained large, and those estrangements seemed not to heal entirely.

Because of historic discrimination and exclusion, many persons of color have lived in poverty as well. Poverty and issues of social class are not unique to persons of color, and social class issues are addressed in chapter 10 of this volume. However, when poverty and racism have combined in people's lives, other forms of endemic trauma exposure are likely to have been present as well.

Some European origin cultural and ethnic heritages carry historical and insidious trauma as well. Irish Americans, as noted earlier in this volume, have an extensive history of trauma exposure arising from the colonization of Ireland by the English. Jews have experienced historical trauma in the Diaspora, with outbreaks of genocide during the Crusades of the 11th and 12th centuries; dispossession and expulsion from England, France, Spain, and Portugal between the late 1200s and 1497; everyday anti-Jewish laws in countries dominated by Christian and Muslim faiths; and the Nazi Holocaust of the 20th century. Moreover, modern aversive anti-Jewish beliefs continue to be present in the United States today. Persons of Armenian heritage in the

United States are almost entirely descended from survivors of the Turkish genocide against the Armenians at the end of World War I. Various countries and cultures within central Europe were at times colonized, with indigenous languages and norms suppressed by the Austro-Hungarian and Russian empires (Poland, which was repeatedly divided up between Austria, Germany, and Russia being one of the best examples of this sort of colonization). Psychotherapists who are familiar with European history will know that the large German migration to the United States at the end of the 1840s was one result of a failed revolution by democrats against a monarchy. French Americans are often the descendants of the original Acadians who invaded Canada as colonizers and then lost control of that space to the English colonizers; some, in exile, form the Cajun communities of Louisiana, whereas others have been culturally marginalized both in Quebec and in the northeastern United States. When a person from these heritages comes into a psychotherapist's office because of a present-day trauma, an exploration of the possible meanings of that event within cultural context may deepen the therapy and assist clients in greater understanding not only of their posttraumatic responses but also of their inner resources and identities, leading to the potential for posttraumatic growth.

Culturally competent trauma practice necessitates gathering information about a client's culture and ethnicity of origin as well as the culture and ethnicity with which an individual identifies; these may or may not be the same. The potential for inter- and transgenerational transmission of trauma in cultures in which trauma exposures are widespread and long standing must be carefully considered in understanding how to approach a survivor's experiences in a culturally competent manner. Variations within a culture are also likely to exist, so taking sufficient time to explore the nature of a person's cultural identifications can be quite salient to understanding how she or he makes sense of or experiences the specific trauma for which she or he is currently seeking therapy. Questions such as "How would you describe your cultural background?" and "What does it mean to you to be part of that culture?" can invite clients in an open-ended way to share information about their sense of their culture and ethnicity.

RACE—A POWERFUL AND FLAWED SOCIAL CONSTRUCT

All humans alive today have their origins in the first homo sapiens who evolved in Africa. Various waves of human migrations from Africa over the millennia have led to variations in human phenotype. Skin rich in melanin pigment, vital for survival near the equator, adapted to the long winters and sparse light of northern hemispheres by losing pigment; closely situated groups reproduced with one another, creating gene clusters leading to tolerance for dairy products, sickled red blood cells that resisted malarial parasites, and other genetic sources of resilience and vulnerability that are now associated with particular ethnicities.

To describe people of a particular sort of phenotype as a race is, however, a social construct that denies within-group variability as well as the actual ethnic identities of those who are arbitrarily grouped within a race. Race is a biological fiction (Smedley & Smedley, 2005) that is treated as a social reality and used as a rationale for oppression. For example, persons of Japanese, Chinese, Vietnamese, Thai, Burmese, Cambodian, Indonesian, Filipino or Filipina, Korean and Hmong, Malay, and Indian ancestries are all categorized as Asian by racial definition. Some of their cultures have influenced each others'; some have colonized one another, as Japan did with Korea, China did with Vietnam, and Vietnam did with the Hmong, leading to enduring hostile themes among these cultures. The cultures are quite different; both the Malay and Indonesian cultures have large Muslim communities. The small Muslim communities of southern Thailand are a target group in the Buddhist-majority country. Korea, Vietnam, China, and Japan are all cultures influenced by Confucian philosophies of hierarchy within family and society. The Hmong people had no written language prior to their mass displacement to the United States after the war in Southeast Asia; in China writing goes back many millennia.

Additionally, each of these various Asian ethnic and cultural groups has, within the United States, its own particular history of immigration and discrimination. Only Japanese Americans were placed in internment camps by the U.S. government, including secret interrogation centers for community leaders, of which the illegal detention centers run by the U.S. government in its war against some aspects of radical Islam are eerily reminiscent. Chinese American history includes episodes of lynching and mass murder; Filipinos have experienced multiple episodes of colonization, with the United States being only the most recent colonizer. Vietnamese and Hmong people are in the United States largely because of the disruptions and dislocations following this country's failed expansionist efforts in Southeast Asia and the massive flight of refugees from there after the fall of the U.S.-controlled puppet government. The long sojourn of many of these people in refugee camps after having been promised safe haven in the United States in return for their loyalty to American interests added betrayal on top of other traumas of war and dislocation.

This brief and extremely cursory description of some of the easily identifiable differences among some Asian ethnic groups will make it clear that culturally competent practice eschews grouping people by the spurious construct of race, and instead invites clients to describe culture, heritage, and ethnicity as the individual defines it for her- or himself. It also requires a psychotherapist to develop a sense with clients of what their family and cultural trauma history has been so as to place current trauma into that context of historical and cultural trauma.

Because racist discrimination and violence has targeted people on the basis of phenotype, people's sense of themselves as belonging (or not) to a particular race may be an important component of their understanding how trauma happens to them today. Psychotherapists must honor the client's internal conflation of culture and phenotype into the construct of race because it is the client's lived experience and must themselves avoid falling into essentialist notions that phenotype governs any particular aspect of behavior. As with gender, which is built onto the biology of sex, so culture, ethnicity, and race have been built onto the biology of phenotype (Smedley & Smedley, 2005). Additionally, because of the nature of racism in the United States, phenotype has a real association with experiences of lack of safety and protection, which are the factors creating insidious trauma in the lives of people of color. As Daniel (2000) noted, it may be incorrect to refer to the distress suffered by people of color as "post"-traumatic because the trauma of racism is an ongoing event rather than one existing in the past.

"I AM BECAUSE WE ARE": COLLECTIVIST CULTURE AND TRAUMA

Many target-group ethnic cultures present in the United States are collectivist rather than individualist cultures. This means that members of such cultures may be particularly vulnerable to insidious trauma because harm done to one extends to others through bonds of family connection. With family often defined well outside the limits of legality or biology, the potential for trauma to be a factor in the distress experienced by persons of target group ethnicities is high indeed. In Paula's story, described earlier in this chapter, the harms done to her extended to her children, her family members, and her entire community. Culturally competent trauma interventions with members of such cultures may involve engagement with families and communities of trauma survivors who are affected by the identified client's specific trauma.

Several years after the lawsuit, Paula's psychotherapist asked her if it might be helpful to meet together with a traditional healer and elders of her community to seek reconnection with her extended family. The psychotherapist, informed by Attneave's (1969) model of whole-systems therapy that was in turn based on experiences working with members of American Indian nations, had come to realize that Paula's individual therapy could only take her so far and that as long as she experienced what the traditional healer identified as *shadow sickness*, a form of distress at the level of soul and spirit, she would likely remain stuck in her healing process. Over a period of 1 year Paula and the psychotherapist met, first with the healer and elders and then with members of Paula's family. Paula participated in several healing rituals, including a women's sweat lodge. It was only after engaging the wounds to the family and her indigenous nation that Paula was able to move fully through her therapy process. In this instance the use of a culturally flavored intervention also led Paula to growth emerging from her trauma experience as her connections to her culture and family, which had always been affected by historical trauma, healed and strengthened.

Members of these target group ethnic cultures are also negatively affected by dominant cultural pressures to assimilate and acculturate into the U.S. mainstream. These pressures can become aggravating factors in the context of trauma exposure because acculturation may strip people of access to culturally based coping or healing systems. Comas-Diaz (2006) noted the higher rates of diagnosed mental illnesses in U.S.-born or long-time U.S.-resident Latino and Latina persons than in ethnically similar persons who were recent immigrants; she commented, however, that these statistics fail to describe the posttraumatic stress disorder present in those Latino and Latina immigrants fleeing war or persecution in their countries of origin. Acculturation trauma, which entails the loss of cultural markers in exchange for apparent greater ease within the dominant culture, often represents an unmourned source of grief for persons of target ethnic and cultural groups. This can in turn serve as an additional vulnerability when trauma exposure occurs. The mourning and remembrance component of trauma recovery should thus be inclusive of mourning and remembrance for cultural losses and traumas as they relate to the client's identities and experiences.

Persons attempting to cope with racism and discrimination by assimilation may find it difficult or embarrassing to be using culturally based healing systems because to do so appears at odds with their assimilated presentations of self. Culturally competent work with trauma survivors requires the psychotherapist to use privilege responsibly so as to initiate the conversation about such resources as a strategy for reducing shame or embarrassment about what one of my clients, a Dominican woman who went to a *botanica*, bought candles, and did novenas to the Virgin, called "that woo-woo stuff," so that these clients living in the liminal identities of assimilation can integrate cultural healing practices into the Western mode of psychotherapy in a direct and transparent manner. Comas-Diaz (2006) described working with Latina women who complemented psychotherapy with visits to a *curandera*; Duran (2007) spoke of both himself and his clients engaging in American Indian healing ceremonies and studying with a traditional healer.

CULTURE AND EXPRESSIONS OF DISTRESS

The experience of distress is universal; the expression of that same distress is highly culturally driven and learned, reflective of cultural understandings of the source of misery in body, spirit, and mind. Culturally competent trauma practice assists psychotherapists in considering the various ways in which people will have the phenomenological experience of posttraumatic distress and not privilege one over another as a real posttraumatic symptom.

Persons of European ethnicities, both dominant and target, are very likely to be influenced by the Cartesian mind–body dichotomy that pervades Western medicine. As such they are more likely to present both with a conventional *DSM–IV–TR* set of posttrauma symptoms and also an equally conventional Western understanding of their distress as psychological in nature. Social class and education mediate this phenomenon, with stigma associated with psychological distress significantly lessened among middle- and higher-class and college or higher educated individuals, and correspondingly still more likely to be present in poor or less educated persons. Because an emotionally minimizing style is present in many Euro-American cultures, clients with these ethnic heritages may be constricted in their expression of affect. Stamm and Friedman (2000) went so far as to suggest that clinicians working with clients from Northern European "stiff upper lip" cultures assume that overt expression of distress by these clients is likely to be evidence of extreme breakdown of coping strategies, given the violation of cultural norms for affect expression.

However, psychotherapists working with trauma survivors from ethnic cultures of color, indigenous cultures, and some immigrant cultures need to be aware of the high likelihood that posttraumatic distress will both be understood and expressed in culture-informed ways. These are cultures in which overt expression of emotion may not be proscribed; however, in many such cultural contexts the causes of the distress being displayed are not seen as psychological but as either physical or spiritual or some combination of these. Patterns of distress labeled *culture-bound syndromes* in the *DSM–IV–TR* are, as noted by Comas-Diaz (2006) and Hinton, Pich, Chhean, Safren, and Pollack (2006), most commonly culturally informed expressions of posttraumatic distress seen through the lens of a culture in which distress unashamedly takes somatic forms. In those cultures informed by spiritualities in which dreams, magic, and other nonrational epistemologies are valued, distress may be both manifested and healed by engagement with these forms of knowing rather than with conventional Western styles of psychotherapy or psychopharmacology.

Castillo (1997) noted that emotional distress is transmitted through the lenses of cultural meaning systems. These systems, which include strategies for understanding and classifying the phenomenology of distress, will be present in the ways in which trauma survivors tell psychotherapists about their pain as well as their healing. As he noted, cultural meanings deeply inform people as to how to respond to events in their lives. He gave as an example the universal human experience of loss of a loved one due to death. Although in some cultures a death is literally cause for weeping and wailing, in others quiet tears and a contained demeanor are prescribed, and in still others a celebration of the person's movement to a better place marks the grieving process. Reading the death notices in a local African American community paper, for instance, I was struck by how often the death was referred to as a joyful homecoming. When that death occurs in the context of trauma, however, the engenderment of helplessness, terror, and shame, which may have attended on the loss, will complicate and confuse people's experiences and expressions of distress, particularly as that loss refutes cultural narratives.

Similarly, culture also lends meaning to all forms of trauma. In the many European and Euro-American cultures and ethnicities centered around a just-world construction of reality, certain kinds of trauma exposure will be perceived as even more meaningless and painful because they were undeserved. In other cultural contexts the precise events will be experienced as sad or painful but not shake meaning-making foundations because their occurrence fits with rather than shatters normative expectations of reality. Finally, in some ethnic and cultural milieus a trauma will be experienced as retraumatizing, cementing hopeless or helpless beliefs about the relationship of a target group to the dominant society and its agents. For culturally competent work to occur with trauma survivors it thus becomes necessary to understand the ways in which clients' culture and ethnicity shape their understandings of the meanings of events.

MAYBE I'M NOT WELCOME HERE

One effect of racist norms is to define ethnic cultures of color as alien and foreign (Sue, Bucceri, Lin, Nadal, & Torino, 2007). Persons whose ancestors came from Asia and the Pacific Rim report being asked, "Where are you from?" and when responding with the name of the suburb in California where they were born and raised being asked again, "No, where are you *from?*" with the interrogator's message being that no matter how thoroughly American a person of a certain phenotype may feel, that phenotype brands them as not from here. In New Mexico, where communities of Spanish heritage have existed since the invasion of the conquistadores in the 1500s, similar questions are asked by phenotypically White Euro-Americans of people whose ancestors arrived there 300 years later after the U.S. conquest of what was then part of Mexico.

In a number of locations in the United States English-only laws have been passed that outlaw the use of languages other than American English in settings such as government. Informal English-only policies are also imposed by employers in a variety of businesses. This kind of experience conveys to members of some cultures of color that they do not look or speak like a "real" American. As a form of insidious trauma, these policies function to create an unspoken but potentially powerful perception that there is a target on one's back.

PHENOTYPE, ETHNICITY, AND SAFETY RESOURCES

When I was a child, I was exposed to the folk music of the American progressive movement, including most memorably, Tom Paxton's 1963 song "What Did You Learn in School Today?" as performed by Pete Seeger. The song is a satire about the just-world consciousness of dominant American culture; a verse that has stayed with me and that informs the remainder of this discussion, went

> I learned the policemen are my friends.
> I learned that justice never ends.
> I learned that murderers pay for their crimes,
> Even if we make a mistake sometimes.[1]

For many people of color in America these lines are not merely a satire; they are lies. The long lists of African American and Latino men executed and sometimes lynched for rapes and murders that they did not commit, the history of unprosecuted crimes of violence against people of color, the ghosts of Emmett Till, the realities of internment camps in which Japanese Americans were incarcerated, the litany is long and apparently never ending.

While finishing this book in the spring of 2007 I had a conversation with a young African American criminal defense attorney of my acquaintance and happened to ask him why he became a lawyer. "I guess it was because of what started happening to me when I was in college," he told me. He had grown up in an upper-middle-class family in the 1970s and 1980s in the Pacific Northwest, the son of a doctoral health care professional who was himself a prominent member of the community and was on the board of regents of the university attended by my young friend. The family lived in a predominantly Euro-American suburb.

> I began to be stopped by the police driving and walking in my own neighborhood. One time they stopped me for littering; they said I'd thrown a cigarette butt out the car window. Well, I've never smoked. But they tore the car apart, looking for drugs, guns, I don't know. Of course they didn't find anything. Another time they came up behind me just as I pulled into my parents' driveway. They told me there'd been a burglary in the neighborhood and I matched the description of the suspect. It finally hit me; I was Black, that was their probable cause. I realized that if this could happen to me, what were they doing to kids from the ghetto. So here I am.

My acquaintance's experiences are so common in the lives of men of color that the concept of "driving while Black" has entered the lexicon of communities of color as both a metaphor for and a reality of the fact that law

---

[1]From "What Did You Learn in School Today," by T. Paxton, 1963. Copyright 1963 by T. Paxton. Reprinted with permission.

enforcement has historically not been a friend to people of non-European phenotype; not only has there been overt persecution in the forms of harassment, false arrests, and sometimes fatal miscarriages of justice but there has also been absence of the sort of protection assumed as a right by members of the phenotypic dominant groups. As we saw in Lisa's experience earlier in this chapter, it can feel like a betrayal of the group to go to law enforcement when one is the victim of a within-group crime; because most crimes of interpersonal violence both by strangers and acquaintances occur between members of ethnically and phenotypically similar groups as a result of simple issues of access and proximity, the trauma of criminal assaults may be complicated emotionally by the historical and present-day realities of differential protection by the justice system. Culturally competent practice with trauma survivors holds these realities in awareness to assist all parties in comprehending how and why a given trauma may be experienced as intensified in its threat level.

A NOTE ABOUT LANGUAGE

For members of some target ethnic groups English is not the language of emotion. Espin (1995), in her study of Latina lesbians, found that for each woman certain topics could only be discussed in her native Spanish, others only in English, and some in both. Culturally competent psychotherapists are sensitive to linguistic issues as they affect the expression of affect and the transmission of information about the experience of trauma. Cultural competence and sensitivity do not require a psychotherapist to be fluent in or even speak a client's mother tongue (I discuss the use of interpreters at length in chap. 11, this volume, on immigration and dislocation). It does require knowing that some things will be better voiced in that mother tongue than in an acquired language or that others will be best described in the idiom of the culture even when English is the mother tongue.

Early in my practice I worked with a woman born in North Africa whose native language was French and who was addressing in therapy issues related to her grief over the death of her mother at a young age. She seemed emotionally distanced as she spoke of this experience in English, which was the language in which she had been raised since around age 6, a language in which she was so accentless as to be taken for someone who'd spoken it all her life. I invited her to consider speaking her grief in French, the language in which her loss had occurred. This serendipitous suggestion opened the door for her to gain access to her affect, consistent with Espin's (1992, 1995) later findings about language and emotion. Inviting clients to speak the truths of their traumas in the language of their heart, whatever that might be, empowers them to decide what the words are in which they will frame the narrative of their pain. It is less necessary for the psychotherapist to comprehend the specific content than to be willing to be present with the affect and support for clients in knowing their experience in a language that makes sense to them and reflects the emotional syntax of their culture.

A NOTE ABOUT INTERGENERATIONAL AND TRANSGENERATIONAL TRAUMA

Throughout this chapter I have commented on the likelihood that a person whose culture of origin has a history of oppression or genocide may be living with effects of trauma exposure that occurred not to that individual but to their forbearers. The concept of historical, intergenerational, or transgenerational transmission of trauma has been studied most carefully with only a few groups of people—Jewish survivors of the Nazi Holocaust, and increasingly, indigenous people in North America.

A culturally competent trauma therapist will approach any psychotherapeutic work with a member of such a culture with an enhanced awareness of the possibility of the impact of historical trauma on functioning. However, no assumptions should be made about the presence of such intergenerational effects. Specific familial resilience factors as well as individual differences in access to resources may function to mostly or entirely ameliorate the effects of historical trauma. However, to the degree that more extended family members and more generations of a family have a history of trauma exposure, a therapist will enhance cultural competence by keeping the possibility of such effects in mind as they invite a client to make sense of whatever distresses them.

Ultimately, culturally competent trauma practice weaves the experience of trauma and its meanings into the complex identities of the client. As a psychotherapist deepens in the capacity to consider gender and culture and mixes these ingredients into the process of knowing the client, deepening will occur with the addition of a next element of identity. In the next chapter, I look at sexuality, another experience of identity that begins at the level of the body and that has multiple social constructions layered on to that lived reality.

8

TRAUMA AND SEXUAL ORIENTATION

In this chapter, I look at definitions of sexual orientation and examine the effects that sexual orientation has on risk for trauma exposure, response to trauma, and resilience in trauma's wake. The impacts of pervasive cultural homophobia and the specific effects of current discriminatory political movements are explored. I also look at risks potentially inherent in dominant sexual orientation.

TARGET SEXUAL ORIENTATION AS A SOURCE OF TRAUMA

Overview

It has been barely more than a century since Western science and psychology have come to conceive of persons having a fixed nonheterosexual orientation and then to define such an orientation as normative for a numerical minority of the population. That century has not sufficed to reduce bias against and stigma associated with nonheterosexual status. Lesbian, gay, and bisexual (LGB) people constitute a target group with a unique status based solely on sexual orientation; unlike many other target groups in the United States, they continue to be subject to legal discrimination and in some arenas increased legal discrimination. This social context lends a unique experience to the intersection of sexual orientation with trauma. For LGB people, having a minority sexual orientation leads to endemic exposure to insidious trauma, frequent exposure to active discrimination and maltreatment, and some risk of hate crimes. Although many discussions of the topic of LGB people include transgender people in discussions of sexual orientation, I have opted to include transgendered people in chapter 6 in the discussion of gender. Transgendered people can be heterosexual, gay, lesbian, or bisexual, and thus issues of sexual orientation will be a component of identity as they are for nontransgendered individuals.

Usually LGB people, unlike members of target ethnic and cultural groups and like people with disabilities, do not share target group status with their immediate family members. Many LGB people thus develop their sexual orientation identities in a vacuum informed by myth, misinformation, and negativity (Garnets & Kimmel, 2002). Although this picture is beginning to change as openly LGB people are becoming more visible in the public sphere, having openly lesbian comic and talk show host Ellen DeGeneres cheerfully appearing on one's television screen daily does not make up for the absence of direct and emotionally intimate paradigms for becoming LGB nor does it counteract the ubiquitous presence of anti-LGB sentiment in dominant culture in which pejorative terms for gay men and lesbians are common epithets. Because bias against LGB people continues to have potentially life-threatening consequences and discrimination against LGB people is active and legal in the United States, I argue here that for most LGB people the social environment has regular potentials to be traumatizing.

Families are sometimes the source of trauma for LGB people as well; even in a family in which no other abuse has occurred, an LGB person growing up may encounter continuous biased commentary and experience the threat of loss of relationship with family simply because of sexuality. As a result of persistent mythologies, some promulgated by mental health professionals, that LGB orientations are chosen freely and thus can be unchosen as well, LGB people frequently receive the message that they are to blame for their own victimization and in control of whether they are targets. Most LGB people are affected by systemic forms of bias, including homophobia, which is an anti-LGB sentiment, and heterosexism, which privileges heterosexual lives and relationships although does not necessarily stigmatize in the manner of homophobia. Like racism and sexism, homophobia and heterosexism can be systemic, institutional, and also individual. Like other forms of bias, homophobia and heterosexism can, and frequently do, become internalized and a source of emotional distress; in fact the bulk of the literature on psychotherapy with LGB people speaks to the importance of addressing internalized homophobia, heterosexism, and biphobia as a core component of affirmative psychotherapies.

Trauma From Family

When LGB people make their sexual orientation known to their families of origin there can be very negative consequences. Even nondisclosure can have negative outcomes arising from the strategies of distancing and disengagement from families used by many LGB people in attempts to conceal their sexual orientation from family, something Pharr (1988) referred to as "internal exile." Higher rates of suicidality and homelessness among LGB youth are attributed in part to extreme negative responses by families to learning of a child's sexual orientation (Hershberger & D'Augelli, 2000). Being kicked out of a family, told that you are no longer their son or daughter, and denied access to younger siblings because you are now seen as a child molester are all varieties of traumatic experience that have been repeatedly reported by LGB people. Some data also document physical or sexual assaults by family members on LGB people when their sexual orientation became known to the family (Garnets, Herek, & Levy, 1993). These events do not occur in a vacuum; these are families in which LGB people have often first been exposed to the insidious trauma of overt verbal expressions of homophobia by family members or cultural systems of authority such as religion that are embraced by the family of origin.

Trauma From Target Ethnic and Cultural Groups

When LGB persons are members of target ethnic and cultural groups they often find themselves facing the racism of the Euro-American LGB communities and the heterosexism and homophobia of their cultures and communities of origin. Kanuha (1990) and Greene (1990, 1992) have each referred to lesbians of color as experiencing "triple jeopardy" psychologically because of risks associated with sexist, racist, and heterosexist oppressions, although Greene (2007) also commented on the special resiliencies inherent in having to successfully navigate the daily challenges of multiple and intersecting oppressions. Espin (2005) and Gock (2007) have each spoken eloquently of the creative synthesis of identities arising from their social locations as lesbian or gay members of ethnic cultures of color and engaged members of often-homophobic communities of faith. Frequently, LGB people of color violate gender-role norms of their target ethnic cultures of origin and may experience exclusion or violence in those cultures due to their transgressive identities. For those ethnic cultures strongly associated with particular faith traditions that are overtly rejecting or stigmatizing of nonheterosexual orientations, the experience of betrayal by those closest to the LGB person is not uncommon and can be traumatic.

Cultural competence with a survivor of trauma who blends these multiple identities will lead a psychotherapist to explore the meaning of the trauma not for each identity alone but for the place of intersection that is the client's life. Such clients may have experienced far more insidious traumatization than a Euro-American LGB client, although she or he may also have, in turn, a more diverse range of coping strategies. These individuals will also potentially have different support networks available to them in times of trauma, some of which will require making one important identity invisible or lesser for the sake of survival.

Trauma for Gay Euro-American Men

For many gay Euro-American men, encountering homophobia and the loss of White male privilege attendant on coming out as gay are experienced as a traumatic violation of just-world beliefs as the privileges of their visible social locations are undermined (Brown, 2003). These men frequently struggle with attempting to hide their orientation, adopting a public persona that includes no personal private life, immersing themselves in work as an avoidance strategy, and frequently engaging in risky sexual activities with unknown partners rather than pursuing stable relationships because to have an ongoing relationship risks being known as gay. Men in this group appear to be at somewhat higher risk of being assaulted by casual sexual partners; the posttraumatic stress disorder (PTSD) and other posttrauma symptoms that emerge for these men are not only about assault and targeting but about the extreme loss of illusions of control and a just world. This group of men is also at high risk of other interpersonal loss; the recent stories of former Congressman Mark Foley and former evangelical preacher Ted Haggard, each apparently a gay man who attempted to conceal his sexual orientation (and in the case of Haggard did so through a strategy that included being virulently antigay in the public domain) illustrate the risks for trauma inherent in the attempt to pass.

Trauma From Religion and Spirituality

Religion and spirituality, which are sources of comfort for many people, are frequently not for LGB people. Some faith traditions are actively anti-LGB, including the one in which Ted Haggard was a pastor and national leader; these traditions single out the sin of homosexuality from among other behaviors that are Biblically proscribed and focus on its eradication as a necessary condition for entrance into the community of believers. Haldeman (2002) has documented the emotional harms, some of them traumalike, experienced by LGB people who, in the context of such faith traditions, have attempted to change their sexual orientations through so-called reparative therapies. Many LGB people in these faith traditions, which include many of the fundamentalist or orthodox versions of several faiths, struggle with the untenable choice of faith versus intimacy and partnership and may in the process experience traumas of betrayal and insidious traumatization.

Other faith traditions are nonrejecting of LGB persons as worshippers but ban LGB individuals from the clergy. In faiths in which clergy experience a divine call to the pulpit, the coexistence of such a call with same-sex attractions can be wrenching and lead to experiences of traumatic loss and grief.

Paul had been an active Methodist his entire life and in his midadolescence experienced a call to ministry. As he later noted to his psychotherapist, he was also busily trying not to notice his call to homosexuality, knowing that the United Methodist church, although increasingly welcoming to LGB members, banned openly LGB people from the clergy. He struggled with these apparently conflicting identities through his late adolescence and through his time in seminary. He was a gifted preacher and a skilled congregational leader and accepted a call to a church in a small Midwestern town. "I did my best to be straight," he later recalled, dating women and using his status as a clergyman to explain his avoidance of nonmarital sexual contact. At the same time he was having high-risk anonymous sexual encounters with men in quasi-public places, always fearing being arrested or otherwise found out. He found it ironic that his congregation voted to name itself "open and affirming," which meant that it welcomed LGB members.

In the mid-1980s after a series of illnesses Paul was diagnosed as HIV positive. "I took this as a sign from God that I could no longer in conscience hide myself. I was going to die from homophobia." He entered therapy after his diagnosis and made the decision to come out to his congregation and to his bishop. His church responded with love and support; the bishop initiated the proceedings to have him dismissed from ministry, which happened within the following year. Although Paul had chosen to disclose his status as a gay man knowing the risk of being rejected by the organized church, the experience of this was extremely traumatic and painful for him. It evoked and made foreground his having been bullied as a child for being slight and effeminate, bullying that had included a large number of antigay slurs. Struggling with his health, without employment or health insurance, he was now also afflicted with nightmares in which the faces of his tormentors changed from those of his boyhood to those of the ministers who had presided at the church hearing, dismissing him from ordained ministry. His loss of his ministry imperiled his relationship with his faith, which had been a source of comfort for him for most of his life, and he went through a several-year period of what he described as "existential nihilism."

Hate Crimes

Hate crimes against LGB persons continue to be common (Garnets et al., 1993). Even in places that are considered friendly to LGB persons as a result of legislation protecting civil rights, such crimes occur. Sometimes the perpetrators of these traumas will travel into LGB communities to find and assault individuals believed to be gay or lesbian by targeting people leaving LGB social settings such as bars frequented by LGB people (Skolnik, 2005). Balsam, Beauchaine, Mickey, and Rothblum (2005), in a study comparing prevalence rates of sexual assault between gay men and lesbians and their heterosexual siblings, found that gay men and lesbians were at significantly higher risk to be the victims of sexual assault. These researchers argued that in these instances the sexual assault may be a form of homophobia-based hate crime.

Absence of Legal Protections

Absence of legal protections can also become a source of trauma or its intensification. Because LGB people may not legally marry their same-sex partners anywhere in the United States outside of the state of Massachusetts, complicated legal arrangements and documentation of relationships are required to create relationship rights accorded to heterosexual married individuals. Aaron's husband Seth, to whom he was married in a religious ceremony, was struck by a car while crossing a busy street and rushed to the emergency room of his local university hospital with a closed head injury, unconscious and unable to speak. Although his wallet, which was apparently searched for an insurance ID card, also contained an easily visible card with Aaron's name, cell phone number, and identification as "holds medical power of attorney," Aaron was not contacted by the emergency room (ER) admissions or social work staff. Distraught when by midnight Seth had not come home from work, Aaron called the police and was told that indeed, Seth had been the victim of a hit-and-run accident and could probably be found at the university hospital.

Aaron, an upper-middle-class Jewish gay man who was a research scientist at a biotech firm, searched frantically for the papers designating him as holding medical power of attorney but could not find them. He rushed to the hospital anyway, only to be turned away when he tried to see his spouse because "you have no proof of your relationship." His begging and pleading were in vain; the hospital called in an administrator who cited federal privacy laws as rationale for denying him any information and threatened to call security to escort him out, so he sat quietly in a corner of the ER waiting room, crying, trying to be as close as possible to Seth. He called his attorney's office and left a message asking if she had a copy of their paperwork. By the time she arrived in the office the next morning to find the message Seth had died in the intensive care unit without Aaron ever seeing him.

Aaron's grief over the traumatic loss of his spouse was intensified dramatically by the hospital's denial of access, a denial founded in cultural homophobia and heterosexism. "I could have held his hand," he sobbed in his psychotherapist's office months later. "I could have comforted him, encouraged him to stay alive. He was completely alone and surrounded by strangers when he died. He was my husband, the love of my life, and I couldn't be with him." The hospital's letter of apology to Aaron was experienced as another level of trauma because it was full of legal justifications for his exclusion from his partner's deathbed framed by a technical apology for "any distress we might have caused you."

Trauma From Laws of Exclusion

Clearly, LGB persons can experience trauma through acts of discrimination or through laws that exclude their participation. Laws excluding LGB people are one source of trauma. The U.S. Department of Defense forbids service in the military by out LGB people under a policy popularly known as "don't ask, don't tell, don't harass, don't pursue." In principle this policy means that LGB people may serve so long as they do not make their sexual orientation known to the military. In practice, this policy has been the cause of numerous abuses.

Colleen, a Cuban American lesbian in her mid-20s joined the Army after the September 11, 2001, terrorist attacks because of her strong desire to serve her country. Her family were vocal patriots and her father, who had come to the United States as a child refugee, had served in the U.S. military with distinction. She had a long discussion with her partner about how they would keep their relationship invisible so that Colleen, a nursing assistant, could lend her medical skills to her country in its time of need. Her partner, a computer programmer who worked from home, agreed to move to wherever Colleen was stationed to support her.

In basic training Colleen did well and was successful in concealing her sexuality from her peers and superiors, although the process of going back into the closet took its toll on her relationship. After basic training she was assigned to work in a military medical facility where her supervisor, a sergeant, began to sexually harass her. She resisted, reminding him that he was married and that sexual harassment was a violation of military law. He told her that if she resisted him he would tell the chain of command that she was a lesbian and have her separated from the service. Recounting this years later, she said,

> My face must have turned all kinds of colors when he said that, like, how did he know? Then I realized, of course, that he hadn't known, it was just his usual threat, and my reaction, well, then he knew he'd hit a nerve.

The sergeant forcibly raped Colleen repeatedly and gave her bad fitness reports. Depressed and despondent, she went to the commanding officer and outed herself as a lesbian, which began the process of her being discharged. She also finally reported the sergeant but was told, "It's your word against his, and he's a respected career military man." He retaliated for her report by finding her family—he knew her father's name because she had proudly spoken of his military service—and outing her to them as well, leaving her with few supports when she returned to civilian life.

In therapy her self-blame for having been raped was thick with internalized homophobia.

> If I weren't a lesbian I could have stopped it right away because he wouldn't have had anything on me. What was I thinking, that a little dyke like me could succeed in the service? This was all my fault.

The trauma of the rapes was complicated by the trauma of discrimination, the threats to career and family ties, and internalized homophobia.

Absence of laws prohibiting discrimination in employment, housing, and public accommodation (the three pillars of all civil rights laws) based on sexual orientation also leave LGB people vulnerable to discriminatory practices that can be traumatizing or can aggravate other trauma. Exclusion is not necessary when inclusion is not protected. As of late 2007, LGB people constitute the only target group except immigrants and refugees not now covered by some sort of federal antidiscrimination law; they are also the only target group covered by a federal law that mandates discrimination, the Defense of Marriage Act. An LGB person fired from a job because of her or his sexual orientation in a jurisdiction where there are no protective laws has added to the helplessness of discrimination the powerlessness of having no legal avenues open for remediation. The combination may aggravate previous insidious traumatization to the point of active posttraumatic symptoms of distress.

Culturally competent trauma practice with LGB people requires that psychotherapists know the legal contexts in which their LGB clients live and work because those contexts may provide more or less support or offer more or less potential for insidious trauma based on what legal protections are available. These LGB trauma survivors may be hesitant to reach out for support to victim's advocacy groups, shelters, or crime victim assistance programs, fearing that if their sexual orientation becomes known they will experience the secondary trauma of being denied or excluded.

In Colleen's case, for instance, even though she clearly had PTSD related to being raped in the military, she had for years not sought disability services from the Veterans' Administration (VA) women's sexual assault program, believing that her lesbianism would disqualify her for services. It was only after she had mentioned this to a friend familiar with the program and its staff that she learned that the VA, unlike the military, did not discriminate on the basis of sexual orientation and that several of the staff of the women's PTSD program near her home were openly lesbian. She then finally felt able to ask for assistance that was legally owed her as a veteran honorably discharged.

Trauma and the Aggravating Effects of Heterosexism

When oppression and homophobia are not themselves the direct cause of a trauma exposure for an LGB person, heterosexism may compound or aggravate the experience of a trauma and its aftermath. After the terror attacks of September 11, 2001, a number of lesbian and gay widows and widowers found themselves excluded from pensions, awards of damages, and other benefits available to legal family members of partners who had died that day; this sort of legal exclusion resulting from heterosexist failures to include LGB partners in inheritance structures is common but was an aggravation of traumatic loss in those instances, similar to what happened in Aaron's story earlier in this chapter. An LGB trauma survivor may also have difficulty accessing resources available to trauma survivors because of a real or perceived sense of unwelcome to LGB people by that resource. In a time when federal funding to support social services is increasingly going to faith-based agencies, which are legally allowed to discriminate against LGB people on the basis of theological principles, the risk that an LGB person may feel unsafe seeking assistance after a trauma has grown.

Aside from these sources of exclusion, an LGB person may, like other members of target groups, be both more vulnerable and more or differently resilient in the face of current trauma exposure because of a history of insidious traumatization. Data indicate that LGB people are the target group most likely to seek therapy of any; as many as 80% of White lesbians and gay men studied in nonclinical samples indicated having sought the services of a psychotherapist at some juncture (Perez, DeBord, & Bieschke, 1999). Other data suggest that the high rates of depression, anxiety disorders, and substance abuse in LGB populations in the United States are persistent consequences of stigma and discrimination (Cochran, Sullivan, & Mays, 2003), an interpretation of the data that would be supported by Russell's (2004a, 2004b, Russell & Richards, 2003) findings of the specific negative impacts on LGB mental health of antigay political discourses. I have previously argued (Brown, 2003) that trauma, particularly insidious and betrayal trauma, is a normative component of identity development for many LGB people and thus should be considered endemic in the LGB population.

Consequently, culturally competent practice with LGB survivors will involve a psychotherapist in considering these various factors as they play into, aggravate, or ameliorate trauma exposure. The effects of internalized homophobia and heterosexism within an LGB person's psyche and the impacts of oppression in the client's immediate and historical social milieus must all be weighed as contributing factors in response to trauma. The interactions between sexual orientation and all other aspects of identity will create powerful possibilities for healing as well as increased risks for pain, both of which a psychotherapist must consider in comprehending the distress experienced by an LGB trauma survivor.

Interpersonal Exclusion and the Trauma of Betrayal

Because of the stigma placed on nonheterosexual orientation, many if not most LGB people have experiences of exclusion. The model of Betrayal Trauma discussed in chapter 4 is an excellent paradigm for understanding how those experiences might be traumagenic or aggravate other trauma exposures for LGB people. The concept of insidious traumatization can also be helpful in understanding the cumulative effects of multiple betrayals.

As noted previously, it is not uncommon for LGB people to have strained relationships with their families of origin that take stances ranging from avoidance to outright rejection regarding homosexuality or bisexuality. Some LGB persons will experience their families countenancing various sorts of bad behavior by other family members who remain welcome in the family so long as they are heterosexual, whereas their own lives are devalued simply because of their sexual orientation.

Yuri, a gay man in his late 30s whose Ukrainian immigrant parents are members of a virulently antigay church, commented that his brother, who was currently serving prison time for assault and robbery, was beloved by his parents, who were supporting his wife and small child while his brother was behind bars. Yuri, who had just been promoted to manager of his department in an engineering firm, owned a home with his committed partner Leon, and was in the process of adopting a child, was not allowed in his parents' home. "They want nothing to do with me. As far as they're concerned I'm the real criminal. They visit Sasha every week; they bring him food; the whole church writes him letters. Me, I'm the pariah, all because I'm gay."

Yuri had come into therapy when the process of filling out the application for adoption plunged him into a depression. "I realized that my child would not have grandparents, that my whole community had cut me off and would condemn me for this act of love, wanting to raise a child." His enhanced awareness of betrayal had triggered acute distress, which then revealed his pain from a lifetime of hearing homophobic comments in his home even before he came out. Although no *Diagnostic and Statistical Manual of Mental Disorders* (4th ed., text rev.; American Psychiatric Association, 2000) Criterion A trauma happened to Yuri, the insidious traumas of devaluation and his sudden awareness of how betrayed he had been by his family were an emotional experience of trauma; he felt exposed, cut off, and threatened by his family's attitudes and rejection.

Child Sex Abuse and Homosexuality: Cause or Effect?

Cultural competence working with LGB survivors of trauma also needs to interrogate mythologies about childhood trauma and the etiologies of homosexuality. Recent research does indicate higher rates of childhood sexual abuse (CSA) among self-identified LGB adults (Balsam et al., 2005), although the majority of those sexually abused in childhood develop a heterosexual orientation as adults. The possibility of a causal relationship between adult homosexuality or bisexuality and childhood sexual abuse is unclear and unproven. Balsam et al. have postulated that some perpetrators are aware of a child's sexual orientation and engage in sexual abuse as an early form of antihomosexual action against the child or adolescent, suggesting an opposite direction of causality, and some LGB adults who were sexually abused in adolescence after their sexual orientation was known to them do report perpetrators who targeted them because of that orientation.

Many LGB people have no history of childhood sexual abuse. However, work with LGB survivors of childhood sexual abuse will often contain questions by the client about whether or to what degree the abuse contributed to the development of their stigmatized sexual orientation. Because data do not support a paradigm of causality, all that can currently be said is that there appear to be higher rates of CSA in some studies of LGB adults and that no inferences of causation can be made. More specifically, the etiology of any sexual orientation is unknown; the persistence of heterosexual orientation in people sexually abused by members of the other sex suggests that sexual trauma is not a factor in the development of sexual orientation but more specifically has effects on sexual functioning.

HETEROSEXUAL ORIENTATION AS A RISK FACTOR FOR TRAUMA EXPOSURE

Although the discourse about sexual orientation and risks for trauma has historically focused on the experiences of LGB individuals, the risks of heterosexuality, particularly for women in relationships with men, need to also be addressed. Heterosexual women are at risk of being physically and sexually abused by male partners. Whitaker-Clark (2005), in an extensive critical review of the literature on abuse in intimate partner relationships, found that for adolescents in heterosexual relationships an average of around 30% of girls reported abuse from their dating partners, and adult women in heterosexual relationships reported abuse approximately 25% of the time at the hands of their male partners (with lesbians reporting about one half that rate from female partners). Heterosexuality appears to be a protective factor for men because heterosexual men report less abuse from female partners than do gay men at the hands of their same-sex partners (suggesting that sex of partner is a stronger predictor for risk of partner violence than sexual orientation per se). The mediating effect of sexual orientation on the sex of one's partner thus places heterosexual women at risk of intimate violence arising from their sexual orientation as well as their sex.

Culturally competent psychotherapy thus takes into account a person's sexual orientation, whether or not it appears to be directly related to the experience of trauma. In so doing, the therapist increases the chances of a deepened understanding of the client's experiences of the world by acknowledging this phenomenon that has so often been tied to shame and danger.

9

LIVING WITH DISABILITIES
IN THE CONTEXT OF TRAUMA

In this chapter, I focus on the relationship of disability to the experience of trauma. Disability as a life-time identity is differentiated from disability as a posttraumatic experience. Discrimination against people with disabilities as a risk factor aggravating trauma exposure is discussed and explored, as are issues of access to treatment with people with disabilities who are trauma survivors is analyzed.

People with disabilities constitute the largest target group in the United States (Olkin, 1999), cutting across sex, phenotype, social class, sexual orientation, and national origin. Although the experience of disability begins in the body, being defined as disabled is a socially constructed category. As noted in chapter 1, this group is extremely heterogeneous, including people with mobility impairments; people who have difficulty seeing, hearing, or speaking; people with learning and cognitive disabilities; and people with psychological disabilities. Some disabilities are developmental or congenital, a component of a person's life and reality from birth or early childhood. Others, especially others arising from illness or injury, are acquired throughout life. No one is exempt from possibly acquiring a disability; disability rights activists refer to the *temporarily able bodied* (TAB) to describe people who have not yet experienced disability.

Being a person with a disability exposes an individual to systemic emotional risks, including higher risks of exposure to certain kinds of trauma. Trauma exposure is also itself directly implicated in the development of disabling conditions. Culturally competent practice entails a comprehension of these intersections and of the specific risk and resiliency variables present in the social location of disability.

ABLEISM

Ableism refers to bias against persons with disabilities. This bias appears most palpably and visibly in the form of denial of access to these individuals as well as in the attitudes and behaviors of TABs interacting with people with disability. Persons with disabilities are referred to in negative or patronizing ways. For instance, the disability rights community has critiqued Jerry Lewis's telethon to raise money for muscular dystrophy because of what is seen as objectifying and infantilizing images of people with muscular dystrophy. As McBryde Johnson (2006) noted, to be referred to as "Jerry's kids" leaves adults with neuromuscular disorders fixed in the minds of the public as helpless children rather than as adults who happen to require more assistance with many activities of daily living than do other adults who do not have such disabilities.

Similarly, hearing people, when communicating with a Deaf (using the capital letter *D* to denote this cultural identification) individual through the services of a sign language interpreter, frequently address the hearing interpreter rather than the Deaf person, as if the inability to hear equates to an inability to comprehend. Slang terms for persons with disabilities, such as retard or lame, are used in daily vocabularies to denote stupidity or incompetence, communicating a negative view of people who are cognitively impaired or have difficulty walking. Persons with disabilities are seen as either lacking in sexuality or are sexually fetishized (Fine & Asch, 1988; Olkin, 1999).

Internalized ableism affects people with disabilities, leading to self-devaluation as well as devaluation of other people with disabilities. Because of the heterogeneity of people with disabilities and the manner in which resources are constricted in dominant culture, struggles for resources and for who is really a person with a disability can occur in this target group just as they do in other target groups affected by realities or narratives of resource scarcity.

When the Americans With Disabilities Act (ADA) was signed into law in 1991 it was the capstone of a lengthy fight by disability rights activists to outlaw overt discrimination against people with disabilities. It was not, however, the end of the line for ableism; the ADA has simply made it more difficult for overt exclusion to occur. Covert exclusion and devaluation continue apace. This has much to do with how the ADA distributes power. Employers and educational institutions may not discriminate and must provide reasonable accommodations, but the right to decide what makes an accommodation a reasonable one is not determined by the person with a disability but instead by the institution of nondisabled society. The very system of support for persons with disabilities is itself inherently discriminatory against the full employment and autonomy of persons with disabilities (Panzarino, 1994). My colleague Alette Coble-Temple, a member of the clinical psychology faculty at a school of professional psychology, uses a wheelchair and requires an assistance dog as well as personal care attendants; she wrote in response to my query,

> Individuals with disabilities who require personal assistance are typically caught in a double bind. They are capable of working, are offered a job, but cannot financially afford to work. Once you start earning money, you no longer qualify for state assistance with personal assistants. Another complicated component is that many states do not allow personal assistants to perform functions in the workplace. (A. Coble-Temple, personal communication, April 5, 2007)

She and other psychologists of my acquaintance with disabilities have described their struggles to be genuinely accommodated during their training and professional lives. Frequently, institutions follow the letter of the ADA, but rarely the spirit; that disconnect can be a source of insidious and betrayal traumas.

Arthur is a Euro-American, 27-year-old graduate student in clinical psychology. He is Deaf, and his native language is American Sign Language (ASL). He reads and writes English about as well as other students for whom English is a second language. He is able to lip-read a little; like most Deaf people of his generation he was exposed to an educational philosophy that encouraged the acquisition of spoken language, and when the light is good and he has close visual access to the speaker he can comprehend about 40% of what is being said, high average for a lip-reader but clearly not enough for classroom participation.

Arthur requested that his school accommodate him under the ADA and provide ASL interpreters for his classes. It did so. But classes are just one part of graduate school in clinical psychology or other mental health professions. There are visiting lecturers, tutoring and prep sessions for comprehensive exams and internship applications, and the many important informal mentoring and social support contacts that occur among peers and between students and faculty. Each time Arthur requested interpreter services for these other sorts of activities he was denied; these are not essential aspects of his education, he was told by the school's student services department, and the school is not obligated to pay for interpreters for anything that is optional and not required of all students because that is not a reasonable accommodation. The school is within its legal rights to make this decision (in fact, the administration consulted an attorney to be certain of precisely what they must offer Arthur and what they might decline to give him by way of accommodations).

Arthur did not have funds to pay for interpreters for these other optional events. He thus missed a nonrequired meeting at which the faculty offered mentoring to students about how to write their comprehensive examinations. Every other student in his program attended. He got notes from an acquaintance; he had not made any real friends in the program because his interpreters were not paid to stay after class and interpret conversations with his peers who did not know ASL. Consequently, he had only cursory and somewhat distant relationships with those peers. He tried to use the notes to prepare his exam papers. He failed his exams, having missed a crucial piece of information about how to respond to the assignment that his acquaintance did not write down although it was mentioned at length in the optional prep meeting that every other student in his cohort attended (and some audiotaped for further review, another option not available to Arthur).

As a consequence of failing this exam, Arthur was put on probation. For him this was an extremely painful experience; he felt not just that he had failed but that perhaps he was a failure. He withdrew emotionally. His advisor had had little contact with him because she too did not speak ASL, and the school would not cover interpreter services for their meetings because he could lip-read in one-on-one settings such as an advising meeting. She did not know that he was depressed and suffering from his loss; she knew only that his attendance at classes was becoming spotty and that his practicum site supervisor had called to voice concern about his apparent drop-off in clinical capacities. After a semester Arthur dropped out of graduate school. No one had illegally discriminated against him, but ableism had been active and functioning so as to exclude him first from the community of his school and then from the discipline he wished to pursue.

A few years passed. Arthur's depression had not lifted. His primary care physician put him on antidepressant medications, which blurred his vision; because seeing was his primary means of communicating with the world he took himself off the medications and felt worse. Finally, he learned of an ASL-speaking psychotherapist who had moved to town. Although she was hearing, he found out through the Deaf community grapevine that she was from a Deaf family, so he thought that he could perhaps trust her to understand Deaf culture. In his initial session with her, he broke into sobs, telling her that graduate school had become a terrible reenactment of his experience of being mainstreamed into hearing classes in elementary and middle school.

> I felt so alone, and so stupid. I know I'm not stupid; I have to be twice as smart as hearing people to do half as much. I just didn't have the heart to

keep struggling with them about what was right. I gave up. That's what makes me really a failure. That I gave up. And that makes me feel stupid all over again, only worse.

Arthur's story illustrates several levels of trauma potentially inherent in the experiences of people with disabilities that arise from ableist attitudes and values in the dominant TAB culture. He has experienced life-long insidious trauma from continuous exposure to devaluation of Deaf and other people with disabilities. He has repeatedly encountered exclusion and discrimination, which have morphed over time into aversive ableism in which exclusionary attitudes and practices can be denied because they are within the parameters of legality. He has internalized ableism, evaluating himself and his abilities as *lesser than*. In addition, he has experienced the more recent trauma of failure in which ableism and exclusion played a significant part.

Culturally competent psychotherapists need to be aware of their ableist attitudes and values. Because psychology's relationship to people with disabilities has long been that of the care provider, people with disabilities are commonly socially constructed into the patient or pathologized position, and many psychologists and other psychotherapists have internalized a medical model of people with disabilities. Ableism takes many forms including offices that are not accessible to people who use wheelchairs or have mobility impairments that preclude climbing stairs; forms that are not available in large-print versions; tests that are not available in taped as well as written versions; and lack of knowledge about the implications of a particular disability for a person's health, resilience, and capacities as well as their distress and difficulties. The stigma associated with disability is very similar to that associated with trauma; thus psychotherapists may unconsciously withdraw from clients with disabilities, not to speak of colleagues with disabilities, as they do from individuals known to be trauma survivors.

Not all disabilities are apparent or visible to a psychotherapist. Much of psychotherapists' training leaves them with a faint, and sometimes not so faint, suspicion of people's complaints of their physical ills as being nothing more than somaticized representations of denied emotional distress. It can be difficult for some TABs to understand how all-encompassing and preoccupying it can be to live with some disabilities (and conversely, how inconsequential it can be to live with others). As one friend of mine who lives with progressive relapsing multiple sclerosis (MS) put it,

> You get up in the morning not sure of what's going to be working today. Which circuits got blown overnight? So you get up hoping that your vision's no worse and your legs no more wobbly. And then you hope that the fatigue doesn't hit you over the head in the middle of the workday because there's no place to lie down, and even if there were no one would look very kindly on your doing that (she is not out at her workplace about her MS). If it's going to be a hot day you scurry into the car and

crank up the air conditioning and run to the office and pull down the blinds (many people with MS have very poor heat tolerance). And then hope that nothing switches off during the workday.

Approximately 2 years ago she lost all vision temporarily from a flare-up of optic neuritis during the course of a workday; her fears of having changes to her functional capacities during the course of a day are reasonable, and they are also posttraumatic. The day she was blinded by her illness she did not and could not know whether her sight would return (it did), and she remains hypervigilant to any diminution in her visual field. My friend is still very high functioning; her gait is only minimally impaired; her vision works more often than not; her mild cognitive slippages can be easily explained as normal aging; and her disability is unknown and thus invisible to her co-workers and her boss, who she fears will slowly freeze her out of her work-place if he knows she has MS. For her psychotherapist to be culturally competent, that person must ignore the apparent absence of functional impairment and genuinely believe what my friend tells her about her experience, which includes regular scolding from TAB people who think that she cannot possibly deserve her disabled parking sticker because she continues to be able to walk without assistance.

Notice how similar the experience of living with disability can be at times to that of a trauma survivor. The experiences of trauma are often not visible. The survivor's phenomenological realities can only be known through her or his narration of existence to others, and if others do not know, wish to know, or believe the survivor's experiences, then she or he becomes invisible (Birrell & Freyd, 2006). An important aspect of culturally competent practice with people with disabilities, trauma survivors or not, is the psychotherapist's willingness to believe and take seriously clients' accounts of their experiences of living in the world with a disability and not pathologize either the accounts of experience or clients' reactions to their social and physical environments.

DISABILITY AS A RISK FACTOR FOR TRAUMA AND VICE VERSA

Disabilities affect functioning and have impacts on how people with disabilities relate to those around them. Some disabling conditions lead to increased dependencies on family and paid caregivers for such basic functions as being fed, toileting, being turned in bed or moved from bed to wheelchair, being guided through traffic, or dealing with others who do not speak sign language. To the degree that any relationships of dependency can engender abusive behaviors on the part of the more powerful person in the dyad (in these instances the TAB person), risks for interpersonal violence seem to be accentuated by some kinds of disability. Olkin (1999) noted that children with disabilities are more likely than their nondisabled age-mates to be sexually abused, with the majority of perpetrators being paid caregivers, particularly in the case of people with developmental disabilities. She also found that women with disabilities are at enhanced risk for violence from intimate partners (Olkin, 2003), again largely because of increased issues of both physical and financial dependency. These findings about increased risk of interpersonal violence are confirmed by other authors (Martin et al., 2006), with one study finding rates of sexual assault four times higher for women with disabilities than TAB women. Data about men with disabilities and abuse are scarce, but it may be reasonable to extrapolate a similar degree of risk for those individuals, particularly men with disabilities who experience cognitive problems or who use the services of personal care attendants for meeting basic needs such as feeding and toileting.

Emotional abuse is an important potential trauma to which people with disabilities are exposed in ways that TABs may not be. One of my clients with moderate mobility impairments, who used the local paratransit system to get to and from her appointments, would frequently come into my office sobbing because the driver had become impatient and raised his voice at her for her disability-caused difficulties and slowness getting in and out of the vehicle. When she complained to the main office, she was told that she could choose not to use the service. My intervention became necessary for her to be taken seriously rather than dismissed. Since the paratransit service was her only option for getting out of the house to shop, go to events, and attend appointments, she felt trapped in the emotionally abusive environment. Contrast this with a TAB riding a bus; if the driver is impolite or a fellow passenger threatening, a TAB can get off, walk, call a cab, or if possessed of a car, decide to drive, an option not open to this woman. A component of what Arthur experienced in his graduate program was the reenactment of earlier experiences of emotional abuse and verbal bullying by peers.

Trauma is also a risk factor for becoming a person with disabilities. Complex trauma of childhood in which an individual experiences physical, sexual, and emotional abuse and/or neglect over an extended period of time has been shown to be associated with an excess rate of a number of physical, potentially disabling chronic illnesses in adulthood, including fibromyalgia, autoimmune disorders, chronic pelvic and other pain, irritable bowel syndrome, and cardiovascular illness. Because some of the coping strategies used by trauma survivors, such as cigarette smoking, excessive use of alcohol, disordered eating, and avoidance of physical activity, have serious health consequences, many trauma survivors also struggle with Type II diabetes, which has the potential to be disabling as a result of neuropathy and/or impairments of circulation to the extremities. Finally, of course, posttraumatic distress can itself be disabling to a person under some circumstances, particularly in the instance of complex trauma resulting from multiple childhood experiences of maltreatment. Many of the people I have worked with in my own psychotherapy practice live on disability payments for just that reason.

Some persons acquire disabilities through traumatic accidents or disasters. For those persons the loss of function associated with physical injury is tied to the traumatic circumstances under which that loss was sustained. For these clients culturally competent practice will focus on the mourning and remembrance component of trauma recovery and then on the process of uncovering and unpacking internalized ableism. As we saw in Sara's story in chapter 4, suicidal thoughts are not unusual in people who acquire severe disabilities as a result of accidents or illness. Some of these self-destructive desires reflect internalized ableism in former TABs who never previously saw value in the lives of people with disabilities and now cannot see value in their own. The development of a disability identity consciousness and a positive disability identity are important components of culturally competent work with this group of trauma survivors with disability to ensure that ableism does not claim a victim.

DISABILITY AND HEALTH CARE DISPARITIES: EMOTIONAL ABUSE BY THE SYSTEM

Disability also intersects with a number of other target group memberships. Because of persistent health care disparities, members of communities of color in the United States are at greater risk of acquiring illness-based disabilities during their lifetimes than are Euro-American people, even with financial resources held constant, with research showing disparate treatment of people of color by all sectors of health care. People who are poor and TAB are at higher risk than middle-class people of becoming people with disabilities because of higher physical risks inherent in many of the lowest-paying forms of work; also, people with disabilities are overrepresented in the poverty class, with education not functioning as a source of upward income mobility as is true for TAB individuals because of exclusionary hiring practices and difficulties obtaining adequate health care coverage in the marketplace. Thus persons with disabilities may experience trauma arising from barriers to health care access, health care that is necessary for survival but that cannot be obtained because of obstacles to access inherent in health care systems for poor people.

George, a working-class heterosexual Euro-American, had acquired paraplegia in his mid-20s as a result of an industrial accident; he had been working as a laborer on a construction project when a structure collapsed on him, injuring his spine at waist level. He had received a settlement payment from his worker's compensation board and was living on Social Security Disability payments, which meant that his health care coverage was through Medicare. His medications had previously been paid for by a state program for low-income people, but when Medicare Part D went into force that program went out of business. George found to his distress that one of the drugs that he depended on to reduce spasticity in his legs was not on the formulary of the Medicare Part D plan to which he had been assigned. He knew from experience that the drugs on the formulary would not help him; he called the plan administrator and pleaded to have his medication covered, to no avail.

Prior to that point George had demonstrated an optimistic attitude about his loss. He had put together a life that was working for him; he was attending a community college to get a general equivalency diploma and acquire skills to become employed in an office job and had joined a wheelchair rugby team. But the denial of medication hit him hard; his disability payments barely covered the costs of his mortgage and food. The denial of necessary health care resources triggered an episode of posttraumatic stress disorder related to the original accident that had never previously surfaced. When 3 months later his mother came to visit and found him playing with his handgun, he came into therapy. His psychotherapist searched for and found a disabilities rights group in a nearby community that was able to assist him with appealing the insurance company's decision by teaching him and the psychotherapist how to navigate the labyrinth of the appeals process.

DISABILITIES AND CULTURE

Each culture has its own social construction of the meanings of disability. Fadiman (1998) described how a Hmong refugee family living in California constructed their daughter's epilepsy as a form of spiritual gift; when the child was sent home to die by a medical community that had repeatedly taken her away from that family because of what was coded as insufficient (Western style) medical intervention, the family gave the unconscious girl a place of honor in the family and continued to relate to her as a vital member of the family system. Contrast this with the advice routinely given to the parents of children born with Down syndrome or other cognitive disorders prior to the past few decades in the same Western culture—institutionalize the child immediately and forget her or his existence. In some cultural settings, a person's disability is framed as evidence of sin in her or his past life, a parent's life, or her or his current life; in others it may be construed as evidence of divine gift. Culturally competent practice requires a psychotherapist to consider the possibility of special meanings for disability in a client's culture, not to know those meanings per se, which requires a level of etic knowledge not available to most psychotherapists but to know to ask about the existence of any such meanings.

In families in which, as a result of poverty, resources are scarce and support services for persons with disabilities even scarcer, a family member with a disability may become a target of abuse because she or he is perceived as threatening the well-being of other family members by virtue of her or his needs for specific forms of care. In other families in which resources are plentiful but TAB family members are affected by malignant narcissism, persons with disabilities may be shunned, stigmatized, or avoided as evidence of undesirable imperfection. The movie *The Other Sister* (Marshall, Rose, Richwood, & Brunner, 1999) portrayed this last sort of family in which upper-class parents attempting to cover up the cognitive impairment of a daughter deny her the special education opportunities that would be available if her developmental cognitive disabilities were recognized; instead she is treated as a flawed TAB by a parent who cannot tolerate the reality of her daughter's "imperfection."

Deaf members of cultures in which English is not the primary language may experience tensions among and between their several linguistic target group statuses. Corbett (2003) described the dilemma of a Deaf Latina woman; her family was Spanish-speaking and her mostly Euro-American Deaf community, although ASL speaking, was referenced to the English-speaking dominant culture. Norms of her family culture, which was hearing and Spanish speaking, and those of her Deaf community clashed and led to tensions and miscommunications for her around important life events. Even though ASL is closer in grammar and syntax to French (being based in French Sign Language) than English, being ASL speaking is perceived in many Latino and Latina families as forcing a child into the linguistically dominant Euro-American community (C. Antuna, personal communication, May 14, 2005). Like lesbian, gay, and bisexual people of color, people of color with disabilities are sometimes placed in the untenable position of having to pick which community they will affiliate with, which negates their multiple identities status.

When people straddling these borderlines experience trauma, the resources available to them for support will be affected by their multiple identities status. Psychotherapists attempting to work in a culturally competent manner with such clients must be careful not to unintentionally aggravate experiences of the insidious trauma of exclusion by ignoring the importance to these people of all components of their identities and by considering how social locations that people might otherwise rely on for support could themselves be sources of betrayal or insidious traumatization.

ACCESS TO PSYCHOTHERAPY
FOR TRAUMA SURVIVORS WITH DISABILITIES

It makes little difference how much a psychotherapist knows about disability issues if access to that psychotherapist is unavailable to people with disabilities. Culturally competent practice means undertaking a systematic review of issues of access and taking steps to reduce any barriers to access that the psychotherapist controls. Because so many people with disabilities are living in poverty and dependent on government disability programs for income and health care, psychologists wishing to adequately serve people with disabilities need to consider becoming Medicare providers, a status available to any licensed psychologist who applies. Although organized psychology fought hard to be included in Medicare in the early 1990s, apparently few psychologists have become providers, stating concerns about low reimbursement rates and high standards of documentation required by Medicare. For psychotherapists who are unable to enroll as Medicare providers, access for people with disabilities may include having lower fee slots in one's practice reserved for individuals with reduced income, some of whom will include people with disabilities who lack other payment resources.

Physical access issues are another component of cultural competence. For reasons both of function and finance many people with disabilities rely on public transportation or paratransit systems. An office situated too far away from public transport lines may be unreachable for some people with disabilities for whom driving is not physically possible or who cannot afford a car because of limitations on income arising from living on disability payments. Wheelchair access, chairs for clients that can be easily entered and exited by a person with neuromuscular or joint problems, and having a teletype device (TDD) or knowing how to use relay services for the deaf are all simple strategies both for ensuring access and also communicating to people with disabilities that a psychotherapist has considered them and their needs in the planning and design of a psychotherapy office.

Growing numbers of persons with disabilities use assistance animals that are trained for a variety of functions. A psychotherapist should be prepared to welcome these four-legged assistants into the office (water bowls are useful) and to know proper etiquette vis-à-vis these assistants. On the other hand, personal care attendants are usually not welcome in sessions because of reasonable concerns about confidentiality; psychotherapists must examine their own feelings evoked by being alone in the room with someone who is visibly disabled and may have difficulties communicating as a result of neuromuscular impairment. Large print and nonprint versions of forms for people with visual disabilities will increase clients' autonomy and reduce greater power imbalances; offering to read out loud regular size print, although helpful, keeps a person with a disability in a more dependent position. Psychotherapists who work with Deaf clients should learn how to work with an interpreter, choose interpreters who are trained in mental health issues when those are available, and know that there are a variety of different sign languages that may be used by a client. Finally, and importantly, psychotherapists working with trauma survivors with disabilities should never assume that the disability is caused by the trauma, that disability is traumatic, or that disability is central to a person's identity. As one Deaf acquaintance said to me,

I'm a woman who loves dogs, works with domestic violence victims, and spends her free time reading mystery novels. And oh yeah, I'm Deaf, so if you want to be my friend you'd better learn ASL or have a lot of money to hire interpreters. But there's not a special Deaf way to walk a dog.

AND WHAT ABOUT TRAUMA?

As noted previously, trauma and disability have a complicated interrelationship. Disability is not traumatic or traumagenic per se but vastly raises the risk of trauma exposure. Trauma exposure can frequently be psychologically disabling. However, people with disabilities can live free of trauma, simply annoyed and frustrated by the obstacles placed in their path by a culture designed by and for TABs.

Culturally competent trauma practice involves teasing out the strands of the relationship for each person, once again avoiding assumptions. Persons who have acquired their disability as a result of accident or illness may not be traumatized by the event that changed their physical capacities nearly as much as they are by the loss of status, power, or identity deriving from those changes. The person whose changed functional capacities lead to little or no decrement in interpersonal safety or who does not experience betrayal by systems or relationships designed to be protective may experience grief and existential challenges arising from illness or injury, but not trauma.

Gary's experience illustrates the complexity of the intersection between trauma and acquired disability. A heterosexual, married, late-20s, formerly able-bodied member of the Army Reserve who worked as a machinist, Gary's unit was called up and deployed to Iraq where he and his colleagues drove supply trucks. Theoretically not in combat, he and his unit were in fact in a highly dangerous situation; their vehicles were insufficiently armored, and the trucks were the frequent targets of roadside bombs. Even before he was wounded he wrote home frequent e-mails in which he spoke of his feelings of being abandoned by the military. "Tell people that we need armor for our trucks," he wrote his wife and friends. He pleaded with them to raise both awareness and money and in fact likely survived the explosion that tore apart his vehicle because he was wearing body armor that his family had bought and sent to him.

Gary lived through the explosion, which sent shrapnel tearing through his head. He lost one eye, and his vision in the remaining eye was compromised. His right hand was also badly injured in the explosion, with two fingers traumatically amputated and one other taken off by the emergency surgical team because it was too mangled to control blood loss. He experienced injury to his brain, primarily on the right side, leading to some problems of motor coordination and affect management.

"But I can live with this all," he told the counselor running a support group a year later. "Or I could if the Army didn't make it so hard for me to live with it." Gary identified his trauma not as the explosion but as what happened before and after. He described the explosion as a predictable hazard of being in a war zone, "But the Army didn't care what happened to reservists. They just sent us out there with old equipment and let us get blown up. Then they treat you like garbage when you get home." Because disparate treatments are available to reserve as opposed to regular Army members, Gary's health care when he returned home was not of good quality, and he had difficulty accessing care that allowed him to live close to home and family. All of this complicated his experience of becoming a person with disabilities. "I look at my face," he said, "And I'm reminded of all the letters I wrote asking for better truck armor." His wounds and his functional incapacities were annoying to him by and of themselves, but because they served as visible, palpable, and inescapable reminders of betrayal they were painful and traumagenic for him in a distinctive manner.

Gary's story illustrates the importance of understanding what a loss-related disability represents to a person. Many individuals who experience the losses attendant on acquired disability experience mourning, and many are individuals who can draw on extant inner and outer resources for the development of coping strategies that are protective against a posttraumatic emotional outcome. When the loss and resulting disability are constant reminders of an experience of targeting or betrayal, those interpersonal violations of safety may come to emotionally trump the actual experience of loss of safety or health. Other identities held by a person may ameliorate or aggravate this process as well. George, who was discussed earlier in this chapter, had his difficulties aggravated by issues of social class status; as a working-class man with little sophistication about health care systems he lacked knowledge as to how to deal with the denial of health care. Persons with disabilities who have excellent health care coverage and skills in working systems are less likely to encounter traumas of betrayal because their preexisting resource structure acts as a protective factor.

When a person who already has a disability is exposed to trauma, these factors will intersect as well. The deaths of a number of people with disabilities during Hurricane Katrina occurred because people's usual systems of care were destroyed by the storm; for example, ventilators could not operate without electricity, and people sitting in wheelchairs drowned by rising waters because no one had developed evacuation plans that included their needs (Karam, 2006).

Sometimes being a visible person with a disability leads to bias-based violence. David, a Euro-American heterosexual man in his early 40s had retinitis pigmentosa, a progressive eye disease; at the time he started therapy he could see colors and shapes but was otherwise visually impaired. He used a cane to assist him in getting around and was in the process of applying for an assistance dog. He was divorced, dating, and worked as a human resources administrator at an architectural firm. One day on his way to the bus stop he was accosted by a group of adolescent young men who screamed epithets at him, grabbed his cane, pushed him down to the pavement, and then began to kick him. A passerby witnessed the attack and called the police, who found David dazed on the ground. "I don't know why they were so offended by my blindness," he later said to his psychotherapist, referring to the content of their shouts.

> Becoming blind gradually hasn't exactly been my idea of a good time, but I think I've done a bang-up job dealing with it. I'd never thought that someone would want to hurt me because I was blind. Or maybe it didn't offend them—perhaps they were just looking for a way to humiliate me. I don't know; all I know is that I suddenly feel distinctly unsafe out there. I told my girlfriend that I should get a pit bull for an assistance dog, and I'm not sure I'm joking.

Other persons with disabilities describe experiencing themselves as more vulnerable to this sort of random assault because the visibility of their disability (e.g., the use of an identifiable assistive device such as a cane, wheelchair, or walker) communicates more vulnerability to predatory violent strangers.

In David's case the trauma had been linked by his attackers' words to his disability. However, trauma occurring in the life of a person with a disability may be simply random and either complicated or made more manageable by the existence of disability. Heather had lived with cystic fibrosis her entire life. A Euro-American woman in her mid-20s, she was driving to meet a date when her car was hit from the side by a vehicle whose driver had fallen asleep at the wheel. She was trapped in the wreckage for several hours and came out with broken legs, a broken arm, cracked ribs, and a mild concussion; she experienced few emotional consequences other than great annoyance at the total loss of a car she loved and had spent time customizing.

Her friends, who included a psychotherapist, were unsurprised by her response to the accident.

> Look, I was supposed to die before I got to 20, so I'm in extra innings. And heck, hospitals are like my second home. I know how to be in a hospital. Broken bones, hah! They don't kill you. Now I have an excuse to be dopey (referring to her concussion), I can get away with stuff.

As a result of Heather's life-long experience of living with disability and chronic illness, she had developed an attitude that allowed her to experience the motor vehicle accident as an unfortunate but not life-threatening blip in her existence. "Hey, the respiratory psychotherapist cracked my ribs when I was 7. Now *that* was scary, let me tell you. This hurts, but I've got some great drugs for that."

THERE BUT FOR FORTUNE:
DISABILITY AND COUNTERTRANSFERENCE

Stigma is often associated with disability, as it is with trauma, and as with trauma, people, including psychotherapists, avoid persons with disability as a strategy for managing their own sense of vulnerability and their unspoken knowledge that being able-bodied is truly a fragile state. Culturally competent practice requires psychotherapists to confront their own ableism and internalized ableism. They can begin with their use of language; how often do psychotherapists thoughtlessly use the slang term *lame* to refer to someone being foolish or *blind* to speak of someone being thoughtless? Colloquial American English is replete with terms that associate forms of disability with devaluation. Psychotherapists can look at how and if they relate to people with disabilities, especially visible disabilities; after race, disability is one of the most powerful segregating factors in American culture today; do psychotherapists know such individuals only as clients or as colleagues and friends? Disability rights activists in psychology such as Rhoda Olkin (1999; Olkin & Taliaferro, 2006) have noted that for most practicing psychologists, people with disabilities are compartmentalized into the client category, with all of the pathologizing implications of that assignment.

Adopting the concept of being temporarily able-bodied as part of one's own identity if one is still TAB can be a powerful intervention in a psychotherapist's own ableism because it foregrounds the reality that one's current able-bodied status is unpredictably mutable. For those psychologists who, like me, have disabilities that are invisible, willingness to come out about the disability also contributes to undermining ableist assumptions and allows one to be privy to the ableism of others.

A brief vignette from my own experience illustrates this last point. I have a moderate case of multiple chemical sensitivity (MCS; Gibson, 2000). When I am exposed to a long list of airborne substances I experience neurological symptoms including transient cognitive difficulties, irritability, muscle spasticity due to nerve misfiring, and sleepiness. During my worst episode, the nerve to my vocal chord went into seizure mode for several months, disabling me from speaking and requiring the use of an assistive device in the form of an electronic larynx to conduct psychotherapy.

When I approached my first term on the American Psychological Association's (APA's) Council of Representatives, I asked a staff person at APA to send a request to the Council membership to refrain from wearing some of those substances (perfumes, colognes, aftershaves, and other highly scented products) to the meeting. She obliged and without identifying me as the source of the request put that information in a premeeting letter to Council members.

On the second day of the meeting, I was sitting at my seat in front of 2 other members and thus overheard the discussion of some "crazy person who wanted us not to wear scents. Some kind of somaticizing disorder, I would imagine." I took a deep breath, turned around, and said, "That would be this crazy person. Thanks for leaving your scents at home." I smiled; they had the grace to look embarrassed; and we went on. Luckily, I am a person with considerable resilience in the face of this sort of ableist attitude and can have a sense of humor when exposed to such low-level bias in action. I was less amused several years later when a campus administrator revoked my accommodations for MCS on the grounds that my need to have a scent-free workplace was "a preference, not a disability," despite a letter from my physician. I was then forbidden to ask any coworker or student to refrain from exposing me to substances that would disable me.

I have the educational and social class privilege to have been able to quit that job, and I had excellent other alternatives, which I proceeded to pursue. The experience was stressful and annoying, not traumatic. However, many people with disabilities who encounter this kind of insidious trauma daily have neither those options nor the social class privilege that informs my sense of entitlement. Their experiences of feeling trapped and powerless create the reality of being traumatized. Psychotherapists working with people with disabilities can enhance cultural competence through attention to the pervasiveness of ableism and its role as a potential source of trauma.

I next turn to social locations that are less embodied, yet no less powerful. I have alluded repeatedly to the interaction of poverty and social class status with sex, phenotype, age, sexuality, and ability as factors contributing to the experience of and response to trauma and take that as my starting point for an examination of these more socially created components of identity.

10

THE GREAT DIVIDE: TRAUMA AND SOCIAL CLASS

In this chapter, I discuss the various definitions and expressions of social class status, examining both socioeconomic status and the possession of social capital as aspects of social class. Passing and assimilation as response to classism and shame are explored. The role of poverty in greatly increasing risk of trauma exposure is examined.

Social class is the great hidden aspect of social location in the United States, one that is hidden in psychology's discourse as well (Lott & Bullock, 2006). Many people living in the United States today were raised to see it as an explicitly classless society, held up in admiring contrast to the highly socially stratified worlds of Europe from whence the original European invaders of this continent came. A discourse of classlessness has had several functions. First, it has operated to obscure the realities of income disparities in the United States, particularly disparities within the broad swath of the population that self-identifies as middle class. Second, it has functioned to cast shame and stigma on the poor, especially those who are chronically caught in poverty, with all of the social and emotional distancing associated with stigma (Lott, 2002). Third, it has upheld the American narrative of rugged individualism, the notion that any one person by her- or himself can "pull oneself up by the bootstraps" and obtain a higher social status and income. This narrative implies the converse as well, that those not successful financially have failed to exercise initiative, work hard, or seek success and are thus solely at fault for their poverty or financial struggles. Finally, the discourse of a class-free society obscures the power resting in the hands of the very rich by making them invisible except as objects of prurient interest in gossip media and thus obscures the extreme difference in resources available to rich people and poor people.

In the past decade this discourse of the classless society has begun to crumble. Some of this reflects social forces at work since the early 1980s. Much of the classlessness narrative of the middle 20th century was derived from the post–World War II successes of unions and the continuing effects of the policies of the New Deal and then the Great Society. Each of these social phenomena had the temporary effect of smoothing out economic differences among social classes by creating more equitable distribution of income and by ensuring good wages for blue-collar unionized workers. Generous veteran's educational and housing benefits available to returned troops of World War II and the Korean War had similar impacts on the landscape of American life.

But with the election of Ronald Reagan and the ascendancy in American politics of social forces whose credo has been the reduction of spending on social programs, education, and health care, the gains made in income equalization have become slowly but surely unraveled, to the extent that discussion of social class advantage and disadvantage are now part of the public domain, with media pundits opining about a "war on the middle class." During the past almost 3 decades many of the social programs that allowed movement within levels of income and education have been undercut or destroyed, leaving poor and working-class people with decreasingly few options for changing their economic circumstances. Unions have shrunk, and the percentage of the workforce represented by unions has diminished in tandem. Because of free trade agreements, formerly well-paying working-class factory jobs have disappeared, with work shipped to developing countries where labor can still be cheaply exploited. Classism also directly affects access to educational resources in the classroom (Lott & Bullock, 2006); because school districts in the United States are tax supported at the local level, poor communities have less money to spend on education than do wealthy ones. As the costs of postsecondary education have risen, funding for students to obtain such education has fallen; more students start college today, but a smaller percentage complete it, and most of those who do succeed in obtaining a bachelor's degree emerge laden with debt. In tandem with the increased frequency of discourse about class in the general media, psychologists are also attending more to the issue of social class, exploring both why it has been neglected and how it affects people's well-being (Lott & Bullock, 2006).

Historically, psychology has been most concerned with mental health issues as they pertain to very poor people and has had some impact as a discipline in reducing stigma associated with poverty (Bullock, Wyche, & Williams, 2001). But *classism*, defined by Bullock (1995) as "the oppression of poor people through a network of everyday practice, attitude, assumptions, behaviors, and institutional rules" (p. 119), as well as *internalized classism*, the presence of bias against oneself for being poor, persists among psychotherapists. Classism is not reserved only for the poor; it also affects people who are working class. This is in part because working-class people frequently live on the slippery slope that can lead to poverty. Because trauma exposure is often implicated in a person's economic difficulties, attitudes toward people of other than middle-class status can infiltrate and negatively affect psychotherapy with trauma survivors. Trauma exposure can undermine a person's shaky status in the middle class, leading internalized classism and classist oppression to become contributing factors in the posttrauma experiences of a survivor.

Social class in the United States does not exist separately from other social locations. Because of racism, sexism, heterosexism, ageism, and ableism and their individual and collective impacts on access to economic resources, education, and high-paying work, social class is not evenly distributed across all groups in American society, nor is absence of social desirability ascribed to working or poverty-class status evenly distributed either. Larger percentages of communities of color in the United States live in the working or poverty classes, although the bulk of working- and poverty-class people are Euro-American. Classist bias thus is frequently tinged by racism, because racist bias often contains classist assumptions. Women are more likely to be poor than are men with similar levels of education because jobs at all levels tend to pay women less than men. Poor women are also more likely than poor men to be parents, which means that poor women's challenges in obtaining material resources affect not only themselves but their children. Research on lesbian, gay, and bisexual (LGB) people shows that holding steady such factors as years of education and other demographic variables, LGB people earn significantly less annual income than their heterosexual counterparts. People with disabilities are disenfranchised from the workforce; if people access government disability benefits, they are constrained from making more than a small amount of additional money, often forcing people with disabilities into the choice between medical coverage linked to disability benefits or entering a workforce in which their medical care needs are unlikely to be met. Age discrimination in employment affects many people under 18 and over 55; children are more likely to be in poverty than any other demographic age group. Thus a range of other forms of oppression operate to conflate poverty and near-poverty status with other target social locations. The stigma and negative biases associated with membership in these other target groups accrue to the stigma associated with poverty or being working class.

Social class has a circular relationship with trauma. People who are poor or working class are more likely to have exposures to some kinds of trauma and also less likely to have the resources with which to respond to a trauma when it does occur. In fact, extreme poverty in the United States means almost certain exposure to endemic forms of trauma such as violence and dangerous housing conditions; if one is poor in this country, trauma of some sort may well be inescapable. Middle- and upper-middle-class people, whose class status is largely dependent on continued participation in the paid workforce, are vulnerable to economic disruptions catalyzed by the aftermath of trauma exposure in ways that very wealthy people, whose financial well-being is not related to their ability to appear at work regularly, are not. Disruption in earning capacity can lead to a fall in class status, which can be experienced by and of itself as traumatic depending on what that class status represents emotionally to individuals and their culture.

Although the film *House of Sand and Fog* (Perelman, Dubus, & Otto, 2003) is also a commentary on immigration and social dislocation, it is largely about how social class and trauma are interrelated. One of the main characters is an Iranian man who has lost his social class status and been forced to flee to America after the 1979 Islamic Revolution; although he works as a day laborer and as a clerk at an all-night gas station, he finds the notion of having his actual poverty exposed so painful that he eventually commits terrible crimes and then kills himself, rather than have the reality of his poverty exposed. The other main character, impoverished because she is a practicing alcoholic and exposed to homelessness and violence as a result, is so undermined in her functioning by the loss of resources and home that she too descends into violence.

Ironically, wealthy people are at some risk of having their trauma exposures ignored or perceived as inconsequential given the apparently shielding effects of financial privilege; the trauma of wealthy individuals can be trivialized or minimized with sometimes deadly consequences (Wolfe & Fodor, 1996). Grethe exemplified that conundrum. She was raised in an upper-class Swedish family, married an older and also wealthy man, and came with him to the United States as a young woman pregnant with her first child when he accepted a job as a manufacturer's representative. Not long after her daughter was born her husband began to beat her. The physical abuse, and accompanying verbal and emotional abuse, continued for the entire 30 years of their marriage. One time she called the police, who came through the guardhouse of her gated community to find her urbane, smiling husband telling them that there had been a misunderstanding. The terrible beating Grethe received after that episode convinced her never to call them again. Her physicians never asked her about her bruises; although all of them worked in a medical community with a high degree of awareness of domestic violence (DV), her wealth and European background seemed to make the violence she was experiencing invisible. She was treated for 15 years by a psychiatrist who tried a variety of antidepressant medications with little success. Finally, after seeing a popular television show on which a famous woman spoke of her own DV history, Grethe felt emboldened to reveal her experience to her psychiatrist. He immediately transferred her care, commenting that he knew nothing about DV. In her work with her subsequent therapist, she processed how abandoned and invisible she had felt. "I am the bird in the golden cage," she said one day. "Lovely designer cage, carpeted with thorns. But all anyone could see were the golden bars."

Culturally competent psychotherapy is conscious of and attends to issues of social class and interrogates it in a complex and sophisticated manner that includes an understanding of both the monetary and nonmonetary aspects of social class status. It is important to note that when working with survivors of any sort of trauma the contribution of class and classism to the experience is used as one means of deepening understanding of the experience of trauma exposure.

WHAT CLASS?

Current critical thinking about class suggests that social class status derives from a person's location on two nonparallel continua and is not simply a matter of income or financial resources. The first is the continuum of actual income or access to real capital resources such as current income, savings, inherited wealth, and other aspects of net financial worth. The second, which can be equally meaningful and is quite powerful psychologically, is the continuum of what has been referred to by some authors as *symbolic* or *cultural capital*. Symbolic capital refers to a person having attitudes, behaviors, values, and knowledge that are associated with education and higher class status or a family history of these. Thus, for instance, a person who is currently living in poverty as a result of a posttraumatic inability to work but who attended an Ivy League college and has an advanced degree is not simply a poor person; she or he is a person with mixed-class status, which can create attendant confusion and shame or attendant resilience and feelings of entitlement. She or he is also a poor person who knows how to work systems, how to dress for job interviews, and how to write a resume and a poor person likely to have contacts with college friends who can help network her or him to a job when she or he is ready.

Conversely, the person who grew up very poor, never attended college, did very well in his work, and is now well-off financially and who, because of an absence of education, lacks sophistication about art and music or which fork to use at a formal dinner, is not simply a wealthy person, she or he is also someone of mixed-class status, which may also lead to confusion and shame. Coffey (2005) noted that "it is unlikely that upward mobility of persons from a lower class to an upper class will be comfortable, or the actual change in financial status will result in a fully realized transformation of class status" (p. 12).

The many psychotherapists who are themselves the beneficiaries of cultural capital have little awareness of the advantage it gives them in their professional education and practice until they encounter colleagues, all capable and intelligent people, who seem confounded by the things that middle-class and upper-middle-class people take for granted. I'm one of those formerly obtuse psychotherapists. Because of my own family's mixed-class status (my parents grew up poor as children of immigrants, went to college and became middle class, and raised their family in an upper-middle- to upper-class neighborhood), I never saw myself as having advantage. The fact that in my public school I could choose to study any one of six languages, take advanced placement courses, and be coached continuously from fourth grade onward about what I needed to do to apply to college and graduate or professional school was simply the reality of life as I knew it. I felt shame because my mother did not know how to dress correctly, understanding only as an adult that she dressed like the working-class woman she had been raised to be and not like the upper-class mothers of many of my schoolmates. So I aspired to look and sound like the teachers and scout leaders who, in retrospect, were those who demonstrated the most markers of upper-middle-class status; their accents, their ways of dressing, their styles of affect expression were all what I emulated.

After attending a small private undergraduate school where most of my peers were from the parallel universe of the Jewish-majority suburbs of cities east of St. Louis, I was accepted into a doctoral program where I met, for the first time, people who lived in trailers. One of my classmates had grown up in a trailer and was pleased and thrilled that the one she was able to rent in Carbondale was larger and more modern than the ones she had inhabited as a girl. I can look back now with embarrassment and compassion on my response to this; why, I wondered, would anyone live in a trailer? When this same classmate struggled with what seemed obvious to me about writing a paper or giving a talk in front of the class, I had no framework for comprehending that she was struggling with class issues. I noticed that her styles of dress and makeup reminded me of my mother's and told myself that my discomfort with my classmate was just a transference-like phenomenon. I did not know then that I was being classist.

Because of this complexity of the meanings of social class, culturally competent practitioners engage the topic best by asking their clients about the economic and educational realities of their lives, both in childhood and adulthood in a descriptive way that will invite information and decrease associated shame. Bullock (Lott & Bullock, 2006) noted the surprise of her college students when she, a Euro-American college professor, revealed to them that although she grew up mostly in the middle class she also spent some time growing up in poverty, intermittently homeless and dependent on welfare payments to survive. Her story exposed the realities of class in America; people do not always spend their lives entirely in one social class location, and middle-class status is a fragile phenomenon for many, even those people who are highly educated as were Bullock's attorney father and social worker mother. Asking clients about whether family income was just enough, less than enough, more than enough, or changed at times, can be a useful strategy for eliciting information about class status in a nonstigmatizing manner. Gathering information about the educational levels and occupations of primary caregivers is also a useful source of data; asking about both formal and practical education will make the picture of social class origins for clients more complete (Wyche, 1996).

The apparent mutability of social class status, especially in the United States, sometimes leads to a discourse about the undeserving nature of poor or working-class people. America's radical individualism preaches that if people are poor it is because they have not worked hard enough or been willing to try hard enough and are lazy or quitters. As Baker (1996) noted, class status, dissimilar to phenotype or sex, superficially appears to be easily changeable through hard work, education, or some combination of both. When trauma enters into this equation and affects a person's ability to work, learn, or participate either in upward mobility strivings or maintain current levels of income, the stigma associated with lower social status becomes woven into the experience of trauma.

Because so many psychologists and other psychotherapists are themselves middle-class persons, they often fail to appreciate the degree of privilege attendant on their class status, similar to the way in which psychotherapists and other persons of European descent often do not see the White-skin privilege that makes life easier. Middle- and upper-middle-class people do not only have financial means. They also are possessed of cultural and symbolic capital that allows for certain assumptions about safety, control, and access to medical, psychological, and educational resources that are not readily available, or available at all, to working class or poor people. Those psychologists who grew up poor and working class and have, through education, moved financially and professionally into a different class status than that of their raising may experience themselves as imposters or frauds not deserving of being taken seriously (Coffey, 2005).

CLASSISM AND THE HIDDEN WOUNDS OF CLASS

Classism, the stigma associated with poverty and working-class status and the overvaluation of wealth and middle-class status, is the form of oppression powering insidious trauma for people who are poor and working class. Like other forms of hierarchical devaluation, classism is ubiquitous and conveyed in a myriad of ways. There are almost as many ways for it to wound people and function as a trauma.

An excellent example of classism at work has to do with the differential value assigned to different sorts of governmental benefits. Money given to poor parents and their children to ensure basic needs for those children such as housing, food, and medical care is generally stigmatized; *welfare*, the umbrella term under which this sort of funding is discussed, is part of a social narrative of laziness, absence of initiative, and unearned entitlement. When in 1996 the Congress passed so-called welfare reform, the ironically named Personal Responsibility and Work Opportunity Reconciliation Act (1996), the emphasis of this reform was to require the poorest mothers to work outside the home for low pay and place their children in the care of strangers. The message conveyed was if one is responsible and works hard then one will not be poor.

Classism denies the presence of institutionalized obstacles to economic well-being and justice; these obstacles can be sources of insidious trauma while the poor person is blamed as the cause of her or his own problems. Caroline is a Euro-American woman in her late 30s. Her parents were college educated; her father, an aeronautical engineer, lost his job in the downsizing of the aerospace industry, and her mother had worked at home as a parent and homemaker for no pay. Her father was never able to find professional employment after being laid off in his mid-40s and had a series of temporary jobs; her mother found work as a retail salesperson. Savings for Caroline's college education were depleted to keep up mortgage payments. She finished high school and went to work as a waitress. There she met and became pregnant by one of the cooks; the pair did not marry, and when their son was 1-year-old they separated. Unable to find adequate childcare, she applied for welfare so that she could support her son.

Over the intervening 12 years Caroline was on and off welfare. When she was on welfare she made money under the table by babysitting to make ends meet. She returned to waitress work when her son entered kindergarten, working less well-paying day shifts where the tips were smaller so that she could be home when he returned from school. During those times when she was off welfare she had no medical coverage for herself, and she would often go to work ill or hurting.

One day at work she slipped and fell on a floor where someone had spilled cooking grease; she injured her back so badly that she could not keep working. Worker's compensation payments covered only two thirds of her actual wage and did not take into account the considerable contribution of tips to her income; thus her actual cash flow was cut by two thirds, not one third. The compensation system paid for some of the medical care required to treat her injuries, but as her pain and disability persisted over several months she was sent to an independent medical examiner who pronounced her malingering and told the state that she was fit to return to work. Worker's compensation cut off her payments. While she had been on worker's compensation she became ill with flu, which deteriorated into pneumonia because the steroidal antiinflammatory medications that she was on had, unbeknownst to her, severely depressed her immune response system. When she finally went to an emergency room for care the physician wished to hospitalize her for intravenous antibiotics, but knowing that she had no health insurance and no one to care for her son she refused and went home with oral medications.

When required to return to work Caroline was still coughing from her bout with pneumonia and in pain from her back injury. She lasted 1 day at the job, quit, and went back on welfare. At that point she was also 3 months behind on her rent, in debt to the hospital for her care and medications, and dispirited about ever being able to get ahead. She became depressed. Creditors called multiple times a day about her past due bills, and she was threatened with eviction from her apartment. Eventually she and her son moved in with a friend of hers from work who allowed them to sleep on her couch while Caroline was applying for low-income housing.

When Congress passed welfare reform, Caroline was informed that she had a time frame during which she had to become employed; she had to demonstrate that she was attempting to get work or have her current benefits reduced by a certain amount each month. By that time Caroline had been living with chronic pain and depression for several years; she had received treatment for neither. Although she had medical coupons since returning to welfare, her requests for pain medication had been viewed with suspicion as "drug-seeking behavior," and the only treatment available for depressed people who used coupons was case management and antidepressants. She found the former demeaning, describing some of the case managers as being "kids like I used to be, middle-class brats who don't know any better. I think I would have been just as cruel if I hadn't had my life experiences." The latter had side effects that were difficult for her to tolerate. It was ironically because of her difficulties complying with the demands of the welfare-to-work program in which she had been enrolled that she finally received access to psychotherapy, which was being mandated for the noncompliant participants in that program.

Caroline's story illustrates the hidden but daily insidious wounds of poverty. Because health care in the United States is not universal, poor people are caught in no-win sets of bad choices; go without, as a member of the working poor, or have access to medical care that often comes with a ration of stigma including restricted access to mental health care and some kinds of medical care (recall George's story in chap. 9, this volume, of losing access to his antispasmodic medication because it was not on the list of those for which he could be reimbursed). Ill health can lead to financial reverses, financial reverses to loss of housing, loss of housing to risk of exposure to unsafe situations, and all of the these factors to trauma exposure. The concatenation of experiences that is systemically present for poor people in the United States resists the efforts of all but the most hard-working, personally responsible, and optimistic poor people. All the while, the stigma associated with poverty plays in the psychological and psychosocial background.

INTERNALIZED CLASSISM

Internalized classism also leaves it marks on the psyche (Russell, 1996). As Coffey (2005) noted, the experience of being *fake* shared by many people who grew up working class or poor and who have achieved professional status through education is accompanied by a range of psychological distress including high levels of anxiety and self-doubt and fears of becoming exposed to professional peers as not being really middle class. Additionally, because of the inequitable distribution of educational resources across the social class spectrum, the achievement of higher education is itself more difficult for many poor and working-class persons. These difficulties are often coded through internalized classism as evidence of being stupid or intellectually inferior to classmates raised by college-educated parents in school and home settings that were rich in education resources.

Helen's story illuminates this phenomenon. Her parents, Slovakian American children of immigrants had less than high school educations and had divorced when she was young. She lived with her mother, who worked as a housekeeper at a local hotel; the family struggled financially. Her mother had 4 young children with 2 different fathers. She did well in her public schools in a lower income urban neighborhood, but her classes left much to be desired, and her teachers frequently communicated to her and other students that they would be unlikely to attend college. She left high school after 10th grade and worked in fast food restaurants to help support her mother and 4 younger siblings, none of whose fathers contributed to the family's finances for long.

In her 20s, after her youngest sister had started high school, Helen, with the support and at the urging of her parish priest, started to take classes at the local community college and got her general equivalency diploma. She continued on to earn an associate's degree, experiencing mounting anxiety as each term passed and she continued to do well academically; she was "waiting for the other shoe to drop," as she commented later, certain that she was insufficiently intelligent to succeed in the nursing program she had entered. She struggled with writing, grammar, and punctuation, subjects that her school had given short shrift; her study skills were absent as well, all of which appeared to validate her view (and those of her high school teachers) of herself as academically incapable. Her mother was critical of her efforts, complaining that Helen was going to think that she was too good for the family now that she had exceeded everyone else's educational accomplishments and expressing irritation that Helen was preoccupied with her studies instead of working more hours.

At a meeting with her mentor the priest Helen broke into tears. "I'm a bad daughter," she said to him, "and who *do* I think I am anyhow? I'm just faking it. I'm going to fail my nursing exam and disappoint all of you. I should just quit now." Her priest comforted her, telling her that she was indeed honoring her mother by staying in school "even if your mom can't see it that way just yet." He also connected her with another mentor in the form of a friend, a woman who had formerly belonged to a religious order, who had herself struggled with internalized classism on her path from poverty. Much like Helen, she too had made great efforts to attain her position as the assistant dean of a local private Catholic college. That woman also recognized Helen's intelligence and interpersonal talents and challenged her to go beyond her associate's degree. She held Helen's hand, literally and symbolically, through the last 2 years of college and onward to Helen's doctorate in psychosocial nursing, coaching her about how to write, do research, speak, and dress, and spending time with Helen and her family helping to assuage her mother's concerns.

As Helen told me, her friend, many years later,

> If Father Jim had responded any other way at all I would have dropped out that moment and gone back to supervising the late shift. It was so incredibly painful, the voice inside me that said that I was a fraud and a phony. My mom didn't really know better; she was afraid that she would lose me, and she was doing what she knew to do to keep me close. And she was afraid I'd get hurt, that I didn't have what it took and would just be bashing my head against the wall. Rosemarie was just as essential; she taught me not to be ashamed of what I didn't get and helped me learn how to get it. But it still scares me to death when I have to present at a conference; the ghost of my inner imposter shows up every time. So I've started doing eye-movement desensitization and reprocessing to deal with that, because I'm tired of being that anxious about my accomplishments.

Helen had luck; she had rich human resources in the form of her priest and her mentor who helped her to fill in the pieces that were missing from her secondary education and who gave her the emotional support that she needed to navigate the complexities of becoming the only doctoral professional in her family. Even with that remarkable assistance she continued to experience anxiety; although no one, including Helen, would call that distress posttraumatic stress disorder (PTSD), in it were the echoes of how internalized classism and the institutional wounds of class served as forms of insidious trauma for her earlier in life.

CLASS: THE NOT-SO-HIDDEN WOUNDS

Poor people also experience the real traumas of risk to basic needs. Poverty can mean going without dependable food, shelter, medical care, or adequate clothing. The numbers of poor people who chronically are in a state of food-related risk has grown in the past decade, with the federal government reporting that in 2002 meals were skipped as a result of lack of money for food in 12 million American families (Lott & Bullock, 2006). In a median cost American city a wage earner must take in more than double the minimum wage to afford market-rate housing, and in hot urban markets affordable housing is being razed and replaced with expensive housing at rates that endanger the viability of those other than middle class (Lott & Bullock, 2006). Housing for poor people is additionally often situated in locations that are physically unsafe because of the presence of toxins in the soil and water, current dumpsites or incinerators, and other forms of environmental hazard (Allen, 2001). According to the *Diagnostic and Statistical Manual of Mental Disorders* (4th ed., text rev.; *DSM–IV–TR*; American Psychiatric Association, 2000) definition of trauma as a threat to life or personal safety, then for many poor people life is a continuous series of potential exposures to trauma related to basic needs.

Poverty increases the risk of exposure to violence in one's immediate surroundings. Poverty is associated with homelessness, which increases the likelihood of exposure to random violent acts by strangers because of the loss of control over one's physical environment. Poverty makes natural disasters more disastrous; having savings and credit cards means that one can find a hotel room to stay in and rent a place to live while one's storm-damaged home is repaired. Having little or no financial margin in the same circumstances means living six to a motel room or in a Federal Emergency Management Agency trailer, with little hope of being able to afford the restoration of one's home.

Poverty is not per se a traumatic stressor; people can live in the poverty and working classes and be joyful and completely emotionally functional. However, the potential for poverty to be a powerful and pervasive risk factor for the range of traumatic stressors is something that needs to be taken into account in a psychotherapist's process of assessing a client's total trauma exposure. The fragility of the social matrix that supports good functioning for poor people can be exposed when trauma of the *DSM–IV–TR* Criterion A type appears and sweeps that social matrix away. If, like racism, psychotherapists consider poverty and the threat of poverty to serve as insidious traumata that can effectively widen a person's vulnerability to other traumatic stressors at any time then their assessment of their clients' suffering and of the resources available to their clients for the amelioration of that suffering will become more culturally competent.

CLASS PLUS TRAUMA EQUALS DIFFERENTIAL IMPACT

The experience of being poor or working class intersects with each and every other aspect of a person's multiple identities to affect how an individual will be affected by trauma exposure. Differential access to resources means differential capacities to respond when trauma happens. Even if someone has changed economic status over her or his lifetime, the memory of poverty may give different meaning to the occurrence of trauma. To understand the impacts of class on the experience of trauma the culturally competent psychotherapist considers both of these variables.

An individual who grew up with not enough or barely enough financial resources is likely to retain a consciousness of scarcity that trumps any current-day realities of apparent economic plenty. For this person, threats to income as a result of trauma exposure will be potentially experienced as more threatening than for a similar person raised in economic safety. Class privilege leaves people with a perception that no matter what the nature of current economic circumstances there is likely to be enough to meet their needs at the end of the day: This belief structure often reflects the fact that they will have access to family sources of capital or have economic resources that are not dependent on their earning a living.

Erin, a fourth-generation Japanese American woman, was raised in a wealthy suburb by parents who were both practicing physicians. She attended private schools and graduated from college with no debt because her parents paid her way. They had also invested money in stocks for her every year while she was growing up so that at the age of 25 she had a considerable portfolio. She joined Volunteers in Service to America (VISTA), lived in a shared household with 5 other people, and drove her parents' old car, a 12-year-old luxury vehicle. While attending a party one night she met a man who apparently drugged her drink; she woke to find herself naked, struggling underneath him to free herself from being sexually assaulted.

In the aftermath of this rape Erin became depressed and developed PTSD; she dropped out of her VISTA job. Because one of her housemates knew the man who had assaulted her she began to feel unsafe in the house, not trusting where his loyalties lay. She turned to her parents, who assisted her by paying first and last month's rent on an apartment close to where they lived. They suggested that she consider drawing on the dividends of her stock fund, the presence of which had been background noise to her life previously. As she told her psychotherapist,

> It's such a relief to know that I don't have to go back to work until I'm ready! My parents did a great job of investing for me, and they're so willing to help me out financially. I don't know what I'd do if I had to try to work feeling the way I do now.

Erin's experiences are those of a person with privilege. Families who are poor and working class care no less about their children than do those of privilege, but the reality of scarcer resources or class-based differences in dealing with finances may be interpreted by a psychotherapist who lacks consciousness of class issues as evidence of less care or poorer quality parenting.

Contrast Erin's experience with that of Joan, Erin's Euro-American age peer. On the surface she appeared solidly middle class, but her consciousness was working class. The first in her family to attend college, Joan graduated with a degree in business and was tens of thousands of dollars in debt. Debt was no stranger to Joan; she had grown up watching her parents, a father who drove a cement truck for the county and a mother who worked in a plant nursery, struggling each month to pay bills and make ends meet. Joan described her family as having "just enough to get by—but my folks were always willing to put something on plastic when it was something we really wanted. We always had a new car, and we took trips every summer." Joan lived with a roommate in an apartment and drove a newish car; her job as a mortgage specialist at a bank paid her very well, but she joked that "I'm a normal American. I live on my credit cards."

When Joan was mugged in a parking garage one evening when she got off work and subsequently developed PTSD, she forced herself to go to work despite her debilitating symptoms. "I wasn't sleeping, so I started drinking before I went to bed. Then I couldn't get up." Her work suffered from her tardiness and her inability to concentrate. "But I had to go to work; I was always one paycheck away from being a bag lady." Her first psychotherapist, to whom she was referred by the company's employee assistance plan, suggested that she quit her job and get crime victim's compensation, not thinking about the fact that this fund offered only about one half of what a individual made and that without her job Joan would have no health care coverage for anything except the direct effects of the mugging. "Your family could always help you out," she offered to Joan who, feeling invisible but not knowing why, quit therapy and decided to try to make it on her own.

Approximately 6 months later, with her nightmares worsening and her job on probation she found her way to a psychotherapist who had himself grown up working poor. His cultural competence about class immediately informed the therapy process; when she recounted her previous experience, commenting that she was not sure why her prior psychotherapist had not seemed very helpful, he was able to validate the realities of social class that informed her understanding of what her options were. "You're feeling trapped, aren't you?" he asked her. Indeed, the trauma of the mugging had become magnified by the anticipated trauma of becoming bankrupt and having nowhere to turn. Joan's ability to solve the problems of her financial situation had become impaired by the terror occasioned by her knowledge that the veneer of middle-class status with which she was viewed by the world was thin indeed. She had learned that financial life was lived on the thin margin of debt but had not learned that trauma could push her over that margin or how not to see herself as a failure when she teetered on the edge.

A psychotherapist's awareness of social class issues can assist clients and psychotherapists alike in making sense of what appears to be added perceptions of threat emerging from trauma exposures. Experiences of poverty, and to an even greater extent of living just on poverty's edge, can leave long-lasting impressions that in turn define an experience of trauma as more or less dangerous. The person who now has money but who grew up without it may, in the absence of class consciousness, not understand her or his panic about the possible financial impacts of a trauma; a psychotherapist without an awareness of class may look for some other form of underlying anxiety disorder, pathologizing the response rather than seeing it as a class-informed understanding occurring in the absence of a consciousness of class. Because the American silence on class issues is an obstacle to the development of class consciousness in working- and poverty-class Americans, it can frequently be the job of the culturally competent psychotherapist to raise the issue of social class and to interpret what is troubling the client through the lens of class, assisting the client in developing class consciousness in the process of trauma recovery work.

SOCIAL CLASS AND PSYCHOTHERAPY

Many persons in poverty- and working-class settings will have cultural norms that make it more difficult to seek psychotherapy, even when and if affordable high-quality resources are available. This is not because, as some authors have posited, poor people are less psychologically minded than those in the middle and upper classes. Rather, avoidance of psychotherapy may be due to continuing shame and stigma associated in those social contexts with mental health care. Because those among the poor who receive such services tend to be only the most psychologically impaired and disabled, the problematic synergy of internalized ableism, especially mental health related ableism, with social class barriers can mean that by identifying oneself as suffering emotionally one will run the risk of being perceived as weak or crazy (McNair & Neville, 1996).

Poverty as it intersects with other components of identity also conveys differential social and emotional meanings that can infuse trauma with emotional valence that is not apparent from the details of the traumatic stressor. Among African Americans even highly educated professionals were often materially poor until the gains of the civil rights movement of the last half century. Material poverty was not per se associated with poverty-class status, and material wealth was not necessarily associated with middle- or upper-middle-class status because the effects of systemic racism often separated those two continua. However, the inability to perform one's job, a job that was the symbol of having achieved middle-class status, was especially threatening. Thus a trauma that interferes with vocational capacities, even though actual threat to life or well-being appears relatively low, may be experienced as more severe by a person to whom doing the job well is core and central to a sense of self and safety.

Sherry was an African American woman in her late 30s, divorced and the single parent of an adolescent daughter. Her father had been a mail carrier and her mother an elementary school teacher; Sherry, with a master's degree in social work, was employed as a supervisor for a Head Start program for high-risk children, which required her to travel from one site to another doing evaluations on children and consulting with staff and parents. She loved her work and was proud of her excellent evaluations and feedback from all of the divergent groups that she served. One winter day she slipped and fell on an icy sidewalk, striking her head on the concrete and suffering a brief loss of consciousness.

In the weeks and months following this apparently inconsequential injury Sherry struggled with cognitive problems; she was fatigued, her memory was spotty, and her vocabulary suffered from holes that she could not explain. Her primary care physician told her that she was depressed and put her on a selective serotonin reuptake inhibitor; this made her feel numb but did nothing to improve her difficulties. She began to receive poor performance ratings at work and after 9 months was placed on administrative leave for failing to remediate. Her physician then referred her to a psychologist for psychotherapy; the psychologist, suspecting minor traumatic brain injury, referred her for neuropsychological evaluation. Although the results of the assessment were in the normal range, the evaluator commented that he could see that Sherry was struggling to do as well as she did and that her results, even though normal, were inconsistent with the scores she had made on the Graduate Record Examination a decade earlier. He suggested that Sherry get vocational counseling to retrain into work that required less cognitive capacities than her job had had.

This news appeared to trigger PTSD-like symptoms for Sherry; learning that her slip and fall had led to possibly long-lasting changes that would affect her ability to function as a high-level professional led to a cognitive reappraisal of the event as a life-threatening one. "My work is my life," she told her psychotherapist. "Without it I don't know who I am anymore. I know that Dr. Prakash thinks that there are plenty of jobs that I can do, but I was proud of my work and my contributions." What emerged in her psychotherapy was the degree to which Sherry's job had satisfied elements of cultural identity about giving back to community and sharing her middle-class privilege with less fortunate and more troubled African American families. The issue of income loss was troubling to her; Sherry's job, although middle class in status, paid as poorly as did many other social services jobs. But the theme of how the accident had come to feel traumatic to her was less about money, "My parents will help me out, and I've been thrifty, so I don't have many bills to worry about," and far more about the loss of middle-class identity that involved being a professional and a contributor.

Poverty, which represents the ultimate trajectory of generations of social injustice, can itself feel traumatizing, and poverty can also come to be a component of cultural identity, making its treatment feel like a threat to cultural connection. This complication can most easily be seen in communities with what Duran, Duran, Brave Heart, and Yellow Horse-Davis (1998) have described as "post-colonial syndrome." In indigenous communities, where poverty is endemic, that phenomenon is well-known to be associated with 3 centuries of genocidal violence aimed at indigenous people by European and Euro-American invaders. The tightness with which genocide and poverty are woven together in these communities is such that internalized colonization and poverty have themselves become intertwined and thus a component of ethnic identification for some. In these communities any individual effort to break free of the effects of multigenerational trauma may be experienced as a threat to the community because of a perception that such individual change can bring unwanted and potentially dangerous attention from the dominant culture. Healing and recovery from trauma by one person can ironically be experienced by the extended social network as betrayals of family and culture. When resources are made available in the form of individual psychotherapy they may go unused or be ineffective in the absence of family or culture-wide interventions that address poverty and trauma as end points of genocidal violence against a group. Healing from trauma in these indigenous communities is best conceived of as a systemwide effort. An example of this phenomenon is the community-healing process engaged in by the Alkali Lake band of indigenous people in Canada in which a community where substance abuse and violence were endemic made a collective decision that these results of genocide would no longer be the identity of their community (*The Honour of All: The Story of Alkali Lake*, 1992).

As these examples illustrate, the issue of class is neither simple nor easily seen when it comes to its effects on trauma. Cultural competence around issues of class in psychotherapy means confronting psychotherapists' own classism and internalized classism and being willing to deconstruct the myths about poverty and wealth that pervade American culture. A psychotherapist's own class consciousness or lack thereof can deeply affect cultural competence by making visible or obscuring the contributions of social class experiences to identity. Understanding how realities of resource scarcity and abundance become experienced through the lenses of multiple social locations and acknowledging that current resources may be inconsistent with self-perceptions about what is available will aide both psychotherapists and clients in seeing a client's distress more clearly.

11

MIGRATION AND DISLOCATION

And home sings me of sweet things, my heart there has its own wings.
                                                          —Karla Bonoff

Home is the place where, when you have to go there, They have to take
you in.
                              —Robert Frost (*The Death of the Hired Man*, 1915)

In this chapter, I address the various experiences of dislocation arising from migration. Distinctions are made between experiences of voluntary immigrants and refugees and between legal and undocumented immigrants in their risk for trauma exposure and differential impacts of trauma in the context of immigration. Refugee status as inherently founded in trauma is analyzed, with a brief description of torture survivors among refugees. The issue of trafficked migrants is also discussed.

An immigrant is never completely home. She or he lives someplace where no one has to take her or him in. The sights, smells, and sounds of the place where she or he lives today will always be off, slightly or vastly foreign, no matter how welcoming that place might be. Home, which poets and lyricists tell us is the place in our hearts where we experience ultimate safety and acceptance, is not quite available. As Espin (1992) poignantly documented, being an immigrant is "a constant reminder of what is not there anymore. It is the loss of this . . . that can be most disorienting and most disruptive of the person's previously established identity" (p. 13).

For the voluntary migrant who leaves home in circumstances that are legitimized by the original and host country alike, the loss of home may be bittersweet, yet it is usually associated with choice, agency, and the movement toward desired goals such as education, employment, or economic betterment. The sense of choice is especially enhanced when such goals lead to a sense of heightened accomplishment, increased economic well-being, and greater access to desired resources. When such migrants are of European ancestry and already conversant in English they are particularly likely to be welcomed into the United States, benefiting both from phenotype and linguistic privilege in how they are accepted into U.S. society. But no privilege and none of that choice and welcome protect an immigrant from the experience of disruption of core senses of the self.

As I was completing this chapter the news was published in my local papers of a tragic murder–suicide committed by a disturbed young man who had been stalking his former girlfriend. As the story emerged, readers learned that he was an undocumented immigrant who had already been stopped several times by the police for drunken driving and domestic violence. He was British. Apparently the spurious association in America between a British accent and legitimacy led no one to question his right to live in America (for American-born citizens of Asian or Latino or Latina ancestries and phenotypes such questions are ubiquitous and have at times led to false arrest and imprisonment by immigration authorities when a citizen of these alien ancestries did not have proof of citizenship in hand). In the discussion about this crime on the local National Public Radio station several callers focused on his undocumented status as if it were relevant to what he did. This story has many of the elements of multiple identities and privilege operating; a young, White-skinned man with a valued accent associated with education and upper-class status is treated kindly by the police. When he commits fatal violence, his immigration status is foregrounded as somehow related to his act. Finally one caller, exasperated, reminded the show's host and listeners that domestic violence was domestic violence and that men who kill women in these circumstances do so when they are citizens and documented. No one pointed out that had he been Latino in the same circumstances he would have been far more likely to have been asked to prove the legality of his residency at the time of his initial arrest and sent to the federal detention center, thus prevented from engaging in fatal violence.

When an immigrant is, like the majority of those coming to the United States today, from Asia or Latin America, her or his phenotype and the accent of her or his speech create immediate exposure to tropes of racism in the dominant culture. A person's identity, which may have been formed in dominant groups in the home country and culture, is thrust by immigration into target status, which combines many facets of marginalization and other-izing, both forms of bias, in a way for which no intellectual understanding is likely to prepare a person. Exposure to insidious trauma in the absence of a reference group that has already developed coping strategies, becoming a target of bias and discrimination that are only partially comprehensible because of language and also of subtleties of social customs, and loss of status and career merge with the experience of social and emotional disruption inherent in immigration.

And these are the privileged immigrants; they are legally resident, frequently well educated, and employed and/or with existing family connections; such are the categories through which the bulk of legal immigration to the United States occurs. Some of these persons have a prior history of trauma exposure, which they have contained and managed within the context of home. When one adds other risk factors to the experience of migration, one adds variables that can be traumagenic or that reflect prior experiences of trauma exposure and that can combine to elicit expressions of distress or dysfunctions of behavior that were invisible or absent in the home country.

Other groups of immigrants have less privilege, in part because of prior trauma exposure; their position in relationship to immigration also greatly increases their risk of trauma exposure during the migration process. These other factors include being voluntary but economically disadvantaged; being voluntary but not documented, a group referred to by most people as illegal aliens; being involuntary because of trafficking; being refugees; and being asylum seekers. Members of each of these groups have historically high rates of *Diagnostic and Statistical Manual of Mental Disorders* (4th ed., text rev.; American Psychiatric Association, 2000) Criterion A trauma exposure and are also more vulnerable to trauma exposure once they arrive in the United States because of their frequently marginal and unprotected status in the society. Immigrants are also not a homogeneous group; issues of age, sex, phenotype, social class, and other social location variables interact with immigrant status; anything that creates the potential for trauma risk in those variables will be a part of the mix for an other-than-voluntary-and-legal immigrant. And finally there are issues of immigration histories in the family heritage of a person who is not her- or himself an immigrant yet who carries family trauma dynamics from the generation of immigration. Each of these issues deserves careful consideration by the culturally competent trauma psychotherapist working with immigrants and their families.

A few overarching issues inform culturally competent treatment for almost anyone who is an immigrant. One of these is language. Although a person may master colloquial American English and speak it with little discernable accent, she or he is likely to always be engaging in translation at some level internally, a process that can create the appearance or reality of distance between self and emotion. A colleague of mine illustrates this reality. Raised in Mexico, she has lived in the United States for half of her life and speaks American English without a discernable trace of an accent. Yet she acknowledged, during a discussion about working with students for whom English is a second language in our doctoral program, that for her writing and speaking in English are always accompanied by the nanosecond of hesitation and translation, visible to no one but very much in her own consciousness.

Additionally, each language has its own strategy for representation of emotion and experience, not all of which translates directly or indirectly into American English. As Espin (1992), herself a doctoral psychologist educated in the United States, wrote, "translated feelings like translated poetry are just not the same" (p. 13). A person who has experienced trauma may be unable to describe it in English, or in her or his mother tongue, depending on how that trauma is represented intrapsychically and when it occurred in the life span. Add to this that for many survivors of severe trauma there is persistent alexithymia, the general inability to speak of the feelings of what has happened, and work with an immigrant or refugee trauma survivor will likely require the psychotherapist's ability to go beyond specific language to nonverbal experiences of affect.

Particularly in the post-September 11, 2001, world any immigrants to the United States are under some degree of threat and suspicion, more so if they are, or are believed to be, of Arab descent. Current federal government policies about immigration are very harsh, making it increasingly difficult for legal residents to gain citizenship and the safety from deportation that this usually offers. Adults who arrived in the United States as child immigrants or refugees and who do not speak the language of their country of birth or have any relationship to it are being deported to those places because of the combination of parental failures to obtain citizenship for their children and criminal conviction.

It is relatively simple for a child to be left behind in this way, as I learned from my own family's experience. My maternal grandmother, who had been left in Poland with her own grandparents when her parents immigrated to America, was unbeknownst to her left out of her father's citizenship filing for himself and his family. She arrived in the United States a few years later, was told that she was a citizen (in the days well before green cards and careful documentation), registered to vote at 21, and voted the straight Democratic party ticket in every subsequent election until her death in 1985. It was only in her early 80s when she applied for a passport for the first time to visit her daughter (my mother) in Israel that my grandmother learned that she had never been a citizen of the United States.

Luckily this was 1983; no one tried to deport her to the Poland she had fled; no one charged her with voting fraud. Her congressperson's office rushed her citizenship and passport through in time for her trip. If this had happened in the post-September 11, 2001, world instead of in 1983 she would likely not have received nearly as much compassion or a fast track to the citizenship that she thought she'd had all along. Immigrants today all live in the climate of extreme anti-immigrant sentiment and xenophobia stirred up under current political leadership of the United States and various media outlets. This climate of fear, even when kept strongly in the emotional background by an immigrant, will shape the experience of trauma exposure and affect that person's ability to seek help.

A final overarching issue is that of alienation from the dominant culture of the host country. Today's immigrants do not face the degree of pressure to assimilate and melt into the pot of American culture that earlier generations encountered. This presents both challenges and opportunities. An immigrant to the United States can maintain strong connections to her or his culture of origin should she or he so desire; the foods, clothing, and now television shows of many other lands are available in urban areas, and it is possible to spend one's life in the United States speaking English only in the workplace but nowhere else in life. Such opportunities to remain connected to the sights, sounds, and smells of home can be deeply comforting and a source of self-care. Yet they may also render it more difficult for an immigrant to receive psychological assistance when exposed to trauma. Although many urban areas now have mental health centers where languages of immigrant groups are spoken by therapists or where qualified interpreters are available, not all these individuals wish to be seen by someone in their own small immigrant community because of concerns about shame to the family or risks to confidentiality. An immigrant trauma survivor may thus become more vulnerable if services are either unavailable in their language or the available services feel unsafe.

Psychotherapy itself is alien to many of the cultures from which today's immigrants arrive. Although psychotherapy is becoming increasingly common in many places in the world where it was formerly unknown, it may still represent an alien entity to trauma survivors from cultures in which body, mind, and spirit are not dealt with separately one from the other or in which the concept of psychotherapy is completely alien. For many immigrants who are not European in origin, psychotherapy is yet another aspect of the experience of life in America that is strange and not like home. Mental health treatment may itself feel traumatizing in some ways because it requires certain kinds of emotional exposure and vulnerability in front of a native-born stranger that constitute reexperiencing the vulnerabilities of being *de-skilled* (e.g., losing access to one's adult linguistic and cultural competencies) by the immigration experience itself.

In addition, of course, there is the omnipresent reality that immigrants are never quite home. If home is safety and the achievement of safety is a basic component of recovery from trauma exposure, then the absence of true home in the life of any immigrant must be figured into the equation and addressed by a psychotherapist who is striving for cultural competence. This will be true even when home is the place from which one has fled in terror; in fact, when home is that terrible mixture of the place that "sings of sweet things" and the place where one was tortured or raped or watched one's family murdered, the confusion experienced over the simultaneous yearning for home and fear of anything reminiscent of home will create specific challenges to recovery from trauma of which a culturally competent therapist will be aware. Immigrants who are refugees from war, forced relocation, and genocide are very similar to children abused by family caregivers, with a complex relationship of attachment, love, terror, and danger informing the connection and thus the identities that emerge from that connection.

Dragica was a Bosnian Muslim woman in her early 50s. Before the breakup of the former Yugoslavia she had been a professor of French literature at a well-regarded university. "I was a civilized European," she told her psychotherapist, describing travels to France and Italy for holidays, her wide circle of similarly educated friends, and her generally secular mode of living her ethnicity. "Of course we were Muslim, but not like Arabs; Bosnians are European first." In the civil war and period of ethnic strife that followed the dissolution of Yugoslavia she was thrust into an identification with her religion that felt entirely foreign and frightening to her; she and her husband were chased out of their home in an ethnically mixed neighborhood by armed thugs who beat him into unconsciousness. Living in internal exile in a Bosnian enclave, she witnessed daily shootings and sporadic atrocities before finally using her contacts with a colleague in the United States to obtain formal refugee status. Her husband, an engineer, found work at a large manufacturing firm; because academic jobs were extremely limited in her field and his work was more certain ("these engineers, they all speak the same language," she noted dryly, "numbers") she found sporadic work tutoring high school students in French.

Dragica had experienced much trauma and many losses, but what felt to her like the most traumatizing experience was the way in which other trauma had undermined her identity at its roots. She struggled with her extreme ambivalence about her ethnic identity as a Bosnian.

> The sound of my language is the sound of my mother speaking to me, but it is also the sound of the men who raped my best friend and murdered her husband in front of her eyes. Because we all spoke the same language, you know, Serb and Croat and Bosnian. There are days, weeks even, when the sound of English is the only thing I want to hear because it is so neutral. No comfort, no mother, but no fear. I hear my husband's voice and I feel terror for just an instant.

She felt even more ambivalent about her religious identity.

> At home I could be secular and a Muslim, it was just another religion that no one practiced. Then suddenly Tito dies and it matters to everyone. And here in America the Muslims are Arabs; we have nothing in common. But then the religion you don't practice is still the one that makes sense to you, so what am I? Not a Muslim like these Arab women, but not a Christian either. I am nowhere.

REFUGEES AND ASYLUM SEEKERS

Refugees and *asylum seekers* like Dragica are by definition individuals who have had negative experiences in their native countries. Their decisions to live in the United States, or even where in this county they are located, are not voluntary or based in an autonomously developed desire to leave home. In many cases they departed because they had been expelled, ethnically cleansed, or in some other manner forcibly relocated from the location where they were reasonably content with their lives. Their experiences have been marked by war, death of loved ones, sexual assault, hunger, thirst, and illness; in the case of asylum seekers there has been political persecution that has at times included torture or the direct threat of death. Although refugees usually enter the United States with a status of legal residence, asylum seekers often do not and may become caught up in the web of being defined as illegally residing in the United States. Issues of trauma that led to their flight from home are frequently entangled in their legal difficulties and in culturally competent assessment and treatment necessary for them to be able to stay safe.

Refugees and asylum seekers frequently have such a high level of trauma exposure that clinicians may have difficulty appreciating the range and severity of what has transpired in their lives. Women and children are at particular risk during the refugee experience, with sexual assault during the flight to refuge being so common as to be endemic (Kuoch, Wali, & Scully, 1992). Additionally, data suggests that women who are sexually violated during the refugee experience become devalued in their cultures, leading to increased targeting for intimate partner violence after resettlement.

Today's refugees to America come largely from the developing world where, as noted earlier, mental health services are uncommon and the separation of mental and physical health does not occur. Emotional distress is more likely to be embodied as physical distress. Although psychotherapists also see high rates of illness in dominant culture trauma survivors the meaning of this physical expression of trauma is likely to be different for an immigrant than for a native-born person because the available avenues for the expression of emotional distress will vary. Traumatized refugees from these countries of origin thus are more likely to come to the attention of a psychotherapist through a consultation request from a primary health care provider who correctly suspects that certain physical symptoms are the somatic expressions of trauma exposure.

For example, Van Boemel and Rozée (1992) documented the phenomenon of posttraumatic nonorganic blindness in a group of more than 100 Cambodian women refugees from the Pol Pot genocide. These women were referred to Van Boemel for ophthalmologic diagnosis when no organic cause for their inability to see could be found; each of them had witnessed horrific atrocities, and each then posttraumatically ceased to be able to perceive that which her eyes registered neurologically. A culturally competent consultation in this or similar situations would begin by understanding the ways in which trauma is being somatically expressed and value those as legitimate expressions of pain rather than as something to be discouraged in favor of dominant normative expression of affect.

Asylum seekers represent a particularly high-risk group for trauma exposure among refugees. Many of them have not only been witness and target to widespread forms of persecution and trauma but have also been individually targeted for harm on the basis of specific personal characteristics such as sex, sexual orientation, family or clan membership, or political beliefs. Some asylum seekers have survived torture, extremely cruel and inhuman treatment. They are asking the U.S. government to give them legal resident status on the basis of their traumatic experiences and as part of doing so are required to recount those traumas so as to prove their worthiness for asylum. The reality that many extremely traumatized people may be unable to speak of their maltreatment without becoming too distressed to function is irrelevant to the workings of immigration courts. Because torturers around the world have become increasingly sophisticated in the use of techniques that leave no visible scars (which are often sufficient proof of trauma), psychic wounds from such tortures as waterboarding, pretend execution, nonfatal electrocution, and threats of harm to loved ones are the only evidence of the acts for which the individual is requesting asylum.

Nina came to the United States on a tourist visa, fleeing her African home country where she was held and tortured by government agents for several months after her father had been killed for his activism with an opposition political party. After her visa expired she stayed on in the United States living and working as a virtual slave in the home of a family who were related to her clan. The man of the family repeatedly raped her, and both adults threatened to report her to immigration authorities. Unfamiliar with rules for asylum seeking, depressed and cut off from contact with most people outside the family with whom she was staying, Nina eventually was befriended by a woman she met at church who had herself sought asylum for other reasons and after hearing Nina's story told her about the process of applying for asylum. However, when Nina put in her application she ran into a double bind; she had overstayed her tourist visa and was in the United States illegally, rendering her subject to deportation, and she had also applied too long after the official deadline for application. The immigration authorities arrested and incarcerated her.

Her attorney engaged me to do an evaluation, hoping that I would find something psychological that would assist her in an appeal of the denial of her asylum claim. Nina's posttrauma symptoms did not manifest themselves in a manner that was easily visible to Americans. Neither did her deference to the family that had virtually enslaved her make sense to the court. She was bright, nearly fluent in colloquial English after months of watching American television, and appeared acculturated to American customs of dress and social exchange, which made her claims of ignorance about how and when to file more suspect to the immigration authorities.

I used Aron's (1992) concept of *testimonio*, a strategy developed for eliciting the stories of asylum-seeking victims of state terror and torture in Latin

America, as an assessment tool with Nina. Aron argued that the appearance of neutrality, which is the normal stance of an evaluator, fails at cultural competence with such survivors of trauma by ignoring the moral outrage inherent in torture. What emerged in the process of assessment was Nina's belief that if those authorities knew how much distress she experienced that they would think her a crazy person and deny her residence in the United States. Not understanding the value placed in this culture on the verbal expression of emotional wounding, she had withheld information from everyone about her nightmares and flashbacks of the torture. Because her trauma had been at the hands of a government, she was particularly terrified of making herself known and visible to any government. Her arrest and imprisonment by immigration authorities was a retraumatizing experience for her and even after months in the federal detention center she found herself cowering, awaiting the torture that had not yet come.

Her deference to the clan members in America who had abused and exploited her had been difficult for her attorney to comprehend; "Why would she put up with being treated like that?" she asked me. To Nina, her compliance and deference was a component of her self-care in the face of threat; if she did as they demanded they would not turn her in to the government, which felt far more dangerous to her than any rapes or verbal abuse could ever be. Her apparent acculturation was a thin veneer under which her ways of understanding the world were entirely African. Cultural competence in this instance meant appreciating the likelihood that an asylum-seeking person would have both a very high trauma load and culturally informed ways of communicating about that pain. Although I also administered a Trauma Symptom Inventory to Nina as a means of having objective findings that would be comprehensible in the epistemic systems of an immigration court, what was more important than the outcome of that testing was to be in the presence of someone who did not require her to conform her communications about her distress to American standards.

Both Nina and Dragica were women who sought asylum, one from the developing world, one from Europe. Cultural competence with each of these required attention to the issue in the foreground, which was their experience of dislocation and terror at home, while acknowledging the interplay of all prior and ongoing aspects of identity. Noticing how privilege and disadvantage mingle in the lives of asylum-seeking immigrants can be especially crucial in assisting both psychotherapist and client in making sense of apparent contradictions and disjunctures in their presentations of self and the phenomenology of their distress. Cultural competence in regard to gender, phenotype and its meanings, culture and ethnicity, sexuality, social class, and ability all play a part in understanding how this individual's experience of migration-related trauma is a component of identity and where the resources will exist in that complex identity for resilience and healing.

A NOTE ABOUT WORKING WITH TORTURE SURVIVORS

A complete discussion of the development of clinical and cultural competence with torture survivors is beyond the scope of this volume. Cultural competence at all levels is necessary for doing psychotherapy with this population, as is deep knowledge of the range of modalities for working with trauma, including verbal, somatic, and expressive therapies (Pope & Garcia-Peltoniemi, 1991). Psychotherapists wishing to develop specific competencies in work with torture survivors are encouraged first to hone their other more general capacities for trauma work and culturally competent practice and then to seek specific training and supervision. An extremely helpful and detailed list of resources for working with torture survivors, compiled by Pope, is available at http://kspope.com/torvic/torture.php. Cunningham and Silove (1992) noted the importance of providing a continuum of services to this population because most have both serious physical and serious psychological sequelae of their extreme maltreatment; outside of a coordinated agency setting it can be very difficult to make this full range of services available. However, for the therapist who advertises a special competence in working with trauma the possibility of encountering a torture survivor should be considered within the range of possibilities; if that person has managed to take the risk to seek psychotherapy, a culturally competent response is not to refer the client away but rather to use this opportunity to seek continuing education and supervision to build on extant culturally competent skills at trauma treatment work with immigrants or refugees. Additionally, because in some places persons who are psychiatrists or psychologists have been parts of torture apparatuses, some torture survivors experience members of the mental health professionals as themselves dangerous.

TRAFFICKED PERSONS

Trafficking in humans is occurring at what appear to be growing rates as globalization, poverty and absence of opportunities in developing countries, demand for cheap and exploitable labor in the developed world, and sexualization of children and women all increase the demands for trafficked individuals (Hidalgo, Hopper, & Okawa, 2006). Trafficked people are not bought and sold solely for sexual purposes, although that form of trafficking is best known to the general public and frequently the concepts of being trafficked and prostituted are conflated. However, large numbers of women and men alike are trafficked from the developing world to be used as domestic servants, laborers in sweatshops and restaurants, and in various low-wage, low-skilled industries in which citizens are increasingly unwilling to participate because of low pay and health risks. Trafficked people are almost always undocumented immigrants; in some instances their migration is voluntary, but they have been tricked or betrayed into being trafficked as a means of achieving their desired transit to the United States. In other instances, especially in the case of sexual trafficking, women apply for what they believe to be work as domestic servants or health care aides only to find themselves imprisoned in brothels. Finally, in some developing nations young children are trafficked into prostitution by destitute families whose need is exploited by a so-called sex tourism industry in which men, primarily those from Europe and the United States, travel to the developing world to purchase the opportunity to sexually abuse children and adolescents (Farley, 2003; Freed, 2003).

Trafficked persons are very unlikely to seek psychotherapy services. They usually do not speak English and are often in virtual imprisonment with their movements restricted by their employers/owners. However, some trafficked immigrants do escape and create lives and families, living as do other undocumented immigrants in a constant state of low-level fear about detection and deportation. An unknown subset of this group has U.S.-born children who are themselves citizens; these families are most likely to come to the attention of mental health providers when problems arise in relation to the well-being of those children rather than of the parents.

Because the possibility that an immigrant who enters therapy in this way may have a history of being trafficked or be otherwise undocumented, culturally competent treatment includes an awareness of the traumagenic potential inherent in having personal history exposed to someone who will be perceived, correctly or not, as an agent of a government that is in an adversarial position with the client. Although informed consent and clarity about the bounds of confidentiality are important with every psychotherapy client, spending time and taking care to explicate these constructs with immigrant clients are particularly necessary steps to begin the process of creating the experience of safety in psychotherapy.

An excellent example of where cultural competence can make the difference for traumatized trafficked immigrants is in regard to the issue of mandated abuse reporting. Many psychotherapists today routinely include language in their informed consent document about mandated reporting of child or elder abuse; although this is entirely appropriate to do, as it is a known and legally required violation of confidentiality norms, it is unwise to simply allow an immigrant client to read these words in an informed consent document. The client who already fears that the psychotherapist will function as an agent of the state will simply never return for care. Cultural competence in this instance extends to clear exposition, preferably in a language and communication modality in which the client is most fluent, about the meanings of mandated reporting statutes and the absence of a relationship between the psychotherapist and immigration authorities. Considering other ways in which the usual and customary practices of psychotherapy in dominant U.S. culture might convey risk rather than safety and developing strategies for modifying those practices so as to combine the highest standards of care with cultural sensitivity and competence allow this at-risk group of people to gain access to mental health care when it is needed and if it is desired.

IMMIGRATION AND GARDEN-VARIETY TRAUMA

Until now in this chapter I have explored trauma exposures that are specific to and derived from experiences of immigration. However, once in America an immigrant, whether an upper-middle-class Englishman who has come to be the new CEO of a local corporation or a trafficked Guatemalan peasant woman working as a domestic servant, has all of the usual opportunities for trauma exposure available to any person. When the car accident victim who is also an immigrant arrives in a psychotherapist's office he or she may be a garden-variety client with posttraumatic stress disorder (PTSD) from a single episode of threat to life or he may be a survivor of childhood physical abuse whose coping strategy of high achievement has been undermined by convalescence from the accident. When the car accident victim who is another immigrant arrives in a psychotherapist's office he or she may be the survivor of sexual assault on the journey to the United States whose PTSD is about that assault, not about the accident, or he or she may be someone who has been exploited yet possesses extraordinary resources of character and resilience developed in a loving and safe family of origin to whom he or she feels deeply connected through the remittances he or she sends home and who is now suffering guilt about the decrease in those funds, not any form of PTSD. In short, a reminder that the multiplicity of identities that any trauma survivor brings to psychotherapy will not necessarily tell psychotherapists where the location of the pain is or what texture ripples through the flashback if such a symptom is present. What is core to cultural competence in work with immigrants is that the psychotherapist remain cognizant of how even the most dominant culture person experiences disruptions as a result of dislocation, no matter how voluntary, no matter how easily accomplished, and no matter how positive and successful the outcome; considering the impact of those dislocations on subsequent or prior trauma will enhance cultural competence in work with immigrants.

12

TRAUMA AND
SYSTEMS OF MEANING MAKING

In this chapter, I speak to the ways in which trauma affects the human capacity to make meaning in life and how meaning-making systems can function as part of the healing process from trauma. The complexity of the relationship between faith, spirituality, and trauma is explored, and the importance of attending to issues of meaning and existential challenges inherent in trauma is discussed.

Human beings are creatures in search of meaning. Although a growing body of research tells us that it is possible and reasonable to admit that nonhuman animals have emotions and theories of mind, the data suggest that what differentiates humans from their mammalian cousins is the capacity to make meaning. My dog, who works in my therapy office comforting traumatized people, can have joy and sadness. He can even be traumatized; his predecessor, the subject of a blitz attack by a larger dog in his adolescence, feared his own species for the rest of his life and would try to bite any other dog that he encountered, a canine sort of posttraumatic stress disorder (PTSD).

However, dogs do not, as far as we know, make meaning, seek to control anything but the hand holding the treat, or develop philosophies of life. Humans do all of these things. In human history people have sacrificed the

227

first crop, the first lamb, their first-born child or his foreskin. People engage in elaborate rituals of sound and movement; they abstain from the pleasures of food or touch or orgasm on certain days or for their entire lives because of their beliefs that such actions will make meaning of their lives and, in the process, ward off the inevitable—death, which is the companion of trauma.

Human life is a constant struggle against knowing what Yalom (1980) described as the existential dynamics: that humans die, that they are powerless, that they are responsible for their lives, that life has no inherent meaning, and that they are alone. Although some reading this would argue with Yalom about the truth of these statements and posit that their system of meaning making gives a divine being power over life and that that same being tells humans how to make meaning, in the larger picture these arguments tend to prove the existential point that humans have strong needs to make sense of things that appear random, senseless, and often frightening and painful. Consequently, each of these issues is core to the existential component of the human experience of trauma in which people experience threats to their lives and safety, powerlessness, the erosion of meaning, and isolation. Trauma is the ultimate challenge to meaning making. People's identities and social locations that speak to meaning making are among the most fully human aspects of their identities, and they are also among those most central to, most affected by, and most powerful in response to trauma in people's lives.

Much of the time most people adequately ward off realities of meaninglessness and randomness, whether they worship at the shrine of Vishnu, pray to Allah, say Our Father or the Shema, keep kosher or a vegan diet, or practice celibacy. Through these and other rituals of being human, they generally find ways to make meaning of their lives in the face of that essential meaninglessness and inject a framework of order onto chaos; they join a religious group, conserve an endangered species, devote themselves to rescuing dogs, or organize a neighborhood watch. For many people the very human activity of parenting offers a daily practice of making meaning.

Trauma deals blows to people's meaning-making processes because it tears them away from the comfort of their meaning-making systems, plunges them into chaos and unpredictability in ways that cannot be denied or ignored, interferes with the practices that embody their systems of belief, and demonstrates the ineffectiveness of their prayers, spells, and charms. It renders hollow the works of their hands, turning them to dust and ashes, leaving them feeling helpless, alienated, and abandoned. It teaches them, in the words of a prayer that Jews recite during their period of atonement each year, that they are "of little merit," in Hebrew *"ayn banu maasim."* Trauma is the great equalizer, the great destroyer of dreams and of beliefs that are the stuff of religious faith and spiritual practice. Trauma leaves people with what the Biblical Prophet Ezekiel, himself a survivor of the traumas of war and forced relocation and displacement, called "a heart of stone," a numbness inside their cores that is antithetical to the aliveness that comes from a sense of meaning. If the reader examines the various definitions of trauma explored earlier in this volume, she or he can see that assaults on meaning are inherent in many of those constructs for understanding trauma.

Culturally aware and competent trauma therapies thus must be rooted in the recovery of meaning. This requires, in part, understanding the role of meaning-making systems, including religions, in the risk for trauma exposure; the ways in which trauma assaults those systems; and the value to both clients and psychotherapists of addressing questions of meaning and spirituality in the healing process. The territory of religion and spirituality is somewhat radioactive for many psychotherapists. Many psychologists and other psychotherapists are trained in traditions that are rationalist and sometimes antireligious. There is, after all, little if any empirical support for the presence of a divine being by whatever name, and research indicates that only a minority of psychologists describe themselves as religious; many of them are agnostic at best or engaged with nonorganized spiritual or meaning-making practices. The evidence base of psychology's practices does not include evidence about the value or efficacy of spiritual interventions qua spiritual interventions, although increasingly some approaches to therapy, calling themselves mindfulness-based (such as dialectical behavior therapy or acceptance and commitment therapy), are integrating spiritual practices of mindfulness meditation from Buddhist thought and finding them empirically sound strategies for responding to a range of human distress. Psychologists are starting to consider the possibility that these nonrational systems have something important to offer that psychotherapy as traditionally constituted does not or cannot provide.

However, trauma also has impacts that are specific to meaning-making systems of the individual to whom it happens. Unlike psychologists, most Americans do describe themselves as religious and find religion to be an important marker of identity and source of solace. If a woman grew up hearing her father say, "In our religious group no one beats his wife," then when her husband beats her that may mean that she is not only a woman beaten but also a failed member of her faith community, perhaps barred from seeking comfort there because she is defined as not existing as a domestic violence target in that community of faith. If a client has believed that her or his steadfast faith in a divine being will protect her or him and those she or he loves so long as she or he follows the rules of good behavior, that system is likely to be badly shaken when her or his child is murdered by random violence or a left comatose by a drunken driver. Persons whose experiences of trauma leave them feeling separated from their divine being may find themselves searching for the hidden or unknown sin that has caused them to suffer this punishment. Feeling abandoned by God, they may lose faith or conversely may redouble in their fervor, trying like the abused child to regain favor through increased efforts at connection. The trauma, in whatever form it takes, may be as much to faith as to body; losses of function and safety may be intensified by the loss of a comforting relationship with a divine being. The path to trauma recovery must in some way address the insult to meaning and identity as well as that to safety. Culturally competent trauma therapists must thus not only make room for faith but actively find ways to foreground the issue of meaning making, be it through formal religious systems, nonreligious systems of spirituality, or forms that do not resemble their understanding of what makes meaning but do so effectively for their clients.

Trauma may also have spiritually or religiously significant meanings because of what its occurrence seems to say about a relationship with a particular version of a higher power. Some of the ways in which trauma assaults meaning come to be because the event lands and lodges in those places in people's lives in which meaning is fermented, places particular to the identities that they bring into and take from experiences of interpersonal violence. When trauma includes disconnection from people's sacred places, its harms seem to go further and deeper. When trauma comes from one's sacred places then those harms are also great.

All kinds of trauma, be they *Diagnostic and Statistical Manual of Mental Disorders* (4th ed., text rev.; American Psychiatric Association, 2000) Criterion A, insidious, just world, or betrayal, carry the capacity to interfere with existential systems. This is because each of these ways in which an experience is felt as traumatic places the meaning of an event in the context of relationship, social context, and power and powerlessness, all of which play large parts in the creation of meaning. Some of these paradigms for understanding what constitutes trauma, as earlier noted, specifically focus on the ways in which relational or interpersonal ruptures constitute the makings of trauma even in the absence of life threat. These diverse visions of trauma allow for an enhanced understanding of how a given trauma might threaten meaning making for a particular survivor.

People's religious affiliations have also historically been the target of persecution, bias, and genocide. Although in the United States today religious-based bias is mostly of the covert and aversive variety, many members of current or formerly target religious groups carry the psychological remnants of that historical trauma and can also be exposed to insidious traumatization based on religious affiliation. Trauma's relationship to belief is complex both because of the importance of systems of belief to trauma response and the function of those systems as a possible risk factor for current and historical trauma.

RELIGION AND DIVINE BEINGS

Humans call the divine by many names; some cultures have one and only one divine being, others a pantheon. People who worship the same divine being have split into scores of iterations of faith, some accusing others of heresy, some escalating those accusations to violence and persecution of one another. Oceans of blood have been spilled over the millennia because of arguments about whose divine being is the true one and whose system of how to worship that divine being is correct. Internecine conflicts between Sunni and Shia Muslims in Iraq, Protestant and Catholic Christians in Northern Ireland, or Roman and Orthodox Catholics in the former Yugoslavia are simply today's most easily identifiable examples of this long-standing tendency for humans to inflict trauma on one another in the name of God.

Many psychotherapists working with trauma survivors will have been raised with one of these systems of belief and may be current adherents of such a system. Others raised in such a system will have modified or rejected their relationship with it. Religion is not a topic about which anyone can honestly describe her- or himself as neutral. And as Greene (2007) recently noted, the efforts of well-meaning psychotherapists to respect and tolerate religious diversity are profoundly challenged when they encounter others who use their faith as a battering ram on members of vulnerable target groups.

It seems a truism to say that the experience of a God or the absence of one is a highly personal event, but it is a truism that bears repeating in any discussion of cultural competence in trauma treatment. This is in part because that experience is so deeply personal and individual that, when people use the available language to discuss it with one another, it is deceptively simple to think that the words in common mean the experience in common. This is an even higher risk when psychotherapists and their clients share a particular faith tradition; ironically, it is probably at the juncture of spirituality that psychotherapists are most likely to know that they are ignorant in the face of obvious difference and less able to grasp the difference present in the context of apparent similarity. I have had the interesting experience in my career of twice working with women raised in precisely the same branch of Judaism in the same city at the same time of the world; each of us had channeled the same religious school texts, the same versions of the prayer book, and the same phenomenon of being Jewish girls in Cleveland Heights, Ohio, in the 1950s and 1960s into entirely unique ways of understanding how it was to be a Jew. Jews joke that there are "2 Jews, 3 synagogues, yours, mine, and the one neither of us will belong to" as a metaphor to communicate the knowledge of within-group difference and conflict. Cultural competence in response to clients' religious meaning-making systems permits psychotherapists to foreground the knowledge that they are most ignorant of the group that worships the same divine being in the same language with the same set of prayers as they do.

Some people were also raised to have contempt or disdain for the divine beings and religious practices of others. Some of that bias comes from dominant groups to target groups; defining someone else's faith as heathen and their pantheon of divine beings as idols and mythology is a clear commu-

refraining from eating dairy or meat until a certain number of hours have passed since the ingestion of the other sort of food.

Kosher prepared foods come with a stamp, called a *hechsher* on the package; many observant Jews will not eat foods that do not carry a hechsher even if all ingredients are clearly kosher. So, for example, the vegan donut shop in Seattle, which does not have a hechsher for its wares, cannot be patronized by most observant Jews even though only neutral, or parve, ingredients, which are by definition kosher, can be found in vegan food. This description of decision rules for eating and shopping is neither full nor inclusive of the rules of kashruth, but in this short version of the basics of food life for an observant Jew the careful reader may detect the faint stirrings of obsessive–compulsive ways of being.

Kashruth, no matter how much psychologically minded Jews may joke about it, is not obsessive–compulsive disorder (OCD). A person with OCD who is also observant is at risk for expressing her or his disorder through increasingly stringent applications of kashruth. The secular Jew who was raised to ridicule observant traditions as old-fashioned and unnecessary or anyone who finds this set of rules ridiculous and happens to be sitting in the role of the psychotherapist who can diagnose others risks enacting bias by conflating kashruth with disorder.

If asked, many thoughtful observant Jews will usually say that keeping kosher is a way of creating sanctity in everyday life through enhanced mindfulness of what is eaten and how it is prepared. When described in that manner almost anyone not misled by bias can agree that creating the sacred in daily life might be a good strategy for making meaning. In a culture that has survived 2 millennia of genocidal violence, having such a quotidian meaning-making strategy can even be seen as a cultural resilience tool in the face of trauma.

However, culturally competent therapists also know when what they are seeing is OCD and not simply keeping kosher or at the very least know how to think through the differential by looking at questions of distress. Keeping kosher can be a challenge, particularly if one forgets to bring one's lunch and no supermarket carrying safe food is nearby, but it is not distressing to those who adhere to it and can become a source of bonding and cultural connection. However, OCD is rife with anxiety and leads to mounting distress and dysfunction. One of the risks of etic knowledge is that it becomes a special pleading in which truly distressing experiences of members of target groups that can impair function badly are trivialized as "that's just their culture." An indigenous person who hears the spirit of her grandmother telling her to kill herself is having command hallucinations, not a spiritual experience in the American Indian tradition; a member of the Latter-day Saints church who is eating disordered is not fasting for spiritual clarity but out of distorted body image, which may itself reflect experiences of embodied or sexualized trauma (Root & Fallon, 1988). Because religion is an area in which many people believe themselves to know more than they do, the psychologist's stance of ignorance has enhanced value for culturally competent and ethically sound practice with people in regard to issues of faith.

Cultural competence in issues of religion also requires at least a passing awareness of the range and diversity that exists within each large religious grouping. Christians can be Orthodox, American or Southern Baptist (two quite different groups), Episcopalians, Methodists or Free Methodists (also very different), Nazarenes, Brethren, Presbyterians, Lutherans, Assemblies of God, and the list goes on. Mormons and members of the Seventh-day Adventist church consider themselves to be Christian, but some other Christians do not agree (witness current public discourse about the faith of presidential hopeful Mitt Romney, a member of the Mormon church). Muslims can be Sunni or Shia and within these larger groupings can have different iterations of interpretation of their faith. Being willing to be ignorant about religion and then willing to know enough to understand its particular meaning and role in the life of a given client are core to culturally competent practice.

PSYCHOTHERAPISTS ARE NOT PROPHETS (EVEN IF THEIR NAME IS JEREMIAH)

In almost every faith tradition, modern and ancient, there exist stories of trauma and redemption. Because trauma exposure has been a constant of human life, the emotional and existential sequelae of trauma are visible in the sacred texts of most religions. Some philosophers of religion have argued that human beings invented the concept of God to assist them in understanding incomprehensible and random loss and pain.

So when trauma survivor clients ask, as they frequently do, "What was God thinking?" or "Why did God let this happen?" cultural competence requires psychotherapists to refrain from answering in a declarative fashion. Even if psychotherapists believe that they hold the answer to this existential plea, their vision is unlikely to be prophetic. If psychotherapists express their opinion, there is a predictable risk of doing harm to a client because the declaration would constitute an exploitation of the power of the role of psychotherapist. However, psychotherapists must also not treat these questions as merely rhetorical because to do so minimizes the very real spiritual agony with which most survivors grapple in the wake of trauma.

Culturally competent practice in regard to faith questions such as these creates opportunities for psychotherapists to empower trauma survivors to find their own answers through means that center authority in the intersection between the client and her or his own experience of the Divinity. These are not opportunities for the psychotherapist to simply refer to a clergyperson; clients may not trust clergy, may not have a relationship with a member of the clergy who they find credible on these matters, or may not practice an organized religion despite still believing in God. Responding well to these existential questions means the ability to hear them as not about God per se or God alone but as a faith-informed version of the more general existential question of "Why me?" that so often accompanies the mourning and remembrance and integration stages of trauma recovery.

If a psychotherapist is an atheist, she or he should refrain from commentary as to the nonexistence of a God in work with clients who are struggling with issues of faith and meaning making. An exchange of letters published in the *Monitor on Psychology* in late 2006 on just this theme underscored the importance of working from a stance of respect and humility about matters God related and of not taking for granted either the good sense or restraint of any clinician. There, one well-regarded psychologist and former president of the American Psychological Association (APA) excoriated another well-regarded psychologist and former president of the APA because the latter described supporting a client in the client's beliefs about God during that client's fatal illness, entering the client's own meaning-making and ontological systems. The first psychologist scolded the second for encouraging the client's belief in the fairy tale of God (the client in question was a young child; Koocher, 2006; Perloff, 2007). Other letter writers weighed in with praise for the clinical response of the second psychologist. Psychologists and other psychotherapists need to remember that although there is little empirical support for the efficacy of faith or the existence of a divine being based on randomized controlled trials, there appears to be a solid evidence base of millennia of practice regarding the value that faith in such a being and spirituality can offer some people when tragedy and loss enter their lives.

Psychologists of faith, conversely, should not assume that in the absence of such a formal system of meaning that a client is lacking in effective meaning-making systems. Religion and spirituality are meaning-making strategies. They are the dominant strategies in American life, and thus the risk is present for those who participate in religion and spirituality to assume that they are the only useful or valuable ones and to express bias toward those who reject the existence of a God. The oft-repeated cliché about "no atheists in foxholes" is a narrative about the presumed inevitability of belief in a divine being when risk of death looms and thus that trauma will inevitably lead to religious belief. There is no more empirical evidence for this than for the belief that no God exists. The reality is that people in terrible circumstances have found meaning through art, music, planting gardens, nurturing children, or doing social justice actions motivated by various other-than-religious ways of knowing. A god figure, a belief in a higher power, or a belief in some mystical transcendent force works well for some and not at all for others as a foundation for responding to the existential challenges that trauma brings.

AVOIDING THE LOSS OF MEANING:
A CHALLENGE FOR TRAUMA THERAPISTS

Psychotherapists working with trauma survivors must also develop their own meaning-making systems to be able to encompass the amount of pain and terror to which they are routinely witness. Psychotherapists' processes of finding those systems that support their work will mirror their clients' struggles; they will discover that their usual existential strategies and rituals may serve them poorly or not at all in the face of the cruelty, injustice, and randomness that are at the core of all trauma. Their images of humans as essentially good, if these are the ones that their existing systems have taught them, will be undermined and threatened by encounters with examples of human evil. If they were raised to see humans as sinful, they will be overwhelmed by the breadth and depth of the human capacity for evil. If they saw nature as benign, they will learn of its destructive power; and if they idealized the family, they will know it as the most dangerous place for children. Everything sacred will be toppled by their repeated witness to trauma in the lives of clients, friends, and themselves. One of the dangerous places that a psychotherapist working with trauma can go to is that of the absence of a meaning-making system; nihilism is an invitation to ethical risk because the traumatic loss of one set of rules can sometimes leave psychotherapists questioning the value of any and all sets of values. Another dangerous movement for a therapist is to a rigid meaning-making system that allows little room to respond to the ever-changing realities of the challenges of trauma practice. Some psychotherapists respond to fear by becoming more rigid, as if overcontrol of themselves and others will protect them against really knowing the fragility of safety for everyone. In these struggles to make meaning for themselves as therapists, they will mirror the struggles of the trauma survivors with whom they work. Like their clients, psychotherapists have no choice but to embrace those struggles because landing in a place of anomie and hopelessness interferes significantly with their capacity to risk connection and feel hopeful about healing and transformation.

WOUNDS FROM RELIGION

For some of the people who come into psychotherapists' offices, the traumatic experiences with which they struggle will have happened at the social location of religion and spirituality. Two types of psychic wounds related to religion are common. One is the wound inflicted within and by one's faith. The other is the trauma perpetrated against a person by others based on bias or hate toward that individual's faith. Each type of religion-related trauma carries its own special challenges to cultural competence.

Although for many people religion or spirituality is a source of comfort or healing, for others it has been the locus of pain and terror. Humans, after all, are the transmitters and practitioners of all faith traditions and thus can distort the most lovely and compassionate of theologies with the cruelties and confusion inherent in human behavior. Abuse by members of the clergy is one now well-known form of abuse by religion (Fortune, 1999; Frawley-O'Dea, 2007), but such abuse need not have been as overt as sexual exploitation. For some people the trauma rests in the terrifying content of a theology intersecting with problematic family or cultural norms.

Zillah was raised in what she called a "fire and brimstone" evangelical and fundamentalist Protestant faith. Her family went to church every Wednesday evening and from early morning until late afternoon on Sundays. Her earliest memories are of the nightmares she would experience after coming home from church and hearing preaching about the sufferings of those condemned in hell. As a child with a vivid imagination and a mild propensity to obsessive thinking, her pastor's words were a source of pure terror for her. Her parents' discussions of hell and damnation frightened her even more; neither parent was particularly warm or comforting, and each tended to use faith as a rationale for disciplining and shaming Zillah. "God won't love you if you talk back to me," her mother would say to her.

By adulthood she was thoroughly averse to anything having to do with religion. She was estranged from her family of origin, who would occasionally send her letters saying that they were praying for her return to faith and reminding her of the torments of hell that she was risking. Her fear of anything religious was such that she was unable to set foot in a Unitarian church to attend a dear friend's wedding, telling her that she knew that the Unitarians did not preach damnation but that anything that even "smelled like a church" frightened her. She was unable to reassure herself that she would avoid hell by embracing atheism, fearing that to reject the existence of God entirely would be too risky, nor did her fear allow her to find a different faith tradition, again running into fear that her family and childhood pastor might be right. For Zillah, religion felt both life threatening and inescapable.

Zillah's experiences can challenge a psychotherapist's cultural competence because they raise the question of how to assist her in healing from being traumatized by her childhood faith while not defining the faith itself as wrong. Greene's (2007) call to psychologists to differentiate between faith and its toxic uses and abuses will inform cultural competence at this and similar junctures. Almost any belief system can be distorted in such a manner as to make it abusive or frightening to its adherents, just as almost any meaning-making system can also be used to assist people to transcend the fear and pain of trauma. Psychotherapists working with individuals who have, like Zillah, been wounded by such toxicity must use care and sophistication, being self-aware in regard to their own biases.

Wounds from religion also occur in adult life. Persons who are shunned by their families because they have left a faith or intermarried or who are expelled from a congregation because of being lesbian, gay, or bisexual have experienced a spiritual dislocation that can feel as traumatic at times as are physical dislocations. These traumas of religious and spiritual separation from faith, family, community, or all of these groups frequently have the dynamics of a trauma of betrayal. Several early authors on the experiences of openly lesbian, gay, or bisexual Christians use the term *exile* to refer to their experiences (Fortunato, 1984; Pharr, 1988) of spiritual dislocation. Culturally competent practice creates space for clients to speak of this sort of trauma and to consider how it has created distress that has often been invalidated or minimized because it arose from choices made by a person to marry, change faith, or come out publicly.

RELIGION-BASED PERSECUTION AND TRAUMA

Being targeted because of one's religious beliefs and identifications or coming from a religious culture with that heritage can endow a person with a trauma-informed identity. As noted earlier, in the United States today there is a diminishing amount of overt faith-related persecution and oppression. Despite this trend, hate crimes against people as a result of their actual or perceived faith, particularly against Muslims and Jews, have risen in the last several years, with bias-based crimes against Jews occurring more frequently in the United States than any other sort of crime except racially motivated violence (Anti-Defamation League, 2006). Although the absolute number of this sort of episode declined from 2003 to 2006, the data indicate that religiously motivated violence against target groups is not only a historical phenomenon.

Aversive bias informs people's collective understanding of these traumas in dominant culture and in turn informs how members of religious target groups are exposed to sources of insidious trauma. When anti-Muslim bias and violence is attributed in part to the terror attacks of September 11, 2001, the narrative of representation is emerging. By this, I mean that all Muslims are considered to be represented by the terrible acts of the terrorists of September 11, 2001; as is true with other situations in which the absences of privilege requires each member of a target group to serve as the representative of that group, so in this instance the terrorists were interpreted by many people in the United States as representing Islam, rather than the terrorists' own extremely disturbed and distorted interpretations of that generally peaceful faith tradition. Contrast this with how members of dominant groups who have committed similarly heinous acts are not turned into representatives of their groups. The best example is that the actions of Timothy McVeigh, the White Christian man who committed the act of domestic terror most directly preceding the September 11, 2001, attacks, the bombing of the federal office building in Okalahoma City, did not lead to an upsurge in violence against Euro-American Christians. As a member of the dominant group his behaviors were seen as aberrant and criminal but not as representative of his faith traditions. When violence against Muslims is rationalized or understood as stemming from feelings about the September 11, 2001, attacks, that narrative conveys the message that the bad acts of one small group of Muslims are somehow representative of all Muslims.

Similarly, when a psychotic man broke into the Jewish Federation of Seattle in August 2006, shooting six women, one fatally, some in the surrounding community "understood" his action as the extension of reasonable anger against Jews because of Israel's policies in Palestine. (This man happened to be a Muslim born in Pakistan; he was also a person who, according to the news media, had a long-standing history of psychosis.) To date there have been no crimes of violence committed against Euro-American Christian Texans because one of that group has led his country into disputed acts and policies in Iraq resulting in the deaths of tens of thousands of noncombatants. Again, the subtexts of aversive bias inform the social context in which experiences of overt religion-based traumas occur.

When overt acts allow covert bias to surface many members of the affected groups who were not directly the targets of the specific violent act will experience insidious traumatization as the presence of threat in their daily lives is exposed to them. In the aftermath of the Jewish Federation shootings in Seattle many members of the local trauma treatment community found themselves working not only with the directly affected women and their co-workers but with many other Jewish community members for whom the events as well as the public response to those events uncovered long-standing experiences of historical and insidious traumatization. The grief and fear that I experienced that day, lingering for several weeks afterward, did not arise to the level of a trauma but were clear and painful reminders of the otherness of that important aspect of my own identity.

MEANING-MAKING SYSTEMS AS PROTECTIVE

For many people, the presence of a meaning-making system serves as a protective factor when trauma strikes. Paradoxically, both a strong religious faith and a rejection of religious belief can be equally protective, depending on how they are applied. The committed existentialist who believes that there is no God and that life is random may find that this belief assists in coping with trauma because it allows for an appraisal of the event as part of the predictable random meaninglessness of existence. As Frankl (1963) pointed out long ago, for an existentialist it is a matter of personal responsibility to uncover and develop meaning out of apparently meaningless and horrific events. Thus his often-quoted passage about finding meaning in the acts of human kindness that he observed among the inmates of Auschwitz during the time he was incarcerated in the death camp; for Frankl, being able to see and participate in his fellow captives' resistance to dehumanization by the Nazis created meaning in the most devastatingly traumatic of circumstances.

Belief systems that separate the kindness of a divinity from experiences here on earth can also be protective at times of trauma. Many groups with historic experiences of oppression and trauma develop God narratives about the heavenly rewards that will accrue to those who bear suffering on earth. Religious beliefs that include a sense of personal connection with a nurturing, parental God can also be protective because many trauma survivors describe being comforted by prayer and the sense that God is listening to them even if their pain and suffering are not immediately relieved.

Some religious belief systems are more ambiguous in the protectiveness. For instance, interviews with survivors of the 2004 tsunami, all of them Indonesian Muslims, yielded expressions of a sense that those who had suffered or died had not caused the disaster; survivors' faith led them to a belief that all of life is predestined by the will of Allah. However, the interpretations given to scripture by religious leaders also suggested to some of those interviewed that the tsunami had been punishment for laxity of religious practice by the community (Bearak, 2005).

In recent years attention has been directed to the phenomenon of post-traumatic growth (PTG; Wilson, 2006). This growing area of research and theory posits that for some persons the process of recovery from trauma does not result merely in a restoration to a premorbid state of functioning but rather that the recovery process moves forward to states of optimal functioning and transcendence. Some controversy exists within the field of trauma studies in regard to this construct, with concerns being raised by clinicians that it will create a new source of shame for those survivors for whom simply functioning adequately remains a struggle. Others have responded that by framing adequate functioning as a triumphant transcendence of fragmentation, those survivors have evidenced PTG as well. The construct of PTG opens fascinating questions about the interaction of meaning-making systems and trauma recovery, suggesting that trauma itself can become a potentially empowering source of meaning as a person challenges the shame, self-blame, and fragmentation resulting from trauma exposure.

Culturally competent responses to issues of faith and meaning making for trauma survivors are complex and multifaceted. The role of a meaning-making system in the development of identity, its relationship to the experience of trauma, and the reality of trauma itself as a powerful existential challenge must all be accounted for in psychotherapists' work with trauma survivors. It is also important to note that the ways in which trauma challenges psychotherapists existentially form a component of their emotional competence to remain engaged in the task of trauma treatment. Trauma does not simply affect the suffering individual; because psychotherapists are human and relational by nature, the distress of one person ripples into the experiences of every life that she or he touches.

III

INTERPERSONAL AND PSYCHOTHERAPIST VARIABLES

13

WEAVING THE WEB OF SUPPORT: WORKING WITH FAMILIES AND COMMUNITIES AND CARING FOR ONESELF

In this chapter, I address the emotional needs of those who work and live with trauma survivors. Strategies for engaging and supporting families of trauma survivors both inside of and collateral to the therapy process are presented. The topic of vicarious traumatization and its effects on psychotherapists is extensively discussed.

Trauma is experienced, survived, and healed in the circles of interpersonal engagement found in every person's life. Trauma can occur in relationships, particularly those of dependency, intimacy, and trust. Trauma and its sequelae are potentially highly disruptive to healthy and loving relationships in which bonds of attachment have not been betrayed; the shame, self-hatred, and problematic coping strategies of traumatized people create high walls between them and those whom they have loved and who love them. Many trauma survivors enter therapy alone and isolated, with neither family nor community available to them. When engaged with and available, however, those relationships of family and community as broadly defined can also be a source of healing and recovery for trauma survivors. Trauma is isolating and alienating; in my experience no one heals from trauma alone, nor does anyone move into posttraumatic growth in isolation. Connection to the human community in new and empowering ways is central to the trauma recovery process. To engage families and social networks or to assist clients to create families and communities of choice as part of recovery, it is important to take issues of social location into account so as to most effectively involve these members of clients' webs of life in their healing processes.

For some trauma survivors the relationship to family of origin is complicated. As noted earlier, families of origin are often a source of trauma exposure, sometimes even constituting a barrier to healing processes. Some survivors of childhood trauma disengage from those families, cutting off contact, changing names, and moving far away to avoid even accidental contact with those who have harmed them. For other trauma survivors, family members are covictims of a natural disaster, genocide, or an accident, with the family dynamic of even the healthiest of family systems being distorted and undermined by the shared experience of trauma that has affected each person uniquely and damaged the family's usual coping resources. For others, family are the passive or unknowing bystanders to trauma, unable to comprehend the changes to their family member, waiting for the survivor to "get over it." In addition, for some others, family is a source of healing, support, and connection during the difficult process of trauma recovery. A psychotherapist can make no assumptions about what kind of family support is likely to be available to a person because of their perceived identities. Having read an etic article about the strength of family support in African American communities will be of little help in conceptualizing how to recruit social support for the African American lesbian healing from a car accident whose family of origin will have little to do with her because of her sexual orientation and whose family of choice of queer people and allies from various cultural and ethnic contexts becomes the one on which she leans.

A culturally competent psychotherapist can and should explore who the people are who constitute family for clients and then consider how and when to involve that network in the healing process. Frequently, particularly for individuals struggling with complex trauma, there will be few or no members of this group; the network will need to be cocreated by therapist and client as one of the projects of trauma treatment. At the very beginning of this book I explored the meaning of an injury to a family member; I then expanded this definition in understanding what constitutes the witnessing of a threat to someone to whom a person is connected; culturally competent practice expands the definition to include whomever clients define as their family when psychotherapists collaborate with clients to strengthen and rebuild their relational world.

One need not adopt a formal family systems approach or directly involve members of clients' families in the therapy. However, in my experience it has been more common than not for trauma survivors to ask to bring members of family, biological and extended, into psychotherapy sessions or to request that I be available for a collateral consultation with family to support a client's healing process. My philosophy of psychotherapy, which focuses on empowerment of clients, leads me to generally respond positively to these requests.

Psychotherapists who do involve family members should be thoughtful as to how to give clear informed consent to these nonclient participants in the process and delineate their professional responsibilities vis-à-vis the family member. Issues of confidentiality of the client's work need to be carefully discussed in advance and, if necessary, releases of information signed so that a psychotherapists does not inadvertently violate confidentiality in a joint session.

Hannah's stepfather had sexually abused her from the time he entered the family when she was 5 until her mother left him when Hannah was 11. She had been estranged from her mother for most of her adult life, blaming her for not having known about and stopped the abuse, which in turn left her distant from the rest of her otherwise close-knit Mexican American family. This estrangement had been particularly painful for Hannah when she herself became a mother of a daughter, which was one of the catalysts for her starting psychotherapy. One of the outcomes of her work in psychotherapy was her deepening appreciation for her mother and her realization of how her beliefs about her mother's capacities were informed by her child's eye view of her mother as all knowing and all powerful. With the assistance and support of her psychotherapist she reached out to her mother by letter and e-mail and eventually invited her mother to join her for several sessions in which the two women were able to speak of their grief and mistrust and take steps toward a different relationship.

One exception to my norm of welcoming family members is when clients desire to stage confrontations with those in their families who have harmed them with the stated goal of being heard or achieving closure. Although a number of psychotherapists working with adult survivors of incest did this during the 1980s and early 1990s, the anecdotal data arising from this practice were that it generally served only to create alienation and experiences of further estrangement of adults from their parents.

Involving the client's own social support network in the healing experience and giving authority and value to the assistance offered in that milieu to the survivor also helps to undercut what I see as a pernicious narrative in American culture today. This is the trend that relegates all emotional caregiving to professionals, for example, psychotherapists, and negates the value of nonprofessional care.

There are many skills and tools that I bring to my work as a psychotherapist; I know a great deal about how to create the conditions under which emotional healing and transformation, both symptom specific and more general, can occur. These are valuable assets that I bring to the table and with them I have been honored to empower many people in the process of trauma recovery. However, there is much that I cannot and should not do in my role as a psychotherapist. All of that nontherapy territory is very rich indeed.

When my oldest friend's sister died tragically and too young during the spring of 2007, her family of choice, most of us practicing psychotherapists like her, did not offer her therapy or suggest that she seek treatment for her grief. We came to her home, cooked her meals, walked the dog with her, and drove her to the airport to fly home to her family across the country for the memorial process. She cried at times, and we listened while she cried and talked about her beloved sister and the pain of her loss. However, we listened as friends, not as therapists, even though I am sure that our skills and training helped as well as interfered with simply being her friends. As her friends we could tell her that we thought that this death was wrong and unfair, commiserate with her about her brother-in-law, and even in some instances talk about God. The Jews among us attended the shiva (mourning) at her home and said Kaddish, the Jewish mourner's prayer, with her. We could hold her and tell her that we loved her. None of these are the tasks of psychotherapy. All of them are part of the healing process.

Identifying and engaging with social support systems is also empirically known to be an important component of well-being and one that trauma itself frequently undermines or weakens. Various components of trauma survivors' identities affect their ability to seek and use social support. Dominant cultural norms for masculine gender roles in the United States have been shown to interfere with help seeking and apparently dependent behaviors in male trauma survivors (Lisak, 2005) because such behaviors are experienced as violations of the masculine imperative to be strong and independent. Lesbian, gay, and bisexual individuals who are not out to families of origin may experience difficulty in requesting support from their families because of fears that their sexual orientation may be inadvertently exposed and lead to even more difficulties during a time of severe posttraumatic distress (Brown, 1988). Persons of mixed phenotype and ethnic heritage who have experienced a hate crime targeted at the visibly non-Euro-American aspects of their identities may find it hard to seek solace from Euro-American family members. Psychotherapist sensitivity to these nuances of how trauma and social location can blend to either enhance or undermine the availability of social support creates the possibility of more culturally competent use and integration of natural support networks into a trauma survivor's healing process.

WHAT ABOUT SUPPORT GROUPS?

Many of the trauma survivors who have worked with me have attended some sort of formal support group concurrent with their psychotherapy. Their experiences have been mixed and sometimes mixed within the same context. Well-meaning therapists commonly refer to support groups, not knowing that there are potential risks inherent in some of these settings. Many survivors I work with entered psychotherapy early in sobriety and have used 12-step programs as support for continuing abstinence. For some of these people Alcoholics Anonymous (AA) and similar groups have been lifesaving, providing continuously available emotional support and companionship that has lifted people out of isolation and into the life of a community. However, as one of my clients said to me, "AA is full of wounded people." There have been times when wounding by peers has temporarily impeded the work of psychotherapy or has threatened a client's then-tenuous connections to sobriety. Psychotherapists who have clients attending 12-step programs need to develop cultural competence about the norms and realities of those programs in their own communities and collaborate with clients on how to effectively use that form of support when clients choose to add it to their coping strategies.

Other people I have worked with have attended non-12-step support groups for combat trauma survivors, sexual abuse survivors, and artists in trauma recovery as well as other sorts of therapeutic and quasi-therapeutic groups. Once again, they and I have found enormous variability in the value added to trauma recovery by such programs. Those that have been carefully designed and led or facilitated by thoughtful, grounded people (not necessarily professionally trained psychotherapists) have been invaluable to people's trauma recovery. Participation in an early dialectical behavior therapy (DBT) skills group that was offered while DBT was in development became a core of one woman's work with me. The specifics of self-care and self-soothing that she acquired and practiced there allowed her to see her autonomous capacities as a resource for herself far sooner than might have otherwise happened had she and I been trying to develop those without the modeling and encouragement of the other trauma survivors in her group.

However, some trauma survivor clients have attended support groups, including some run by psychotherapists, that they found destructive, destabilizing, or disrespectful of issues of culture and identity. An insistence that people tell all details of their trauma stories whether they are emotionally ready or not and whether this is retraumatizing or not, an absence of clear boundaries regarding out-of-group friendships or sexual relationships between group members, an absence of protection for more vulnerable group members in the face of emotional outbursts by other members who have poor impulse control, and other problematic experiences have been part of people's encounters with the support group world. As a consequence it is important for any given psychotherapist and client to carefully evaluate the value and potential risks of engaging with formal support groups. Before referring to a particular support group it is incumbent on a therapist to learn what group norms are on these and other issues of safety and self-care for group members.

Some of the etic literature on work with members of various target groups, particularly ethnic target groups of color, has prescribed group psychotherapies for those clients as particularly well suited to members of collectivist cultures, and some of the early feminist therapy literature similarly prescribed group therapy as a strategy for reducing imbalances of power between women in therapy and their psychotherapists. However, more accurate culturally competent practice does not prescribe a particular therapeutic modality for a trauma survivor on the basis of social locations or identities. Instead, nurturing some kind of relational context that supports the healing process in addition to psychotherapy and attention to shaping that context to be responsive to individual and cultural needs of a client can inform treatment. An art class, a group climbing lesson, singing in a choir, or volunteering for a cause valued by a client are all strategies for achieving support and connection that do not require a person to foreground her or his identity as a trauma survivor and that may be as or more valuable in healing than a formal support group.

DIVERSELY VICARIOUS: CULTURALLY COMPETENT SELF-CARE FOR TRAUMA PSYCHOTHERAPISTS

Laurie Anne Pearlman and Karen Saakvitne (1995) proposed the construct of *vicarious traumatization* (VT) to explain the experiences of many psychotherapists working with trauma survivors. Pearlman and Saakvitne defined VT as the expectable consequences of engaging empathically with trauma survivors during the course of one's work as a psychotherapist. They differentiated it from two other phenomena, *secondary traumatic stress* (STS) and *burnout*. Unlike STS, VT does not entail having posttraumatic stress disorder-like symptoms arising from exposure to information from clients about their *Diagnostic and Statistical Manual of Mental Disorders* (4th ed., text rev.; American Psychiatric Association, 2000) Criterion A traumatic stressors. Unlike burnout, VT does not reflect general stressors in the workplace.

Also, VT is not isomorphic with countertransference, although it inhabits a similar emotional territory. Countertransference can be extremely powerful in working with trauma survivors because of the intensity of painful emotions that emerge in the work of psychotherapy with this population (Dalenberg, 2000). Countertransference, however, occurs in a specific therapeutic relationship and responds to the particular variables present in the unique encounter between a given therapist and individual client or family. As examined in the earlier discussion of issues of representation and privilege, cultural competence in managing countertransference dynamics lies greatly in understanding what psychotherapist and client represent to one another within their multiple identities and relationships of privilege and disadvantage relative to one another.

In addition, VT is a larger and more pervasive experience than is countertransference, reflecting not simply the specific client–therapist relationship but rather the cumulative impact of a psychotherapist's exposure to, and both conscious and nonconscious responses to, the stories and feelings of many trauma survivors. A psychotherapist's VT comes with her or him to every encounter in life, not only those in the therapy office, and is powerful in large part because its effects cannot be compartmentalized within the confines of professional life.

Moreover, VT develops in almost every psychotherapist who works consistently and intentionally with trauma survivors because these stories of harm and betrayal evoke emotions related to a psychotherapist's own identities and social locations. It also occurs because psychotherapists' experience of witnessing these lives acts on and changes their identities and their meanings in a lasting manner. Specifically, VT reflects a profound transformation in the psychotherapist's own consciousness and sense of self. In that transformative process, through the experience of genuine emotional encounter with clients who have survived trauma, psychotherapists experience a change of worldview, identity, and self-view and find themselves reevaluating their needs, feelings, and interpersonal relationships. As Pearlman and Saakvitne wrote, "we view it (VT) as an occupational hazard, an inevitable effect of trauma work" (1995, p. 31).

Additionally, VT is not a passing experience; if a psychotherapist stays engaged in work with trauma survivors, then VT becomes another component of self. This is not necessarily a bad thing; in fact, when VT is acknowledged, embraced, and integrated into a psychotherapist's sense of self rather than denied and disowned, it becomes a source of resilience and an inner place from which a psychotherapist can join empathically with trauma survivors in ever more profound ways. If I can become aware of and know how simply witnessing stories of trauma affects me I have an experiential base that allows me to validate the transformational power of direct trauma exposure in an emotionally truthful manner; when my clients hear and feel my responses to their stories, they can hear and feel a resonance that has its roots in VT. Looking at VT from this perspective makes it an avenue for the therapist's own posttraumatic growth, a process of transcendence and increased personal wholeness that emerges from the encounter with the emotional abyss. Dealing with VT enhances a therapist's capacity to maintain emotional competence (Pope & Brown, 1997; Pope, Sonne, & Greene, 2006; Pope & Vazquez, 2007), which supports ethical practice.

Because it can enhance empathy and the capacity for genuine connection between psychotherapists and trauma survivor clients, VT can become a catalyst for enhanced cultural competence in therapists. This is because, in my experience, the heightened capacities for empathy engendered by successful integration of the VT experience make psychotherapists more attuned to possible ruptures in the relational field and thus more willing to notice if they may be acting in a culturally other-than-sensitive manner with clients. Just as, for many trauma survivors, the experience of trauma has given them the coping strategy of heightened awareness of other humans' subtle emotional cues, so too can VT be a path toward a more nuanced awareness by therapists of where meaning lies for their clients and how to best be fully present in their relationships with them. This sort of deepening of awareness and connection is foundational to a variety of cultural competencies that go beyond an intellectual grasp of the value of greater sensitivity to diversity to an embodied, felt, and committed relationship with that sensitivity.

Left unaddressed, however, VT has the potential to undermine a psychotherapist's cultural competence because of its impact on a psychotherapist's relational and empathic capacities. The risks inherent in VT are similar to those arising from direct trauma exposure. Psychotherapists who cannot identify or acknowledge their VT may find themselves becoming numbed and distanced from the stories that they hear. They may begin to use a variety of affect-control strategies, such as overwork, substance abuse, or intellectualization, to contain the distress that is an inevitable and normal human response to the work of listening to trauma stories. The us–them split in the field of trauma practice in which trauma survivors become the disturbed other from whom professionals create emotional and cognitive distance reflects a professionwide failure to adequately acknowledge and metabolize our collective VT. The more I need to assert how I am not "one of them," and the more exotic and different I make the narrative of posttraumatic distress the more likely it is that I will lose attunement to clients, ignore or minimize issues of culture, and be adversely affected by my own VT.

In part VT occurs because of what psychotherapists working with trauma survivors witness in their work. Even if a psychotherapist were to restrict her- or himself to seeing only those trauma survivors who have experienced natural disasters, that psychotherapist would still be a witness to knowledge of extreme human suffering, loss, and grief. There is simply not a trauma known to humankind the realities of which are not threatening to our illusions about the safety and stability of the world. Psychotherapists who work with the survivors of interpersonal trauma, combat, genocide, and discrimination will have, in addition to confrontations with the random and chaotic nature of the world, emotionally intimate encounters with the realities of human cruelty. As a specialist in therapy with survivors of childhood maltreatment I know that I sometimes feel as if I am surrounded by evidence of unspeakably horrible things that adults have done to children, behaviors beyond my capacity to have ever imagined until my clients gave me this painful education. It is impossible to work with trauma survivors and remain in a state of naïve hopefulness about the world and its human inhabitants.

Yet hope is a necessary ingredient of therapy, something psychotherapists and clients know intuitively and can demonstrate empirically (Snyder,

Michael, & Cheavens, 1999). The trauma psychotherapist's nonnaïve, grounded hope for the client's healing process and her or his expectation that what is offered will be of assistance to the survivor are essential ingredients of what psychotherapists do for the people with whom they work. Ironically, some of the same experiences that give psychotherapists hope, the pleasures of having had the time to watch many people heal from trauma, also expose psychotherapists to increased realities of VT as they spend more time in the presence of survivors.

Because VT is a profound and sometimes hidden experience for trauma psychotherapists, it touches on all aspects of the psychotherapist's multiple identities and social locations and may aggravate a therapist's hidden wounds of insidious trauma, betrayal, or cultural experiences of danger. Thus, just as cultural competence is of importance in working with clients so that psychotherapists can hear and know the multiple meanings of their trauma experiences in light of their various identities, so such competence is a necessary component of responding to VT in themselves. Knowing the meanings of their own identities as they create both vulnerability and resilience allows them, as psychotherapists, to more accurately understand what VT is acting on and how it is likely to manifest.

Although VT involves a transformation of the self of the psychotherapist at a deep level, the signals to psychotherapists that they are experiencing unaddressed VT commonly emerge behaviorally and interpersonally, both with their clients and with their emotional and social networks of support. Saakvitne, Gamble, Pearlman, and Lev (2000) have identified a variety of signs and symptoms that are common in psychotherapists experiencing VT. These include emotional numbing and withdrawal, feelings of hopelessness and despair, loss of meaning making and spiritual connection, loss of respect for survivors and one's own profession, and distancing from intimate relationships. Persons experiencing VT also note that they feel engulfed by their work; "Trauma is everywhere," said one psychotherapist who consulted with me about the emotional numbness that was encroaching on her ability to function in her work.

> Everywhere I turn, I feel surrounded by it. I can't escape it. I look at families and see perpetrators. I can't watch television; every show seems to be about violence and trauma. I want to hide, and then I feel ashamed because nothing has happened to me.

Feelings of loss of safety and loss of the just world figure heavily in VT for some psychotherapists, whereas others may experience a lighting up of previously quiescent insidious traumatization.

Because VT, like trauma itself, does not happen to a generic psychotherapist, issues of power, social location, and identity all play out in how VT is experienced and expressed and in the strategies available to a psychotherapist to respond to and integrate VT. Giller, Vermilyea, and Steele (2006) found that exposing psychotherapists to the Risking Connection curriculum (Saakvitne et al., 2000), which is a structured strategy for introducing the concept of VT and teaching methods of responding effectively to the experience, reduced problematic VT responses for the participants. The emphasis on psychotherapists' own self-care, which is a theme that is countercultural in the usual context of trauma treatment, seems to be a central aspect of the effectiveness of that training.

Self-care is also countercultural for many of the larger cultures informing a psychotherapist's identities. As I have explored throughout this volume, the social constructions of psychotherapists' identities frequently contain prohibitions on care for self, on seeking support, or on using scarce resources if psychotherapists are not in dire need.

Estella's struggle with self-care exemplifies the impact of culture on VT. The eldest daughter of a Dominican American family, she lived simply on her good salary as a psychiatrist running an inpatient trauma unit, sending much of her income to her parents in the Dominican Republic. When Euro-American friends urged her to spend money on her self-care she felt uncomfortable trying to explain to them that it would be a violation of her cultural norms to privilege her own welfare over that of her parents. "A good daughter cares for her parents; that's just our way. I'm always shocked when I hear about White people putting their old folks in nursing homes; it seems so selfish."

A friend and colleague finally assisted Estella to find a balance between self-care and care for her parents by framing self-care as an ethical issue. "If you don't take care of you, you'll burn out, and if you burn out, you can be impaired, and then what happens to your patients?" her friend asked her. Estella fumed at her friend for "putting me in this stupid bind," then complimented her for having done a masterful paradoxical intervention. She decided to discuss her dilemma with her siblings, all of whom were also quite financially successful and all of whom were also sending money to their parents. They encouraged her to allow them to carry a little more of the load, teasing her that even though she was their big sister that she did not have to keep treating them like babies. She found that she was able to do better self-care just by allowing herself to shift out of the role of ever-responsible oldest sibling. She also signed up for a belly-dancing class.

Those who work as consultants and supervisors to colleagues who treat trauma survivors need to integrate cultural competence into the understanding of the challenges that colleagues face when they encounter VT. When psychotherapists extend their awareness of how identity affects their values and choices both personally and professionally into the process of professional development then they will inevitably deepen their cultural competence in every aspect of their work.

CONCLUSION: LOOKING FORWARD

The charge to any author of a book is to say at the end, "Now where do we go from here?" In this case, what is the vision of how culturally competent trauma practice can be deepened and expanded? How does the reader move forward from insights and awareness sparked by this volume to transformation of her or his practice to greater levels of competence in regard to both trauma and cultural competence? How can the field of trauma psychology become more attuned to issues of human diversity? In addition, how can those who focus on diversity become more integrated into the field of trauma studies?

Faced with these lofty questions my first urge is to return to the advice given earlier to readers to adopt a stance of ignorance and to invite each reader to claim her or his own knowledge. In fact, let me do so, and then let me share my vision for the future, clear that it is mine and not the truth about where the field and each psychotherapist's practice needs to go.

In the year and a half between proposing this concept and writing these words I have seen a flourishing of books and articles addressing the intersection of trauma and diversity. The first self-help book for trauma survivors of which I am aware that intentionally merges trauma recovery with themes of multiculturalism and diversity (Bryant-Davis, 2005) has been published. The Diversity Special Interest Group of the International Society for Traumatic Stress Studies and the Diversity Committee of the American Psychological

Association's Division of Trauma Psychology have both become active, thriving groups sponsoring conference programs on a wide range of topics addressing the interface between trauma practice and competence in psychotherapy with diverse populations. This upwelling of interest and energy reflects the forces that led me to write this book—the awareness by those who have been professionally straddling these two worlds that the time has come to bring them together for the benefit of both.

These are all initial steps on what promises to be a long journey, and that is itself a bittersweet reality. In my ideal world I awaken to find that violence and hatred have ended; that children are safe in their homes; and that adequate and high-quality medical, emotional, spiritual, and material support are available to all of those in need. A distinctly utopian vision; and in this world my services as a psychologist are no longer needed. The specialty of trauma treatment has been retired. I take a job as a barista and make people happy with caffeine or even better as a baker for people who cannot eat wheat and sugar, creating lovely tasty cookies and muffins for those who have been deprived until now. I am quite aware that this vision is unattainable within my lifetime, nor do I seriously believe that it will occur in the lifetimes of my nieces and nephews, some of whom may live to see the next century arrive if they have inherited their great-grandparents' tendencies toward longevity and humans do not blow up the planet in the interim. The continuing need for psychotherapists who understand trauma and are willing to stand witness to the healing process is a bitter reality for me. As grateful as I am to my clients for everything they have taught me, I wish that they had never had the experiences that have made each one such an excellent teacher. My sadness over their pain and my anger at the injustices that they have suffered can be considerable. I frequently find myself walking into the dojo where I study the martial art of aikido aware that what I am there to do is not master a particular technique of throwing people but find a place where I can allow the pain that I have absorbed that day to flow out of me as I struggle to find my center.

What sweetens the reality of the pervasiveness of trauma is my knowledge that trauma practice is becoming increasingly effective and that some aspect of that enhanced value derives from the synthesis of knowledge about human diversity and culturally competent treatment with specific information about ameliorating the psychic wounds of trauma exposure. Psychotherapists know more today about how to invite people to heal and more about how to accurately see, hear, know, and witness in ways that evoke people's narratives about their trauma experiences. Increasingly the professions that work with trauma survivors grasp how to respect the diversity and complexity of human experiences threading through the realities of trauma survival.

This increasingly culturally competent and culturally aware trauma practice rests on a too-small and too-shaky empirical foundation. It has become a cliché for authors to call for further research, but in this case that call is necessary. Psychotherapists and researchers in the field of trauma have just begun to scratch the surface of creating etic knowledge about trauma and human diversity. There is a too-small literature that gives psychotherapists piecemeal glimpses of themes and possibilities but as yet no large-scale work that takes as its premise the need to understand culture and identity as factors in the experience of trauma (Stamm & Friedman, 2000). Psychotherapists are even further from developing evidence-based emic methodologies of culturally competent trauma practice. Researcher–clinician collaborations are particularly necessary if high-quality emic knowledge about effective culturally competent trauma treatment is to be developed. Many of those who focus on diversity are practicing clinicians, and the representation of interest in and knowledge about human diversity as a broad epistemic construct among research scientists in the field of trauma is still inadequate.

It is my hope that clinicians who read this book come away from it feeling ignorant and inspired. One of the challenges I encountered in attempting to complete this volume was my awareness at each step that there were more things that I could say, other examples I could give, and more theoretical issues that needed to be considered. At some point I needed to allow this book to be simply adequate and reflective of what I could say in the allotted space rather than complete and all encompassing. Thus, if psychotherapists' appetite for more knowledge has been whetted but not satisfied and if they are aware of how ignorant they have become through reading this book, then my wish is for them to want more. If psychotherapists are inspired to make more meaning in their lives through empowering trauma survivors in increasingly culturally competent ways, then I will have made a step toward meeting the goals of writing this book. If they have come to the place where they understand that when psychotherapists speak of trauma survivors they are not addressing themselves to a damaged other but are describing the varieties of shared human experiences, then I have gone a step further in erasing the artificial distinctions between healthy and unhealthy responses to this endemic human reality. As my colleague Margo Rivera (1996) pointed out in her description of programs for dissociative survivors of complex trauma, humans are more alike than different. It is easy for psychotherapists to hide behind a title and distance themselves from the possibility that they could be faced with terrible trauma; they too would go to extreme lengths to manage their pain. However, if psychotherapists take that easy way, they will have to ignore the richness of experience and the varieties of identity that humans use to engage in coping with the challenges of trauma.

Because of space limitations I spent little time in this book discussing trauma as an embodied phenomenon. The study of the neurobiology of trauma is one of the fastest growing sectors of this field as advances in brain imaging technology allow researchers to watch the posttraumatic brain at work (Mueller, 2005). It is also one of those topics least touched by the cultural competence movements affecting psychology. Even though brains and hormones are consistently human across the species, researchers already have sufficient data from research on drug effects and interactions to know that sex and phenotype have an impact on response to psychotropic and other medications. How possible is it that these biological factors also play a role in the biological component of the trauma response in diverse groups of people? Research on diversity and complexity of the biological component of the trauma response will allow psychotherapists to more carefully tailor somatic interventions to posttraumatic distress.

Researchers also need to develop data that will help understand why certain somatic modalities appear to work so well in certain cultural contexts and why others appear to have little efficacy in the same context. If a pill is a pill is a pill then it should work as well for one human as another, but this is not the case. We know that expectancy effects likely play a role in this phenomenon; Western medicine creates expectancies of healing from certain types of somatic interventions, whereas the patients of *curanderos* or *curanderas* have an entirely other set of expectations. Each group reports being helped. Studying in greater depth the culture by biological interaction in responses to trauma and somatic interventions may illuminate in greater detail not only the diversity of responses to trauma but other variations in human manifestations of psychic distress and behavioral dysfunction.

I have paid little attention to the somatic and body psychotherapies in this volume. There are a number of trauma specialists who are integrating direct work with the body into the treatment of trauma, and that too could fill an entire book. What I have found interesting as I watch colleagues include yoga poses and Buddhist meditation and tai chi in their treatment packages is how infrequently we consider that these non-Western techniques may have in fact developed as part of cultural responses to historical realities of trauma in the cultures from which they derive. The future of culturally competent trauma treatment will likely include an increased appreciation by Western healers for the long-standing evidence base of trauma treatments available outside of the official canon of Western medical and psychological sciences.

Trauma is trauma is trauma. The texture of pain, the color of fear, and the melody of cries are all human and shared. They are all, also, uniquely configured and ordered by humans' identities, cultures, heritages, and networks of relationships. The great Jewish sage Hillel once said that the essence of wisdom was simple but required constant study. The essence of cultural competence in trauma treatment is simply a lifetime of opening oneself to understanding those colors, textures, and melodies as one participates in the process of healing.

APPENDIX:
GUIDELINES TO INFORM CULTURAL
COMPETENCE IN PRACTICE

The American Psychological Association (APA) has developed several guidelines that inform cultural competence in practice. Each is available for downloading from the APA Web site, where most current updates of the document are available.

- Guidelines for Psychological Practice With Girls and Women: http://www.apa.org/about/division/girlsandwomen.pdf
- Guidelines for Psychotherapy with Lesbian, Gay, & Bisexual Clients: http://www.apa.org/pi/lgbc/guidelines.html
- Guidelines for Multicultural Education, Training, Research, Practice, and Organizational Change for Psychologists: http://www.apa.org/pi/multiculturalguidelines/formats.html
- Intimate Partner Abuse and Relationship Violence: http://www.apa.org/pi/iparv.pdf

Other organizations have developed guidelines for treatment of various posttraumatic disorders. The best, in my opinion, are as follows:

- Guidelines for Psychotherapy With PTSD: information for ordering at http://www.istss.org. This Web site also has a host of other useful and credible Web and print resources about trauma research and treatment.

- Guidelines for Treatment of Adults and Children with Dissociative Identity Disorder: http://isst-d.org/education/treatmentguidelines-index.htm.

REFERENCES

Allen, D. W. (2001). Social class, race and toxic releases in American counties, 1995. *The Social Sciences Journal, 38*, 13–25.

Alpert, J. L. (2006, Summer). Nightmares, traumas, and jumping over hurdles. *The Trauma Psychologist, 1*, 1, 3.

American Psychiatric Association. (1980). *Diagnostic and statistical manual of mental disorders* (3rd ed.). Washington, DC: Author.

American Psychiatric Association. (2000). *Diagnostic and statistical manual of mental disorders* (4th ed., text rev.). Washington, DC: Author.

Anti-Defamation League. (2006). *2006 audit of Anti-Semitic incidents*. New York: Author.

Armstrong, J. G. (2002). Deciphering the broken narrative of trauma: Signs of traumatic dissociation on the Rorschach. In A. Andronikof (Ed.), *Rorschachiana: Yearbook of the International Rorschach Society* (pp. 11–27). Cambridge, MA: Hogrefe & Huber.

Aron, A. (1992). Testimonio, a bridge between psychotherapy and sociotherapy. *Women and Therapy, 13*, 173–189.

Attneave, C. L. (1969). Therapy in tribal settings and urban network intervention. *Family Process, 8*, 192–210.

Auerbach, C. F., Mirvis, S., Stern, S., & Schwartz, J. (n.d.). *From trauma to tragedy: The resolution of structural dissociation among Holocaust survivors*. Unpublished manuscript.

Baker, N. L. (1996). Class as a construct in a "classless" society. *Women and Therapy, 18*, 19–23.

Balsam, K. F., Beauchaine, T. P., Mickey, R. M., & Rothblum, E. D. (2005). Mental health of lesbian, gay, and bisexual adults and their heterosexual siblings: Effects of gender, sexual orientation, and family. *Journal of Abnormal Psychology, 114*, 471–476.

Barbara Bush calls evacuees better off. (2005, September 7). *The New York Times.* Retrieved August 25, 2007, from http://www.nytimes.com/2005/09/07/national/nationalspecial/07barbara.html

Bearak, B. (2005, November 27). Apocalypse on the horizon. *The New York Times Magazine*, pp. 47–66, 70, 97, 100–101.

Bem, S. L. (1989). *The lenses of gender*. New Haven, CT: Yale University Press.

Bertolino, B., & O'Hanlon, W. (2001). *Collaborative, competency-based counseling and psychotherapy*. Boston: Allyn & Bacon.

Birrell, P. J., & Freyd, J. J. (2006). Betrayal trauma: Models of harm and healing. *Journal of Trauma Practice, 5*, 49–65.

Bonoff, K. (1976). *Home*. Los Angeles, CA: Sky Harbor Music

Bowes, T. (2007). *Shame's role in aversive racism—Implications for competent clinical practice: A theoretical analysis of the literature.* Unpublished doctoral dissertation, Argosy University, Seattle, WA.

Brasted, T. K., Cruz, R., & James, C. (2005, October). *The coping structure employed by fire-based paramedics.* Poster session presented at the annual meeting of the Washington State Psychological Association, Lynnwood, WA.

Briere, J. (1995). *Trauma symptom inventory.* Odessa, FL: Psychological Assessment Resources.

Briere, J. (2000). *Inventory of altered self-capacities.* Odessa, FL: Psychological Assessment Resources.

Briere, J. (2001). *Detailed assessment of posttraumatic states.* Odessa, FL: Psychological Assessment Resources.

Briere, J. (2004). *Psychological assessment of adult posttraumatic states: Phenomenology, diagnosis, and measurement* (2nd ed.). Washington, DC: American Psychological Association.

Briere, J., & Scott, C. (2006). *Principles of trauma therapy: A guide to symptoms, evaluation, and treatment.* Thousand Oaks, CA: Sage.

Brooks, G. R. (2005). Counseling and psychotherapy for male military veterans. In G. E. Good & G. R. Brooks (Eds.), *The new handbook of psychotherapy and counseling with men: A comprehensive guide to settings, problems, and treatment approaches* (pp. 109–120). San Francisco: Jossey-Bass.

Brown, L. S. (1986). From alienation to connection: Feminist therapy with post-traumatic stress disorder. *Women and Therapy, 5,* 13–26.

Brown, L. S. (1988). Lesbians, gay men and their families: Common clinical issues. *Journal of Gay and Lesbian Psychotherapy, 1,* 23–32.

Brown, L. S. (1991a). Not outside the range: One feminist perspective on psychic trauma. *American Imago, 48,* 119–133.

Brown, L. S. (1991b). Therapy with an infertile lesbian client. In C. Silverstein (Ed.), *Gays, lesbians, and their psychotherapists: Studies in psychotherapy* (pp. 15–30). New York: Norton.

Brown, L. S. (1994). *Subversive dialogues: Theory in feminist therapy.* New York: Basic Books.

Brown, L. S. (2003). Sexuality, lies, and loss: Lesbian, gay, and bisexual perspectives on trauma. *Journal of Trauma Practice, 2,* 55–68.

Brown, L. S. (2004). Feminist paradigms of trauma treatment. *Psychotherapy: Theory, Research, Practice, Training, 41,* 464–471.

Brown, L. S. (2006a). The neglect of lesbian, gay, bisexual, and transgendered clients. In J. C. Norcross, L. E. Beutler, & R. F. Levant (Eds.), *Evidence-based practice in mental health: Debate and dialogue on the fundamental questions* (pp. 346–352). Washington, DC: American Psychological Association.

Brown, L. S. (2006b, March). *If I'm not for myself—But which self? Living in multiple identities.* Invited keynote lecture presented at the annual meeting of the Association for Women in Psychology, Ypsilanti, MI.

Brown, L. S., & Bryan, T. C. (2007). Feminist therapy approaches to working with self-inflicted violence. *In Session: Journal of Clinical Psychology, 63*, 1121–1133.

Bryant-Davis, T. (2005). *Thriving in the wake of trauma: A multicultural guide*. New York: Praeger Publishers.

Bryant-Davis, T., & Ocampo, C. (2006). A therapeutic approach to the treatment of racist-incident-based trauma. *Journal of Emotional Abuse, 4*, 1–22.

Buchanan, N. T., Mazzeo, S. E., Grzegorek, J., Ramos, A. M., & Fitzgerald, L. F. (1996, March). *Use of the computerized MMPI–2 in sexual harassment litigation: Time to use your head instead of the formula*. Paper presented at the annual meeting of the Association for Women in Psychology, Portland, OR.

Bullock, H. E. (1995). Class act: Middle-class responses to the poor. In B. Lott & D. Maluso (Eds.), *The social psychology of interpersonal discrimination* (pp. 118–159). New York: Guilford Press.

Bullock, H. E., Wyche, K. F., & Williams, W. R. (2001). Media images of the poor. *Journal of Social Issues, 57*, 229–246.

Castillo, R. J. (1997). *Culture and mental illness: A client-centered approach*. Pacific Grove, CA: Brooks/Cole.

Chase, C. (2003). What is the agenda of the intersex patient advocacy movement? *Endocrinologist, 13*, 240–242.

Cherepon, J. A., & Prinzhorn, B. (1994). Personality Assessment Inventory (PAI) profiles of adult female abuse survivors. *Assessment, 1*, 393–399.

Cherry, K. E. (2006, August). Responses of the "old-old" to disaster. In A. L. Santiago-Rivera (Chair), *Intersecting dimensions of multicultural issues in disaster response: Aging, disability, ethnicity and SES*. Symposium conducted at the 114th Annual Convention of the American Psychological Association, New Orleans, LA.

Cloitre, M., Cohen, L. R., & Koenen, K. C. (2006). *Treating survivors of childhood abuse: Psychotherapy for the interrupted life*. New York: Guilford Press.

Cochran, S. D., Sullivan, J. G., & Mays, V. M. (2003). Prevalence of mental disorders, psychological distress, and mental services use among lesbian, gay, and bisexual adults in the United States. *Journal of Consulting and Clinical Psychology, 71*, 53–61.

Coffey, R. L. (2005). *Beyond all expectations: The impact of working-class background on professional identity and development of women psychologists*. Unpublished doctoral dissertation, Argosy University, Seattle, WA.

Cole, E., & Daniel, J. H. (2005). *Featuring females: Feminist analyses of media*. Washington, DC: American Psychological Association.

Comas-Diaz, L. (2006). Latino healing: The integration of ethnic psychology into psychotherapy. *Psychotherapy: Theory, Research, Practice, Training, 43*, 436–453.

Comas-Diaz, L., & Jacobsen, F. (2001). Ethnocultural allodynia. *Journal of Psychotherapy Practice and Research, 10*, 246–252.

Corbett, C. A. (2003). Special issues in psychotherapy with minority deaf women. *Women and Therapy, 26*, 311–329.

Courtois, C. A. (1999). *Recollections of sexual abuse: Treatment principles and guidelines*. New York: Norton.

Cunningham, M., & Silove, D. (1992). Principles of treatment and service development for torture and trauma survivors. In J. P. Wilson & B. Raphael (Eds.), *International handbook of traumatic stress syndromes* (pp. 751–771). New York: Plenum Press.

Dalenberg, C. I. (2000). *Countertransference and the treatment of trauma*. Washington, DC: American Psychological Association.

Dana, R. H. (2000). Culture and methodology in personality assessment. In I. Cuellar & F. A. Paniagua (Eds.), *Handbook of multicultural mental health: Assessment and treatment of diverse populations* (pp. 98–120). San Diego, CA: Academic Press.

Daniel, J. H. (2000). The courage to hear: African American women's memories of racial trauma. In L. Jackson & B. Greene (Eds.), *Psychotherapy with African American women: Innovations in psychodynamic perspective and practice* (pp. 126–144). New York: Guilford Press.

Danieli, Y. (Ed.). (1998). *Intergenerational handbook of multigenerational legacies of trauma*. New York: Plenum Press.

Dass-Brailford, P. (2006, August). Ignore the dead! One year of the storms. In A. L. Santiago-Rivera (Chair), *Intersecting dimensions of multicultural issues in disaster response: Aging, disability, ethnicity and SES*. Symposium conducted at the 114th Annual Convention of the American Psychological Association, New Orleans, LA.

Davidson, J. R. T., & Foa, E. (Eds.). (1993). *Posttraumatic stress disorder: DSM–IV and beyond*. Washington, DC: American Psychiatric Press.

Dawkins, R. (2006). *The God delusion*. New York: Houghton Mifflin.

Dovidio, J. F., Gaertner, S. L., Kawakami, K., & Hodson, G. (2002). Why can't we just get along? Interpersonal biases and interracial distrust. *Cultural Diversity & Ethnic Minority Psychology, 8,* 88–102.

Duran, E. (2007, January). *Liberation psychology: An ongoing practice in American Indian country*. Invited keynote address presented at the annual National Multicultural Conference and Summit, Seattle, WA.

Duran, E., Duran, B., Brave Heart, M., & Yellow Horse-Davis, S. (1998). Post colonial syndrome. In Y. Danieli (Ed.), *Intergenerational handbook of multigenerational legacies of trauma* (pp. 341–354). New York: Plenum Press.

Dutton, M. A. (1991). *Empowering and healing the battered woman*. New York: Springer Publishing Company.

Englar-Carlson, M. (2006). Masculine norms and the therapy process. In M. Englar-Carlson & M. A. Stevens (Eds.), *In the room with men: A casebook of therapeutic change* (pp. 13–47). Washington, DC: American Psychological Association.

Ephraim, D. (2002). Rorschach trauma assessment of survivors of torture and state violence. In A. Andronikof (Ed.), *Rorschachiana: Yearbook of the International Rorschach Society* (pp. 58–76). Cambridge, MA: Hogrefe & Huber.

Epstein, H. (1988). *Children of the Holocaust: Conversations with sons and daughters of survivors*. New York: Penguin.

Espin, O. M. (1992). Roots uprooted: The psychological impact of historical/political dislocation. *Women and Therapy, 13*, 9–20.

Espin, O. M. (1995). "Race," racism, and sexuality in the life narratives of immigrant women. *Feminism and Psychology, 5*, 223–238.

Espin, O. M. (2005, January). *The age of the cookie-cutter has passed: Contradictions in identity at the core of therapeutic intervention.* Keynote address presented at the Fourth National Multicultural Conference and Summit, Los Angeles, CA.

Essed, P. (1991). *Everyday racism: Reports from women of two cultures.* New York: Hunter House.

Estrich, S. (1988). *Real rape.* Cambridge, MA: Harvard University Press.

Fadiman, A. (1998). *The spirit catches you and you fall down.* New York: Farrar, Straus & Giroux.

Farley, F. (1991). The Type T personality. In L. P. Lipsett & L. L. Mitnick (Eds.), *Self-regulatory behavior and risk taking: Causes and consequences* (pp. 371–382). Norwood, NJ: Ablex Publishing.

Farley, M. (2003). Prostitution, trafficking, and traumatic stress. *Journal of Trauma Practice, 2*, xvii–xxviii.

Fine, M., & Asch, A. (Eds.). (1988). *Women with disabilities: Essays in psychology, culture, and politics.* Philadelphia: Temple University Press.

Fischer, A. R., Jome, L. M., & Atkinson, D. R. (1998). Reconceptualizing multicultural counseling: Universal healing conditions in a culturally specific context. *The Counseling Psychologist, 26*, 525–588.

Fitzgerald, L. F. (1993). Sexual harassment: Violence against women in the workplace. *American Psychologist, 48*, 1070–1076.

Foa, E. B., Keane, T. M., & Friedman, M. J. (Eds.). (2000). *Effective treatments for PTSD: Practice guidelines from the International Society for Traumatic Stress Studies.* New York: Guilford Press.

Fortunato, J. (1984). *Embracing the exile: Healing journeys of gay Christians.* San Francisco: HarperSanFrancisco.

Fortune, M. M. (1999). *Is nothing sacred? The story of a pastor, the women he sexually abused, and the congregation he nearly destroyed.* Hartford, CT: United Church Press.

Fox, D., & Prilleltensky, I. (Eds.). (1997). *Critical psychology: An introduction.* Thousand Oaks, CA: Sage.

Frankl, V. (1963). *Man's search for meaning.* New York: Washington Square Press.

Franklin, A. J., Boyd-Franklin, N., & Kelly, S. (2006). Racism and invisibility: Race-related stress, emotional abuse, and psychological trauma for people of color. *Journal of Emotional Abuse, 6*, 9–30.

Frawley-O'Dea, M. G. (2007). *Perversion of power: Sexual abuse in the Catholic church.* Nashville, TN: Vanderbilt University Press.

Freed, W. (2003). From duty to despair: Brothel prostitution in Cambodia. *Journal of Trauma Practice, 2*, 133–146.

Freyd, J. J. (1996). *Betrayal trauma: The logic of forgetting abuse*. Cambridge, MA: Harvard University Press.

Freyd, J. J., DePrince, A. P., & Zurbriggen, E. L. (2001). Self-reported memory for abuse depends upon victim–perpetrator relationship. *Journal of Trauma and Dissociation, 2*, 5–17.

Frost, R. (1915). Death of the hired man. In *North of Boston* (pp. 3–4). New York: Henry Holt & Company.

Gaertner, S., & Dovidio, J. (1977). The subtlety of white racism, arousal, and helping behavior. *Journal of Personality and Social Psychology, 35*, 691–707.

Gaertner, S., & Dovidio, J. (1986). The aversive form of racism. In J. Dovidio & S. Gaertner (Eds.), *Prejudice, discrimination, and racism* (pp. 61–89). Orlando, FL: Academic Press.

Gaertner, S., & Dovidio, J. (2005). Understanding and addressing contemporary racism: From aversive racism to the common ingroup identity model. *Journal of Social Issues, 61*, 615–639.

Garnets, L., Herek, G., & Levy, B. (1993). Violence and victimization of lesbians and gay men: Mental health consequences. In. L. D. Garnets & D. C. Kimmel (Eds.), *Psychological perspectives on lesbian and gay male experiences* (pp. 579–598). New York: Columbia University Press.

Garnets, L. D., & Kimmel, D. (2002). *Psychological perspectives on lesbian and gay male experience*. New York: Columbia University Press.

Gibson, P. R. (2000). *Multiple chemical sensitivity: A survival guide*. Oakland, CA: New Harbinger.

Giddings, P. (1996). *When and where I enter: The impact of race and sex on Black women's lives*. New York: Amistad.

Gilfus, M. E. (1999). The price of the ticket: A survivor-centered appraisal of trauma theory. *Violence Against Women, 5*, 1238–1257.

Giller, E., Vermilyea, E., & Steele, T. (2006). *Risking connection*: Helping agencies embrace relational work with trauma survivors. *Journal of Trauma Practice, 5*, 65–82.

Gock, T. S. W. (2007, January). *Asian, Christian and gay: From incompatibility to integration*. Invited lecture presented at the Fifth National Multicultural Conference and Summit, Seattle, WA.

Gold, S. N. (2000). *Not trauma alone: Therapy for child abuse survivors in family and social context*. Philadelphia: Brunner-Routledge.

Good, G. E., & Brooks, G. R. (Eds.). (2005). *The new handbook of psychotherapy and counseling with men: A comprehensive guide to settings, problems, and treatment approaches*. San Francisco: Jossey-Bass.

Greene, B. (1990). What has gone before: The legacy of racism and sexism in the lives of Black mothers and daughters. In L. S. Brown & M. P. P. Root (Eds.), *Diversity and complexity in feminist therapy* (pp. 207–230). New York: Haworth Press.

Greene, B. (1992). Still here: A perspective on psychotherapy with African American women. In J. C. Chrisler & D. Howard (Eds.), *New directions in feminist psychology: Practice, theory, and research* (pp. 13–25). New York: Haworth Press.

Greene, B. (2000). African American lesbian and bisexual women in feminist-psychodynamic psychotherapy: Surviving and thriving between a rock and a hard place. In L. Jackson & B. Greene (Eds.), *Psychotherapy with African American women: Innovations in psychodynamic perspectives and practice* (pp. 82–125). New York: Guilford Press.

Greene, B. (2007, January). *The complexity of diversity: Multiple identities and the denial of social privilege.* Invited keynote address presented at the Fifth National Multicultural Conference and Summit, Seattle, WA.

Guthrie, R. V. (1976). *Even the rat was white: A historical view of psychology.* New York: Harper & Row.

Haldeman, D. (2002). Gay rights, patient rights: The implications of sexual orientation conversion therapy. *Professional Psychology: Research and Practice, 33,* 260–264.

Harris, S. (2007). *Letter to a Christian nation: A challenge to faith.* New York: Bantam books.

Harvey, M. R. (1996). An ecological view of psychological trauma and trauma recovery. *Journal of Traumatic Stress, 9,* 3–24.

Hass, A. (1996). *In the shadow of the Holocaust: The second generation.* New York: Cambridge University Press.

Hathaway, S. R., & McKinley, J. C. (1942). *Minnesota Multiphasic Personality Inventory.* Minneapolis: University of Minnesota Press.

Hathaway, S. R., & McKinley, J. C. (1989). *Minnesota Multiphasic Personality Inventory—2.* Minneapolis: University of Minnesota Press.

Hays, P. A. (2001). *Addressing cultural complexities in practice: A framework for clinicians and counselors.* Washington, DC: American Psychological Association.

Hays, P. A. (2008). *Addressing cultural complexities in practice: Assessment, diagnosis, and therapy* (2nd ed.). Washington, DC: American Psychological Association.

Hershberger, S. L., & D'Augelli, A. R. (2000). Issues in counseling lesbian, gay, and bisexual adolescents. In R. M. Perez, K. A. DeBord, & K. P. Bieschke (Eds.), *Handbook of counseling and psychotherapy with lesbian, gay, and bisexual clients* (pp. 225–248). Washington, DC: American Psychological Association.

Herman, J. L. (1992). *Trauma and recovery: The aftermath of violence from domestic abuse to political terror.* New York: Basic Books.

Hibbard, S. (2003). A critique of Lilienfeld et al.'s (2000) "The scientific status of projective techniques." *Journal of Personality Assessment, 80,* 260–271.

Hidalgo, J., Hopper, E., & Okawa, J. (2006, November). *Human trafficking: Trauma and resilience in modern day slavery.* Workshop presented at the annual meeting of the International Society for Traumatic Stress Studies, Los Angeles, CA.

Hinton, D. E., Pich, V., Chhean, D., Safren, S., & Pollack, M. (2007). Somatic-focused therapy for traumatized refugees: Treating posttraumatic stress disorder and comorbid neck-focused panic attacks among Cambodian refugees. *Psychotherapy: Theory, Research, Practice, Training, 43,* 491–505.

Hobfoll, S. E. (2001). The influence of culture, community, and the nested-self in the stress process: Advancing conservation of resources theory. *Applied Psychology, 50,* 337–370.

The honour of all: The story of Alkali Lake [Motion picture]. (1992). Secwepemc, British Columbia, Canada: Alkali Lake Indian Band.

Hyde, J. S. (2005). The gender similarities hypothesis. *American Psychologist, 60,* 581–592.

International Society for the Study of Trauma and Dissociation. (2005). Guidelines for treating Dissociative Identity Disorder in adults. *Journal of Trauma & Dissociation, 6,* 69–149.

Janoff-Bulman, R. (1992). *Shattered assumptions.* New York: Free Press.

Johnson, H. M. (2006). *Too late to die young: Nearly true tales from a life.* New York: Holt.

Jordan, P. (2005). *Perceptions of adolescent males aged 12–17 who have been convicted of homicide or aggravated assault.* Unpublished doctoral dissertation, Argosy University, Seattle, WA.

Kamphuis, J. J., Kugeares, S. L., & Finn, S. E. (2000). Rorschach correlates of sexual abuse: Trauma content and aggression indexes. *Journal of Personality Assessment, 75,* 212–224.

Kanuha, V. (1990). Compounding the triple jeopardy: Battering in lesbian of color relationships. In L. S. Brown & M. P. P. Root (Eds.), *Diversity and complexity in feminist therapy* (pp. 169–184). New York: Haworth Press.

Karam, J. L. (2006, August). Impact of Rita and Katrina on communities. In A. L. Santiago-Rivera (Chair), *Intersecting dimensions of multicultural issues in disaster response: Aging, disability, ethnicity and SES.* Symposium conducted at the 114th Annual Convention of the American Psychological Association, New Orleans, LA.

Kardiner, A., & Spiegel, H. (1947). *The traumatic neuroses of war.* New York: Hoeber.

Kimerling, R., Ouimette, P., & Wolfe, J. (Eds.). (2002). *Gender and PTSD.* New York: Guilford Press.

Koocher, G. P. (2006). Psychotherapy and faith. *Monitor on Psychology, 37/11,* 5.

Koss, M. P. (1988). Hidden rape: Sexual aggression and victimization in the national sample of students in higher education. In M. A. Pirog-Good & J. E. Stets (Eds.), *Violence in dating relationships: Emerging social issues* (pp. 145–168). New York: Praeger Publishers.

Krystal, H. (Ed.). (1969). *Massive psychic trauma.* New York: International Universities Press.

Kuoch, T., Wali, S., & Scully, M. F. (1992). Forward. In E. Cole, O. M. Espin, & E. D. Rothblum (Eds.), *Refugee women and their mental health: Shattered societies, shattered lives* (pp. xi–xii). New York: Haworth Press.

Langer, E. J. (1975). The illusion of control. *Journal of Personality and Social Psychology, 32*, 311–328.

Lee, S. (Writer/Director). (2006). *When the levees broke: A requiem in four acts* [Motion picture]. United States: HBO.

LeGuin, U. K. (1969). *The left hand of darkness*. New York: Ace.

Lerner, G. (1987). *The creation of patriarchy*. New York: Oxford University Press.

Lerner, M. J. (1980). *The belief in a just world*. New York: Plenum Press.

Levant, R. F. (1996). The new psychology of men. *Professional Psychology, 27*, 259–265.

Levant, R. F. (1999). *Traditional masculinity may be bad for your health*. Unpublished manuscript.

Levant, R. F., & Silverstein, L. B. (2006). Gender is neglected by both evidence-based practices and treatment as usual. In J. C. Norcross, L. E. Beutler, & R. F. Levant (Eds.), *Evidence-based practice in mental health: Debate and dialogue on the fundamental questions* (pp. 338–345). Washington, DC: American Psychological Association.

Levin, P. (1993). Assessing posttraumatic stress disorder with the Rorschach projective technique. In J. P. Wilson & B. Raphael (Eds.), *International handbook of traumatic stress syndromes* (pp. 189–200). New York: Plenum Press.

Linehan, M. (1993). *Cognitive behavioral treatment of borderline personality disorder*. New York: Guilford Press.

Lisak, D. (2005). Male survivors of trauma. In G. E. Good & G. R. Brooks (Eds.), *The new handbook of psychotherapy and counseling with men: A comprehensive guide to settings, problems, and treatment approaches* (pp. 147–158). San Francisco: Jossey-Bass.

Lott, B. (2002). Cognitive and behavioral distancing from the poor. *American Psychologist, 57*, 100–110.

Lott, B., & Bullock, H. E. (2006). *Psychology and economic injustice: Personal, professional, and political intersections*. Washington, DC: American Psychological Association.

Marsella, A. J., Friedman, M. J., Gerrity, E. M., & Scurfield, R. M. (Eds.). (1996). *Ethnocultural aspects of posttraumatic stress disorder: Issues, research, and clinical applications*. Washington, DC: American Psychological Association.

Marshall, G. (Writer/Director), Rose, A., Richwood, B., & Bruner, B. (Writers). (1999). *The other sister* [Motion picture]. United States: Touchstone Pictures.

Martin, S., Ray, N., Sotres-Alvarez, D., Kupper, L. L., Moracco, K. E., Dickens, P. A., et al. (2006). Physical and sexual assault of women with disabilities. *Violence Against Women, 12*, 823–837.

Matarazzo, J. (1986). Computerized clinical psychological test interpretations: Unvalidated plus all mean and no sigma. *American Psychologist, 41*, 14–24, 94–96.

Mazelis, R. (2003, October). Understanding and responding to women living with self-inflicted violence. *Women, Co-Occurring Disorders and Violence Study*. Retrieved September 15, 2007, from http://www.healingselfinjury.org/SelfInjury%20Fact%20Sheet%20Final.pdf

McFarlane, A. (2006, November). Is there a growing conservatism in the field of traumatic stress? In A. McFarlane (Chair), *Past presidents' symposium*. Symposium conducted at the annual meeting of the International Society for Traumatic Stress Studies, Los Angeles, CA.

McIntosh, P. (1998). White privilege: Unpacking the invisible knapsack. In M. McGoldrick (Ed.), *Re-visioning family therapy: Race, culture and gender in clinical practice* (pp. 147–152). New York: Guilford Press.

McNair, L. D., & Neville, H. A. (1996). African American women survivors of sexual assault: The intersection of race and class. *Women and Therapy, 20,* 107–118.

Mio, J. S., & Rhoades, L. A. (2003). Building bridges in the 21st century: Allies and the power of human connection across demographic divides. In J. S. Mio & G. Y. Iwamasa (Eds.), *Culturally diverse mental health: The challenge of research and resistance* (pp. 105–117). New York: Brunner-Routledge.

Millon, T., & Davis, C. (2001). *Personality disorders in modern life.* New York: Wiley.

Morey, L. (1996). *An interpretive guide to the Personality Assessment Inventory.* Lutz, FL: Personality Assessment Resources.

Mueller, F. A. (2005). *The biological component of trauma response: A Web-based survey of clinicians' training, attitudes, beliefs, and practices.* Unpublished doctoral dissertation, Argosy University, Seattle, WA.

Naifeh, J. A., Elhai, J. D., Zucker, I. S., Gold, S. N., Deitsch, S. E., & Fueh, B. C. (2003, November). *The MMPI–2 Fptsd Scale: Detecting malingered and genuine civilian PTSD.* Poster session presented at the annual meeting of the International Society for Traumatic Stress Studies, Chicago, IL.

Najavits, L. M., & Strupp, H. (1994). Differences in the effectiveness of psychodynamic therapists: A process-outcome study. *Psychotherapy, 31,* 114–123.

Norcross, J. C. (2000). *Psychotherapy relationships that work.* New York: Oxford University Press.

Norcross, J. C., Beutler, L. E., & Levant, R. F. (Eds.). (2006). *Evidence-based practice in mental health: Debate and dialogue on the fundamental questions.* Washington, DC: American Psychological Association.

Norcross, J. C., & Lambert, M. J. (2006). The therapy relationship. In J. C. Norcross, L. E. Beutler, & R. F. Levant (Eds.), *Evidence-based practice in mental health: Debate and dialogue on the fundamental questions* (pp. 208–217). Washington, DC: American Psychological Association.

Ochberg, F. M. (1988). *Post-traumatic therapy and victims of violence.* New York: Brunner/Mazel.

Olkin, R. (1999). *What psychotherapists should know about disability.* New York: Guilford Press.

Olkin, R. (2003) Women with physical disabilities who want to leave their partners: A feminist and disability-affirmative perspective. *Women and Therapy, 26,* 237–246.

Olkin, R., & Taliaferro, G. (2006). Evidence-based practices have ignored people with disabilities. In J. C. Norcross, L. E. Beutler, & R. F. Levant (Eds.), *Evidence-based practice in mental health: Debate and dialogue on the fundamental questions* (pp. 353–358). Washington, DC: American Psychological Association.

Padden, C., & Humphries, T. (1988). *Deaf in America: Voices from a culture*. Cambridge, MA: Harvard University Press.

Pagels, E. (1996). *The origins of Satan*. New York: Vintage Books.

Panzarino, C. (1994). *The me in the mirror*. Seattle, WA: Seal Press.

Paxton, T. (1963). What Did You Learn in School Today? On *Ramblin' Boy* [Record]. New York: Elektra Records.

Pearlman, L. A. (2003). *Trauma and Attachment Belief Scale*. Los Angeles: Western Psychological Services.

Pearlman, L. A., & Saakvitne, K. W. (1995). *Trauma and the therapist: Countertransference and vicarious traumatization in psychotherapy with incest survivors*. New York: Norton.

Peirce, J. M., Newton, T. L., Buckley, T. C., & Keane, T. M. (2002). Gender and psychophysiology of PTSD. In R. Kimerling, P. Ouimette, & J. Wolfe (Eds.), *Gender and PTSD* (pp. 177–204). New York: Guilford Press.

Perelman, V. (Writer/Director), Dubus, A., & Otto, S. L. (Writers). (2003). *House of sand and fog* [Motion picture]. United States: Dreamworks.

Perez, R. M., DeBord, K. A., & Bieschke, K. J. (Eds.). (2000). *Handbook of counseling and psychotherapy with lesbian, gay, and bisexual clients*. Washington, DC: American Psychological Association.

Perloff, R. (2007). Psychotherapy beyond faiths. *Monitor on Psychology, 38/1*. 4.

Personal Responsibility and Work Opportunity Reconciliation Act of 1996. (1996). Retrieved September 29, 2007, from http://thomas.loc.gov/cgi-bin/query/z?c104:H.R.3734.ENR:

Pharr, S. (1988). *Homophobia: A weapon of sexism*. San Francisco: Jossey-Bass.

Pheterson, G. (1986). Alliances between women: Over coming internalized oppression and internalized domination. *Signs: Journal of Women in Culture and Society, 12*, 146–160.

Pope, K. S., & Brown, L. S. (1997). *Recovered memories of abuse: Assessment, therapy, forensics*. Washington, DC: American Psychological Association.

Pope, K. S., & Feldman-Summers, S. (1992). National survey of psychologists' sexual and physical abuse history and their evaluation of training and competence in these areas. *Professional Psychology: Research and Practice, 23*, 353–361.

Pope, K. S., & Garcia-Peltoniemi, R. (1991). Responding to victims of torture: Clinical issues, professional responsibilities, and useful resources. *Professional Psychology: Research and Practice, 22*, 269–276.

Pope, K. S., Sonne, J., & Greene, B. (2006). *What therapists don't talk about and why: Understanding taboos that hurt us and our clients*. Washington, DC: American Psychological Association.

Pope, K. S., & Vasquez, M. J. T. (2007). *Ethics in psychotherapy and counseling: A practical guide* (3rd ed.). San Francisco: Jossey-Bass.

Puller, L. B., Jr. (1991). *Fortunate son: The healing of a Vietnam veteran.* New York: Grove Press.

Putnam, F. (1989). *Diagnosis and treatment of multiple personality disorder.* New York: Guilford.

Raine, N. V. (1998). *After long silence: Rape and my journey back.* New York: Crown House Publishing.

Rasmussen, A. M., & Friedman, M. J. (2002). Gender issues in the neurobiology of PTSD. In R. Kimerling, P. Ouimette, & J. Wolfe (Eds.), *Gender and PTSD* (pp. 43–75). New York: Guilford Press.

Rivera, M. (1996). *More alike than different: Treating severely dissociative trauma survivors.* Toronto, Ontario, Canada: University of Toronto Press.

Rivers, W. H. R. (1918). *The repression of war experience.* Retrieved March 1, 2006, from http://net.lib.byu.edu/~rdh7/wwi/comment/rivers.htm

Robin, R. W., Chester, B., & Goldman, D. (1996). Cumulative trauma and PTSD in American Indian communities. In A. J. Marsella, M. J. Friedman, E. T. Gerrity, & R. M. Scurfield (Eds.), *Ethnocultural aspects of posttraumatic stress disorder: Issues, research, and clinical applications* (pp. 239–254). Washington, DC: American Psychological Association.

Rogers, C. R. (1957). The necessary and sufficient conditions of therapeutic personality change. *Journal of Consulting Psychology, 21,* 95–103.

Root, M. P. P. (1992). Reconstructing the impact of trauma on personality. In L. S. Brown & M. Ballou (Eds.), *Personality and psychopathology: Feminist reappraisals* (pp. 229–265). New York: Guilford Press.

Root, M. P. P. (1998). Preliminary findings from the biracial sibling project. *Cultural Diversity and Mental Health, 4,* 237–247.

Root, M. P. P. (2000). Rethinking racial identity development: An ecological framework. In P. Spickard & J. Burroughs (Eds.), *We are a people: Narrative in the construction and deconstruction of ethnic identity* (pp. 205–220). Philadelphia: Temple University Press.

Root, M. P. P. (2004a). From exotic to a dime a dozen. *Women and Therapy, 27,* 19–32.

Root, M. P. P. (2004b, August). *Mixed race identities: Theory, research, and practice.* Continuing education workshop presented at the 111th Annual Convention of the American Psychological Association, Honolulu, HI.

Root, M. P. P., & Fallon, P. (1988). The incidence of victimization experiences in a bulimic sample. *Journal of Interpersonal Violence, 3,* 161–173.

Rosewater, L. B. (1985a). Feminist interpretation of traditional tests. In L. B. Rosewater & L. E. A. Walker (Eds.), *Handbook of feminist therapy: Women's issues in psychotherapy* (pp. 266–273). New York: Springer Publishing Company.

Rosewater, L. B. (1985b). Schizophrenic, borderline, or battered? In L. B. Rosewater & L. E. A. Walker (Eds.), *Handbook of feminist therapy: Women's issues in psychotherapy* (pp. 215–225). New York: Springer Publishing Company.

Russell, G. M. (1996). Internalized classism: The role of class in the development of self. *Women and Therapy, 18*, 59–71.

Russell, G. M. (2004a). The dangers of a same-sex marriage referendum for community and individual well-being: A summary of research findings. *Angles, 7*(1), 1–4.

Russell, G. M. (2004b). Surviving and thriving in the face of anti-gay politics. *Angles, 7*(2), 1–8.

Russell, G. M., & Richards, J. A. (2003). Stressor and resilience factors for lesbians, gay men, and bisexuals confronting anti-gay politics. *American Journal of Community Psychology, 31*, 313–328.

Russell, M. D. (1996). *The sparrow*. New York: Villard.

Saakvitne, K. W., Gamble, S., Pearlman, L. A., & Lev, B. T. (2000). *Risking connection: A training curriculum for working with survivors of childhood abuse*. Baltimore: Sidran.

Sanchez-Hucles, J. V. (1998). Racism: Emotional abusiveness and psychological trauma for ethnic minorities. *Journal of Emotional Abuse, 1*, 69–87.

Sarlund-Heinrich, P. (2007). *Measuring therapeutic effectiveness in treating post-trauma symptoms with the Rorschach: An exploratory study*. Unpublished doctoral dissertation, Argosy University, Seattle, WA.

Schore, A. N. (2003). *Affect regulation and disorders of the self*. New York: Norton.

Shay, J. (1995). *Achilles in Vietnam: Combat trauma and the undoing of character*. New York: Simon & Schuster.

Siegel, R. J. (1990). Turning the things that divide us into the strengths that unite us. In L. S. Brown & M. P. P. Root (Eds.), *Diversity and complexity in feminist therapy* (pp. 327–336). New York: Haworth Press.

Skolnik, S. (2005, March 31). Three found guilty of hate crime for assaulting gay man. *Seattle Post-Intelligencer*. Retrieved January 31, 2007, from http://seattlepi.nwsource.com/local/218252_painter31.html

Smedley, A., & Smedley, B. D. (2005). Race as biology is fiction, racism as a social problem is real: Anthropological and historical perspectives on the social construction of race. *American Psychologist, 60*, 16–26.

Snyder, C. R., Michael, S. T., & Cheavens, J. (1999). Hope as a psychotherapeutic foundation for nonspecific factors, placebos, and expectancies. In M. A. Hubble, B. Duncan, & S. Miller (Eds.), *The heart and soul of change: What works in therapy* (pp. 179–200). Washington, DC: American Psychological Association.

Stamm, B. H., & Friedman, M. J. (2000). Cultural diversity in the appraisal and expression of trauma. In A. Shalev, R. Yehuda, & A. McFarlane (Eds.), *International handbook of human response to trauma*. New York: Kluwer Academic/Plenum Publishers.

Strickland, B., Russo, N. F., & Keita, G. P. (Eds.). (1989). *Women and depression*. Washington, DC: American Psychological Association.

Sue, D. W. (2003). *Overcoming our racism: The journey to liberation*. San Francisco: Jossey-Bass.

Sue, D. W., Bucceri, J., Lin, A., Nadal, K. L., & Torino, G. C. (2007). Racial microaggressions and the Asian American experience. *Cultural Diversity and Ethnic Minority Psychology, 13*, 72–81.

Sue, S., & Zane, N. (2006). Ethnic minority populations have been neglected by evidence-based practices. In J. C. Norcross, L. E. Beutler, & R. F. Levant (Eds.), *Evidence-based practice in mental health: Debate and dialogue on the fundamental questions* (pp. 329–337). Washington, DC: American Psychological Association.

Swanson, L. K. (2007). *A profile of domestic violence: The responding of female abuse survivors on the Personality Assessment Inventory (PAI)*.Unpublished doctoral dissertation, Argosy University, Seattle, WA.

Terr, L. (1979). Children of Chowchilla: A study of psychic trauma. *Psychoanalytic Study of the Child, 34*, 547–632.

Terr, L. (1983). Chowchilla revisited: The effects of psychic trauma four years after a school bus kidnapping. *American Journal of Psychiatry, 140*, 1543–1550.

Terr, L. (1990). *Too scared to cry: Psychic trauma in childhood.* New York: HarperCollins.

Tsai, M., Feldman-Summers, S., & Edgar, M. (1979). Childhood molestation: Variables related to differential impacts on psychosexual functioning in adult women. *Journal of Abnormal Psychology, 88*, 407–417.

Van Boemel, G. B., & Rozée, P. D. (1992). Treatment for psychosomatic blindness among Cambodian refugee women. *Women and Therapy, 13*, 239–266.

van der Hart, O., Nijenhuis, E. R. S., & Steele, K. (2006). *The haunted self: Structural dissociation and the treatment of chronic traumatization.* New York: Norton.

Vasquez, M. J. T. (2007, January). *The challenge of conflict among allies: Risks and opportunities.* Invited keynote address presented at the Fifth National Multicultural Conference and Summit, Seattle, WA.

Walker, E. A., Gelfand, A., Katon, W., Koss, M., Von Korff, M., Bernstein, D., & Russo, J. (1999). Adult health status of women HMO members with histories of childhood abuse and neglect. *American Journal of Medicine, 107*, 332–339.

Walters, K. L., & Simoni, J. M. (2002). Native women's health: An "indigenist" stress-coping model. *American Journal of Public Health, 92*, 520–524.

Weber, M. (1930/2001). *The Protestant ethic and the spirit of capitalism.* London: Routledge Classics.

Weisstein, N. (1970). Kinder, kuche, kirche as scientific law: Psychology constructs the female. In R. Morgan (Ed.), *Sisterhood is powerful* (pp. 205–219). New York: Vintage Books.

Whitaker-Clark, H. (2005). *Critical review of feminist and communication perspective literature on women's experiences of verbal abuse in intimate interpersonal relationships.* Unpublished doctoral dissertation, Argosy University, Seattle, WA.

Wilson, J. P. (2006). *The posttraumatic self: Restoring meaning and wholeness to personality.* New York: Routledge.

Wolfe, J. L., & Fodor, I. G. (1996). The poverty of privilege: Therapy with women of the "upper" classes. *Women and Therapy, 18*, 73–89.

Wyche, K. F. (1996). Conceptualizations of social class in African American women: Congruence of client and therapist definitions. *Women and Therapy, 18,* pp. 35–43.

Yalom, I. D. (1980). *Existential psychotherapy.* New York: Basic Books.

Zimberoff, A. K., & Brown, L. S. (2006). "Only the goyim beat their wives, right?" *Psychology of Women Quarterly, 30,* 422–424.

INDEX

religious belief-based behaviors, 233–235

sexism effects, 138

social class issues, 202–203, 210–211

structured clinical interviews, 71–72

of surgical experiences, 143

therapist–client shared culture or experience and, 66–69

therapist representation considerations, 65–66

torture victims, 222–223

trauma considerations in intake, 64

trauma in persons with disabilities, 29–30

See also Manifestations of trauma

Assimilation, 32

Asylum seekers, 220–223

Ataque de nervios, 8

Attachment experience, 118–119

Attachment therapy, in STAIR/NST, 73

Attractiveness, as social location variable, 25

Aversive bias, 9, 136–138, 239

Avoidance behaviors, 83

Betrayal Trauma, 107–108, 178

Bias(es)

classism, 32–33, 199, 203–208

cultural assimilation and, 32

hidden, 9

historical trauma, 32

against persons with disabilities, 29

power of privilege, 41

psychotherapist, 9

religious, 31, 231–323, 240

sexual orientation, 35

social location variables, 25

against women, 132, 133

See also Ageism; Oppression; Racism; Target groups

Biology of trauma, 138–142

research needs, 257–258

See also Phenotype

Blindness, posttraumatic nonorganic, 221

Bonoff, Karla, 215

Buddhism, 100

Bullock, H. E., 199

Burnout, 250

Bush, Barbara, 6

Capital punishment, 165

Case examples, 20

Catholicism, 100

Child and adolescent trauma, 20

age bias against victim, 27, 123–124

Betrayal Trauma, 107–108

caregiver as trauma source, 117, 118, 119

cohort effects, 127–129

delayed recall, 89–90, 107–109

dependence needs, 119

homosexuality and, 178–179

intersexed persons, 142–143

later risk of injury and disability, 187–188

manifestations in later life, 120–122, 126

prevalence among psychotherapists, 13

research base, 116–117

self-care strategies, 119–120

sexual abuse in adolescence, 123

shame feelings in, 119

STAIR/NST treatment model, 90

trafficked persons, 225

See also Development

Childbirth, 141–142

Children

in poverty, 33–34

of trauma perpetrators, 14, 126–127

of trauma survivors, 13, 84–85, 121–122

Children with disabilities, 186–187

Chowchilla kidnapping, 116

Classism, 32–33, 199, 203–206

internalized, 206–208

Cloitre, M., 73. *See also* Skills Training in Affective and Interpersonal Regulation/ Narrative Story Telling

Coble-Temple, A., 183

Coffey, R. L., 201–202

Cohen, L. R., 73. *See also* Skills Training in Affective and Interpersonal Regulation/Narrative Story Telling

Collectivist cultures, 161–162

group therapy and, 250

Colonization experience

clinical consideration, 89

of Europeans, 158, 159

identity as perpetrator or victim, 10

long-term effects for cultures and individuals, 156–158

as social location variable, 25, 36–37

sources of trauma in, 156

Communication of trauma experience, 4–5

Competency-based orientation, 18, 45–46

meaning-making as protective factor, 240–241

Dovidio, J., 9

Eating behavior, 64
    coping strategy, 86–88
Ecological model of development, 51–52
Ecological model of trauma therapy, 72
    concept of safety in, 73–79
    conceptual basis, 73
    mourning and remembrance stage, 80–85
    reconnection stage, 85–88
Education, access to, 198
Effective Treatments for PTSD: Practice Guidelines From the International Society for Traumatic Stress Studies, 91
Emic discourse of cultural competence, 11–12
Emotional abuse, 187
Empirically supported psychotherapy relationships, 91–93
Epidemiology, trauma, 3–4
    prevalence among psychotherapists, 13
Espin, O. M., 215
Ethnicity
    clinical significance, 154, 159
    concept of diversity in psychology science and research, 10
    culture and, 31–32, 154
    definition and meaning, 154
    mixed ancestry or association, 156
    phenotype variation and, 31, 154
    race and, 160
    as social location variable, 24, 31
    trauma and, 32
    trauma risk for lesbian, gay or bisexual members, 171–172
Etic psychotherapy approaches, 10
    in education and training of psychologists, 23–24
    limitations, 11–12, 24
Expectations
    body norms, 147
    gender and sex role, 132–133, 134–136, 145–150
    trauma as violation of just world expectations, 99–103
    See also Just world expectations
Exposure therapies, in STAIR/NST, 73

Families of origin
    assessment, 246
    relationship to trauma experience, 246

    therapeutic role, 246–247
Family trauma
    Betrayal Trauma, 107–108
    cultural trauma and, 89
    definition of family, 96
    insidious trauma in collectivist cultures, 161
    for lesbian, gay and bisexual people, 170, 171, 178
    therapeutic confrontation, 247
Female genital mutilation, 141
Feminist psychology, 5, 10, 19, 55
Flashback memory, 140
Foley, Mark, 172
Fortunate Son: The Healing of a Vietnam Vet (Puller), 82–83
Frankl, V., 240–241
Freud, S., 62
Freyd, J. J., 107
Friedman, M. J., 139
Frost, Robert, 215

Gaertner, S., 9
Gender and sex
    biology of trauma, 138–142
    body norm expectations, 147
    as cultural construct, 131, 132–133, 145
    definitions, 38, 131
    emotional expressivity, 148
    female role expectations, 146–147
    gender-related trauma risk, 39, 145–150
    identity and, 38–39, 131
    interaction with other social location variables, 129
    intersexed persons, 38, 142–145
    male role expectations, 133, 134–136, 146, 248
    obstacles to recovery, 148–150
    role nonconformity, 39, 132, 150–151
    sex-related trauma risk, 131–132
    as social location variable, 24
    transgender persons, 39
    trauma perceived as feminizing experience, 146
    See also Sexual orientation
Genocide, 10, 13
Gilfus, M. E., 45
Gold, S. N., 72. *See also* Trauma Resolution Integration Program
Greene, B., 171
Grieving, mourning and remembrance stage of ecological therapy, 80–85

Group therapy, 249–250
    for mourning and remembrance, 85
Guilt
    in child trauma victim, 119
    feelings among privileged persons, 42–
        43
Guthrie, R. V., 24

Haggard, Ted, 172
Hate crime, 173–174, 239
Hays, Pamela, 12, 24, 28, 29
Health
    disability and, 27–28
    health care for persons with disability,
        188–189, 193
    institutional obstacles to well-being and
        justice, 204–206
    refugees and asylum seekers, 221
    somatoform manifestations of trauma,
        63–64
    traditional healing techniques, 79–80,
        162
Help-seeking behavior
    gender role expectations, 248
    lesbian, gay and bisexual persons, 177
    obstacles for immigrants, 219
    social class and, 211
    trafficked persons, 225
Herman, Judith Lewis, 4, 5, 72, 73
Heterosexism, 170, 177
Heterosexuality as trauma risk factor, 179
Hindu cultures, 100
Historical trauma, 32
    religious oppression, 230
Holocaust survivors, 83–85, 122
Homophobia, defined, 170
Hope, 252–253
Hormonal system, 138–139, 140–141
House of Sand and Fog, 200
Housing, 208
Hurricane Katrina, 5–7, 13, 109, 193
Hypothalamic–pituitary–adrenal axis, 138

Identity
    collectivist cultures, 161–162
    concept for culturally sensitive practice,
        15–16, 49–50, 52–53, 59
    concept of diversity in psychology sci-
        ence and research, 10
    cultural narrative and suppression of,
        82–83
    culture and, 153–154

definition, 49–50
development, 17
disability and, 28–29, 191–192
ecological model of development, 51–
    52
ethnicity and, 31–32
formation strategies in response to
    trauma, 53–58
gender and, 38–39, 131, 145–146
immigrant, 216, 226
internalized oppression, 43, 51, 82, 106,
    182, 206–208, 211
invidious comparison of harm, 84–85
liminal states, 52–53
meaning, 228
mourning and remembrance stage of
    ecological therapy and, 80–81
multiple identities model, 52
multiple sources, 13–14, 16, 50
poverty as, 212–213
racial self-identification, 161
rationale for emic approach to trauma
    psychotherapy, 12
reconnection stage of ecological therapy
    and, 85–88
rejection of societal expectations in, 55–
    57, 58
religious, 30
self and, 50
social location and, 49
societal expectation coherence, 53–54
symbolic, 57–58
target and dominant groups, 26
therapist self-knowledge, 12–15
trauma effects, 15–16, 50–53, 58
trauma in adolescence, 123
as trauma perpetrator, 14
values and, 50
in vicarious traumatization, 251
See also Social location variables
Ignorance, 16–17
Immigrants
    access to mental health services, 219
    culturally competent practice with,
        217–218, 226
    expectation of return, 37
    government policies and practices, 218
    intergenerational transmission of
        trauma, 217
    national origin as social location vari-
        able, 24, 37–38
    other social location variables, 38, 217

The Other Sister, 190

Parenting skills, trauma experience and, 121–122
Patriarchal culture, 132, 133
Paxton, Tom, 165
Pearlman, L. A., 9, 250, 251
Perpetrators of trauma, 14
Personality Assessment Inventory, 70
Personality disorder, trauma diagnosed as, 99
Personal Responsibility and Work Opportunity Reconciliation Act, 204
Phenotype
    assessment considerations, 159
    culture and, 31–32
    ethnicity and, 31, 154
    immigration status and, 216
    mixed ancestry or association, 156
    racism and, 154, 161
    as social location variable, 25
    See also Culture; Ethnicity; Race
Phobias, trauma and, 63
Police, 164–165
Post-colonial trauma syndrome, 36–37
Posttraumatic growth, 241, 251
Posttraumatic stress disorder
    biological effects on expression of, 140–141
    clinical conceptualization, 8
    comorbid disorders, 63
    evolution of psychology theory, 61–62
    sex differences, 131–132
Power relations
    class-free society narrative of United States and, 198
    coerced behavior as trauma experience, 99
    feminist psychology, 5
    obstacles to multicultural practice, 8–9
    status of privileged groups, 41
    in therapeutic relationship, 44
    trauma perpetrators, 14
Privilege
    access to protective resources, 209–210
    acknowledging privileged status, 9, 41–43
    advantages of, 41
    definition, 41
    guilt and, 42–43
    implications for therapy, 41–44, 203
    trauma and, 42, 43, 45
    trauma for gay Euro-American men, 172

Projective assessment, 70
Protestantism, 100
Psychometric instruments, 69–72
Puller, Lewis, Jr., 82–83

Race
    concept of diversity in psychology science and research, 10
    ethnicity and, 31
    as flawed concept, 159–160
    individual self-identification, 161
Racism
    age cohort differences, 127–128
    assessment considerations, 72
    classism and, 199
    communication of, 164
    daily threat as trauma source, 98
    definition, 154, 155
    ethnicity and, 32
    insidious forms, 155
    against persons of mixed phenotype, 156
    as source of trauma, 154, 155
    trauma experience mediated by, 6, 155
    trauma risk for perpetrators, 156
    in United States, 154–155, 158–159, 160, 164
Raine, Nancy, 51
Rasmussen, A. M., 139
Reactive attachment disorder, 119
Recovery
    cultural competence and, 7
    family participation, 246–248
    gendered obstacles to, 148–150
    interpersonal variables, 19, 245–246
    self-care strategies, 254
    social support systems in, 247–250
    See also Therapeutic process and technique
Recreational choices, as social location variable, 25
Refugees, 37, 215, 220–223
Religion and spirituality
    antireligious expression, 232
    as basis for oppression, 230, 239–240
    clinical considerations, 30, 31, 229
    concept of trauma in, 235
    culturally competent practice, 30, 229, 230, 232–233, 235–236
    discrimination and bias based on, 231–232
    divinity beliefs, 230–233, 241
    existential meaning-making and, 30

human desire for meaning and, 227–228
individual differences in experience of, 231
protective factors, 240–241
sexual orientation and, 172–173
as social location variable, 24, 30–31
as source of conflict, 231
source of trauma located in, 237–239
therapist background and beliefs, 231, 233, 237
in therapist training and education, 229, 233–235
trauma effects, 229–230
Representation, 39–41, 65–66
Repressed memories. *See* Delayed recall of traumatic experience
Resiliency, 117
Retirement age, 126
Risking Connection curriculum, 254
Risk-taking behavior, 97, 133, 135, 146
Root, M. P. P., 51–52, 53, 104
Rush, Florence, 5
Russell, G., 75
Russell, M. D., 110

Saakvitne, K. W., 9, 250, 251
Safety, 87
ecological model of trauma and healing, 73–79
experience of racism as threat to, 98
insidious traumatization, 103–107
trauma as violation of just world expectations, 99–103
Schemata, Gender, 146
Secondary traumatic stress, 4, 7, 250
Self-awareness, therapist
ableist attitudes and values, 185, 195
age bias, 129
aversive bias, 9
for culturally sensitive practice, 4, 12–15, 40
issues of privilege, 9, 41–44, 203
issues of representation, 39–41
meaning-making and religious belief, 237
vicarious traumatization, 253, 254
Self-care strategies, 77
of traumatized children, 119–120
Self-harm behaviors, 64
September 11 terrorist attacks, 218, 239
Sexism
assessment of effects, 138

insidious traumatization in, 134, 136–138
patriarchal culture and, 133
trauma perceived as feminizing experience, 146
in treatment of intersexed persons, 145
Sexual assault
acquaintance rape, 107–108, 147
with added negative value, 110–111
assessment instruments, 71
biological component of trauma response, 141
disability and, 187
heterosexuality as trauma risk factor for women, 179
intake, 64
refugee experience, 221
trauma risk, 109–110, 132
Sexual harassment, 98, 132
Sexual orientation
bias and oppression, 35
childhood sexual abuse and, 178–179
clinical considerations, 35, 177, 180
concept of diversity in psychology science and research, 10
current social environment, 169–170
definition and psychological conceptualizations, 34–35
heterosexuality as trauma risk factor, 179
kinky sex, 35–36
as social location variable, 24, 34–36
trauma risk and, 36, 170
See also Gender and sex; Lesbian, gay and bisexual persons
Shame feelings, 156
caregiver abuse and development of, 119
as obstacle to help-seeking, 211
in perpetrators of racism, 9
privileges status and, 9
Shay, J., 14
Skills Training in Affective and Interpersonal Regulation/Narrative Story Telling, 73, 90
Slavery in United States, 14, 37–38
Social capital, 33
Social class
abuse in wealthy households, 118, 200–201
attitudes toward psychotherapy, 163, 211
classism, 32–33, 199, 203–206

ABOUT THE AUTHOR

Laura S. Brown, PhD, received a doctorate in clinical psychology in 1977 from Southern Illinois University at Carbondale and has been in practice as a clinician and forensic psychologist in Seattle since 1979. She has served on the faculties of Southern Illinois University, University of Washington, and the Washington School of Professional Psychology. A diplomate in clinical psychology and a fellow of 10 divisions of the American Psychological Association (APA), Dr. Brown has received numerous awards from her peers for her work in the fields of feminist therapy theory and trauma treatment. These honors include the Distinguished Publications Award of the Association for Women in Psychology, APA's Award for Distinguished Professional Contributions to Public Service, the Sarah Haley Award for Clinical Excellence from the International Society for Traumatic Stress Studies, and the Carolyn Wood Sherif Award from the Society for the Psychology of Women. Her books include *Subversive Dialogues: Theory in Feminist Therapy* and (with Kenneth S. Pope) *Recovered Memories of Abuse*. She is the therapist featured in two videos on trauma treatment in the APA video series and is a founding member of APA's Division of Trauma Psychology.

Currently, Dr. Brown directs the Fremont Community Therapy Project, a training clinic that she founded in 2006 to provide low-cost psychotherapy and psychological assessment. She is a student of aikido and lives in Seattle with her partner and her canine cotherapist.